alternative
medicine
MAGAZINE'S

Definitive Guide
to Sleep Disorders

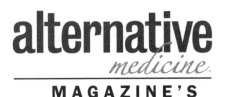

alternative medicine MAGAZINE'S

Definitive Guide to Sleep Disorders

7 Smart Ways to Help
You Get a Good Night's Rest

SECOND EDITION

Herbert Ross, DC,
with Keri Brenner, L.Ac.

CELESTIAL ARTS
Berkeley | Toronto

Many of the designations used by manufacturers and sellers to distinguish their products are
claimed as trademarks. Where the publisher is aware of a trademark claim, such designations,
in this book, have initial capital letters.

CELESTIAL ARTS
an imprint of Ten Speed Press
PO Box 7123
Berkeley, CA 94707
www.tenspeed.com

Distributed in Australia by Simon and Schuster Australia, in Canada by Ten Speed Press
Canada, in New Zealand by Southern Publishers Group, in South Africa by Real Books, and in
the United Kingdom and Europe by Publishers Group UK.

Cover design by Chloe Rawlins
Text design by Chris Hall

Library of Congress Cataloging-in-Publication Data

Ross, Herbert.
Alternative Medicine Magazine's definitive guide to sleep disorders : 7
smart ways to help you get a good night's rest / Herbert Ross, with Keri
Brenner.—2nd ed.
p. cm.
Rev. ed. of: Sleep disorders. 2000.
Includes bibliographical references and index.
ISBN 978-1-58761-263-3
1. Sleep disorders—Alternative treatment. 2. Insomnia—Alternative
treatment. I. Brenner, Keri. II. Ross, Herbert. Sleep disorders. III.
Title.

RC547.R66 2007
616.8'498—dc22

2007011405

1 2 3 4 5 6 7 8 9 10 — 11 10 09 08 07

Contents

	Important Information for the Reader	vi
Introduction	Bringing Home the Goods	1
one	The Basics of Sleep	4
two	Sleep Disorders and Their Causes	21
three	Step 1: Improve Your Diet	42
four	Step 2: Detoxify Your Body	72
five	Step 3: Reset Your Body Clock	102
six	Step 4: Resolve Emotional Issues	127
seven	Step 5: Protect Yourself from Environmental Factors	155
eight	Step 6: Balance Your Hormones	178
nine	Step 7: Correct Structural Imbalances	201
Conclusion	Good Night	226
	Quick Definitions	227
	Resources	233
	Endnotes	240
	Index	259

Important Information for the Reader

Your health and that of your loved ones is important. Treat this book as an educational tool that will enable you to better understand, assess, and choose the best course of treatment when a health problem arises. It will also help you understand how to prevent health problems such as sleep disorders from developing in the first place.

Remember that this book on sleep disorders is different. It is about alternative approaches to health—approaches generally not understood and, at this time, not endorsed by the medical establishment. We urge you to discuss the treatments described in this book with your doctors. If they are open-minded, you may actually educate them. We have been gratified to learn that many of our readers have found their physicians open to the ideas presented here.

Use this book wisely. As many of the treatments described in this book are, by definition, alternative, they have not been investigated, approved, or endorsed by any government or regulatory agency. National, state, and local laws may vary regarding the use and application of many of the treatments discussed. Accordingly, this book should not be substituted for the advice and care of a physician or other licensed health-care professional. Pregnant women, in particular, are urged to consult a physician before commencing any therapy. Ultimately, you must take responsibility for your health and how you use the information in this book.

InnoVision Health Media Inc. and the authors have no financial interest in any of the products or services discussed in this book, with two exceptions. Pure Energies is a company that sells EMF-protection devices, and Dr. Herb Ross is the CEO of Pure Energies. The book also makes references in the text to other InnoVision Health Media Inc. publications.

All of the factual information in this book has been drawn from the scientific literature. To protect privacy, all patient names have been changed. Branded products and services discussed in the book are evaluated solely on the independent and direct experience of the health-care practitioners quoted. Reference to them does not imply an endorsement nor a superiority over other branded products and services, which may provide similar or superior results.

Bringing Home the Goods

If you've picked up this book, chances are you have some sort of problem with your sleep. You're certainly not alone in that. As you'll learn in this book, most Americans don't get enough sleep, and the number of hours we spend sleeping each night continues to decline.

If your sleep problem isn't severe, you may view it as less important than other health issues. But, as we'll explain, a sleep problem can be like the tip of an iceberg—it may indicate underlying imbalances or conditions, such as an overload of toxins, a desynchronized body clock, hormonal imbalance, or even a structural problem. All of these have the potential to create serious health problems, so your troubled sleep may be a wake-up call to address an underlying health issue. It's also possible for disrupted sleep to cause serious health problems. Insufficient sleep has been implicated in everything from cardiovascular disease to obesity to impaired immune response. It can also create stress, disrupt relationships, and make a person more accident-prone.

Because this book is about alternative approaches to helping you sleep better, we won't be discussing that last side effect of sleeplessness—being accident-prone—but suffice it to say, it can have a huge impact on health and well-being, both for you and for others that you put at risk by driving when drowsy. And while alternative medicine can be very effective for helping you sleep better, conventional medicine and intensive interventions may be necessary if you're involved in a serious accident. We won't harp on it, but we do want to be emphatic about it at least once: *If you feel sleepy or drowsy, pull over and take a short nap.*

We will give you some basic background science on sleep. Having an understanding of sleep cycles could actually be therapeutic. For example, the nightly sleep pattern naturally involves several periods of lighter sleep during the night, when you're more easily awakened. Understanding this may help you feel less anxious if you awaken in the middle of the night, and if you don't worry about it, you may just fall back to sleep more easily. We'll also discuss the most common sleep disorders and their causes. If you have an actual sleep disorder, it's probably a good idea to work with a medical professional to obtain a definitive diagnosis.

That background brings us to the heart of the book: seven key factors that may play a role in sleep problems, and how alternative medicine can help you address problems in each of these areas:

1. Diet

2. Toxicity

3. A desynchronized body clock

4. Stress and emotional issues

5. Electromagnetic radiation

6. Hormonal imbalance

7. Exercise and structural imbalance

A key tenet of alternative medicine is using an individualized approach and recognizing that each person's symptoms and health problems arise from a unique set of factors. Therefore, treatment approaches must be similarly individualized. As you read through this book, consider which of these factors may be involved in your sleep problem, and also be sensitive to the interconnections between them. Because our focus is on providing alternative therapies you can start using right away, we won't spend a lot of time drawing out the interconnections between all of the various physiological systems addressed in this book. However, as you read, you'll begin to see these connections for yourself and understand how they may be affecting your situation.

For example, many alternative practitioners believe that detoxification is fundamental for optimum health. This is hardly surprising, given that our modern world assaults all of us with a daily flood of pollutants and toxins. But this isn't a stand-alone topic. The food you eat can be a major source of toxins (or of detoxification), so diet is interrelated to toxicity. By stimulating the lymphatic system, exercise can help keep the body's detoxification processes functioning more smoothly, so exercise, too, is involved. And certain environmental pollutants can have profound effects on hormonal balance, so these two topics cannot be looked at in isolation from one another.

Although we could continue to draw out these connections and relationships, we know you're eager—maybe desperate—to get into the book and start finding some solutions to your sleep problem. All of the therapies described in this book have proven helpful for some people with sleep problems. Though there are few cautions to observe, we've mentioned those where relevant. Best of all, most of these are approaches you can experiment with on your own. That said, you'd be well advised to find an alternative health-care practitioner with some expertise in sleep problems. A sympathetic medical professional can offer guidance and will probably be able to refer you to other practitioners for specific therapies.

One final word on the benefits of the therapies we describe: In addition to helping you sleep better, all have the potential to enhance your overall health and well-being. Curing specific conditions is certainly a worthwhile goal. But beyond that there's the greater goal of feeling good and experiencing more balance and harmony in your day-to-day life. Three common-sense daily practices can create a positive feedback loop of health, which will set your body up for greater general health, better sleep at night, and more alertness during the day. I call these three elements THE GOODS:

1. Getting a good night's sleep every night

2. Having a good early morning bowel movement

3. Eating a good breakfast

Chronically ill patients often have three things in common: they are poor sleepers, they have digestive problems and chronic constipation, and they usually skip breakfast or eat a sugary pastry and coffee. This triad of physiological insults can have grave consequences over the course of a lifetime, including lack of energy, irritability, a compromised immune system, obesity, and loss of focus and concentration. When the body hasn't had a restful and nutritive night and morning, the rest of the day is filled with the effects of poor health, from playing catch-up at work to being constipated, from a dangerously tired commute to a late-night snack that leads to insomnia—starting the cycle once again.

Addressing digestive problems through detoxification and proper nutrition can help you achieve "goods" numbers 2 and 3. By putting your body on the right nutritional schedule, you can increase your energy during the day and avoid the midmorning as well as the midafternoon slump. Subsequently, your body will be better prepared to get a good night's sleep—"goods" number 1. Sticking to a set bedtime and wake-up time will help. Keeping "the goods" in mind while applying the specific health and lifestyle changes detailed in the rest of the book is a recipe for success—not just for sleep, but for your entire health status. Indeed, once you can follow a restful night with a healthy breakfast and an early morning bowel movement—all changes you can make before 9 A.M.—the quality of the rest of your day will increase. So turn the page and let's get started.

one

The Basics of Sleep

We spend up to one-third of our lives asleep. Although some hard-driven people may view sleep as an inconvenience that curtails productivity and leisure activities, slumber is certainly no waste of time. In fact, sleep may play a more crucial role than diet or exercise in fostering optimal health.

Sleep is a natural restorative, an antidote to the damage done to our bodies during the course of the day. It allows the body to replenish its immune system, eliminate free radicals, and ward off heart disease and mood imbalances. The mechanisms of sleep are as remarkable as its physiological function. You may think that merely closing your eyes signals the slumbering instinct, but the process of falling asleep—and staying asleep—requires an elaborate cerebral orchestration of hormones, biological rhythms, and environmental cues. And as with any other bodily function, sleep requires a balance of all factors to ensure proper health.

When sleep is disrupted—whether due to lifestyle factors, insomnia, sleep apnea, narcolepsy, restless legs syndrome, jet lag, sleepwalking, night terrors, hormonal imbalance, or other disorders—emotional and physiological health suffers. If you're among the 60 million Americans suffering from chronic or intermittent sleep disorders each year,[1] tossing and turning all night has likely beset you with a host of potentially debilitating conditions, including an inability to concentrate, fatigue, and poor immune function. But you don't have to accept sleep deprivation and the ills that accompany it. And you don't have to resort to pharmaceutical sleeping aids, which generally bring on their own set of disabling symptoms in the form of side effects.

This book provides practical alternative therapies proven to induce and maintain a deep, regenerative sleep. Before you take a tranquilizer, which will invariably mask your symptoms, consider trying natural remedies that treat the underlying causes of your disorder. Dietary changes, detoxification, stress management, hormonal balance, and environmental controls can gently and effectively help you snooze your way back to health.

success story

Lifestyle Changes Restore Sleep

JERRY, A 47-YEAR-OLD PRINT SHOP OWNER, had not slept more than 3 hours a night for years. Then he started having spasms in his legs at night, which further interfered with his sleep. During his waking hours, he was tired all the time and looked 10 years older than his actual age. He was also irritable and often snapped at his employees and his family. He had chronic bloating and gas, and he frequently alternated between constipation and diarrhea. His energy level was erratic; sometimes he was frenetic and other times he was listless. He was very concerned about falling asleep while driving (25% of auto accidents are linked to sleep deprived drivers).

Jerry had tried many types of sleeping pills, but nothing had worked. He was desperate to get some sleep. Before scheduling any tests, we looked at Jerry's lifestyle. He started every day by drinking the first of many cups of coffee. He worked straight through lunch, grabbing a sandwich at his desk. Then he worked through dinnertime, finally quitting around 10 P.M. After that, he had dinner, washing it down with two or three glasses of wine. After dinner, Jerry immediately fell sound asleep, only to awaken at 2 A.M., unable to fall back to sleep for the rest of the night. Jerry never exercised and was under constant stress from the deadlines and schedules that were the nature of his business. He had become totally driven by the business and left no time for himself.

We told Jerry that the only way we could work with him was if he were willing to change his lifestyle. We made it clear that his sleeping problems were only a sign that all of his vital body functions—his circulatory, digestive, nervous, and hormonal systems—were beginning to fail. It had been so long since those systems were supported with proper nutrition and rest that they could no longer maintain the internal balance necessary to good health. Jerry initially resisted our suggestions but finally agreed, realizing that another sleeping pill was not the answer. He agreed to begin an exercise program (exercise will be discussed at length in chapter 9, on page 204). We referred Jerry to a personal trainer who had him begin with aerobic exercise and resistance training using weights. We also referred him to an acupuncturist for a series of treatments to help balance his system.

We discovered that Jerry had leaky gut syndrome, a condition in which the intestinal wall becomes semipermeable and allows toxins and partially digested food to leak from the intestines and enter the body's bloodstream, tissues, cells, and lymph fluid. Also, Jerry's digestive system was deficient in hydrochloric acid and enzymes, both of which are needed to break down nutrients in food so they can be absorbed. In addition, he didn't have enough of beneficial bacteria in his intestines to digest his food properly. To counter this digestive dysfunction and ease the toxic load on his body, we started Jerry on a liver detoxification program (chapter 4 is devoted to detoxification). A saliva test showed that Jerry was low on the hormone DHEA (dehydro-epiandrosterone), which is important for metabolism, so we prescribed DHEA supplements.

"Jerry was very concerned about falling asleep while driving."

We also examined Jerry's diet, looking for stimulants that impair sleep (chapter 3 is an in-depth discussion of dietary issues related to sleep). We suggested that Jerry reduce his consumption of caffeine. He agreed and started substituting decaffeinated coffee for regular coffee in gradually increasing proportions until he was drinking only decaf. He stopped consuming wine and adding salt to his food and agreed to eat three balanced meals a day and not eat snacks on the run. Jerry also began eating dinner between 6 P.M. and 7 P.M., and he started going to bed by 10 P.M.

For many insomniacs, stress management is very important, encouraging the body to heal and allowing it to respond to its natural internal cues. For Jerry, stress management involved hiring a consultant to organize his business and teach him how to communicate better with his employees and his family. To further reduce his daily stress levels, Jerry learned how to meditate and committed to meditating twice a day for 15 minutes at a time (chapter 6 will explore meditation and other mind-body approaches). Jerry also received weekly chiropractic treatments to correct structural imbalances that were affecting his nervous system (chiropractic and other methods of addressing structural issues are addressed in chapter 9). And, importantly, Jerry was counseled, supported, and encouraged in all of his lifestyle changes.

By the end of three weeks, Jerry was sleeping through the night. In addition, he enjoyed renewed energy and vitality. In a short time, he had lost 20 pounds, was no longer irritable, and found that his business could still thrive even when he started leaving the office at 5 P.M. At the end of three months, Jerry's digestive system was normal and he was feeling relaxed and happy. He had regained his spark and was more youthful. Jerry's sleep continues to be deep, uninterrupted, restful, and restorative.

The Physiological Function of Sleep

For years, scientists have debated the purpose of sleep. According to some evolutionary scientists, sleep evolved primarily as a survival mechanism. Before the discovery of fire, our early human ancestors were unable to see dangers at night, such as stalking animals or precarious cliffs, and avoid approaching them. Thus, humans—as well as all other animals—slept to keep themselves safe.

While this evolutionary approach partly explains the reasons for when we sleep, it doesn't answer why we sleep. The obvious answer is to ameliorate feelings of exhaustion. But researchers have struggled with the missing link between the desire for sleep and the purpose of it: Why can't the body replenish its vitality without delving into a netherworld of dreams and diminished consciousness? What is it about sleep that enables the body to fix itself? At present, it appears that sleep—particularly the sleep-inducing hormone melatonin—plays a crucial role in keeping the brain free of free radicals and stimulating the immune system. Studies prove that without sleep, the body would break down and die.

ZZZs against Free Radicals

During both waking and sleeping hours, our bodies are exposed to numerous free radicals. Free radicals are normal products of metabolism and are also derived from pesticides, industrial pollutants, smoking, alcohol, viruses, most infections, allergies, stress, and even certain foods and excessive exercise. Because free radicals have an unpaired electron, they're highly reactive. The process whereby they "steal" electrons from other substances is known as oxidation; this is the same process that turns iron to rust and the exposed surfaces of sliced apples brown. Free radicals are "free" in the sense of being unattached—molecular loose cannons that combine with oxygen in the air to initiate the process of spoilage. Internally, the same sort of deterioration occurs.

Although certain free radicals actually play an important role in metabolic processes, excessive or undesirable free radicals contribute to many health problems: they attack cell membranes, can interact with DNA to create mutations that may lead to cancer, and have been implicated in various degenerative diseases and the aging process itself. To counter the effects of free radicals, our bodies manufacture antioxidants or rely on outside sources of antioxidants, which serve the function of scavenging for free radicals, binding with them, and eliminating them. Toxins, however, impede this process by creating too many free radicals, which quickly deplete the body's reserve of antioxidant nutrients.

If free radicals are left to roam unimpeded throughout the body, the brain suffers many of the consequences. The brain, which consumes approximately 20% of the oxygen we breathe, is composed mostly of unsaturated fatty acids, complex molecules that are highly susceptible to free radical damage because they have a "loose" hold on their electrons. Also, brain tissue is rich in iron, which can transform hydrogen peroxide, a byproduct of oxygen metabolism, into hydroxyl radicals, which are particularly dangerous forms of free radicals.[2] Damage to brain cells can lead to memory impairment, loss of motor control, Alzheimer's disease, Lou Gehrig's disease, multiple sclerosis, Parkinson's disease, and other neurodegenerative conditions.[3]

Fortunately, the brain is protected by the blood-brain barrier, a layer of modified capillaries of limited permeability that makes it more difficult for substances in the bloodstream to enter the brain. This barrier keeps many toxins out of the brain, reducing (but not eliminating) the load of free radicals. However, it also prevents many antioxidants from entering the brain, allowing free radicals to accumulate.

Sleep can stem the influx of free radicals. When we sleep, the pineal gland (pronounced pie-NEEL), located in the brain, produces the hormone melatonin. Melatonin is best known for its hypnotic or sleep-inducing powers (see "The Role of Melatonin," page 17), but numerous scientific studies have shown that melatonin is a powerful antioxidant as well. And because melatonin is produced within the brain, it does not have to contend with the blood-brain barrier.

Melatonin is a highly effective scavenger of hydroxyl radicals and peroxyl radicals, another type of toxic free radical. In fact, melatonin has been shown to be more effective in scavenging hydroxyl radicals than other well-known antioxidants, such as glutathione.[4] Melatonin appears to inactivate free radicals on a subcellular level, reaching the free radicals that may attack DNA, proteins, and lipids within cells.[5] It also seems to stimulate important antioxidant enzymes within the body, including superoxide dismutase, glutathione peroxidase, and glutathione reductase.[6]

In experiments, melatonin has reduced the neuronal damage associated with Alzheimer's disease and Parkinson's disease.[7] It has also been shown to prevent cataracts (caused by free radical damage in the eye lens), as well as counteract the free radical effects of toxins such as paraquat, carbon tetrachloride, and safrole.[8] Production of melatonin is elevated during sleep, and studies have shown that prolonged periods of sleep deprivation cause neuronal damage in animal subjects.[9]

The Immune System: If You Don't Snooze, You Lose

Antioxidants are not the body's only defense against harmful substances roaming the body. The body is equipped with a potent immune system that identifies, attacks, and ultimately eliminates invading pathogens (antigens). During an immune response, white blood cells called T cells neutralize pathogens and B cells, another type of white blood cell, produce antibodies (protein molecules that bind with specific pathogens and other foreign substances to help destroy them). Other immune cells release chemicals (such as histamine) into the bloodstream to aid in the removal of antigens from the body.

In the context of sleep, it is important to understand the immune function of T cells. Though they are produced in the bone marrow, T cells mature in the thymus gland. The thymus programs each of the billions of T cells for a special immune duty. Some T cells are trained to become killer cells, which engulf or attack invading antigens. Types of killer cells include natural killer (NK) cells, which destroy hard-to-detect virus-infected and cancer cells; phagocytes, which immobilize and kill antigens through ingestion; and cytotoxic cells, which inject a poison into the cell membrane of foreign cells to kill them. Other T cells, called helper cells, act as mission control for the immune system. When antigens invade the body, helper T cells coordinate the activation and deactivation of killer cells and other immune cells by producing intercellular signaling chemicals called cytokines. The major cytokines are interleukins, interferons, colony-stimulating factors, and tumor necrosis factors.

Research has found that helper T cells contain receptors specifically designed to fit melatonin molecules. During sleep, melatonin attaches to these receptors and stimulates the production of a substance similar to interleukin-4. This substance then stimulates the activation of NK cells, phagocytes, and cytotoxic cells, as well as immune cells found in the bone marrow.[10] One study found that increasing nighttime melatonin levels by supplementing with 2 milligrams (mg) of melatonin led to a 240% increase in production of NK cells.[11] Another study found that the amount of melatonin normally found in the bloodstream during sleep increased the ability of a certain phagocyte to destroy skin cancer cells by 73%.[12]

The immune-stimulating properties of sleep may explain why we feel like sleeping more when suffering from an infectious disease, such as a cold or flu.[13] Experiments have shown that animals deprived of sleep for prolonged periods become severely ill and generally die from common viral infections that ordinarily have no effect on animals allowed to sleep.[14]

Other Health Benefits of Sleep

Researchers have also found melatonin to significantly reduce levels of low-density lipoprotein (LDL; "bad" cholesterol). In fact, one study showed that melatonin could decrease LDL cholesterol by up to 42%, and melatonin has also been proven to lower high blood pressure.[15] Sleep also gives your hardworking cardiovascular function a rest, allowing heart rate and blood pressure to decrease by as much as 10%. When sleep is insufficient, you may not experience this benefit, which has significant ramifications. Several studies have indicated that those who don't experience lower blood pressure at night are at greater risk of angina, heart attacks, congestive heart failure, and strokes.[16]

Low blood levels of melatonin have been implicated in patients with manic depression and schizophrenia; in these cases, restoring the person to normal nighttime levels of melatonin may be helpful.[17] Stress and the adrenal hormone cortisol, which is associated with stress, may have been contributing factors in reducing the patients' amounts of melatonin.

The pineal gland isn't the only gland functioning during sleep. It is just one among the glands in the endocrine system, which regulates and normalizes the body's complex systems, and includes the testicles, ovaries, pancreas, adrenals, thyroid, parathyroid, and pituitary, along with the pineal gland. All of these glands secrete hormones during sleep. Also, physiological processes that occur during the dream stage of sleep have been shown to improve cognitive health (see "In Dreams: Memory and Forgetting," page 14).

The Stages of Sleep

In the early days of sleep research, scientists believed that all but the most essential bodily and cerebral functions shut down during sleep. It wasn't until the advent of the electroencephalograph (EEG) in the late 1920s that researchers began to realize that sleep involves a startling amount of brain activity. By monitoring brain waves (see "Types of Brain Waves," page 12), scientists discovered five cyclic stages of alternately low and high brain wave function. It generally takes 90 to 110 minutes for the brain to complete one cycle.

The first four stages are called non–rapid eye movement sleep (NREM sleep); the fifth stage is rapid eye movement sleep (REM sleep). The NREM phases comprise approximately 75% of the sleep cycle (50% in infants) and are characterized by very restful sleep in which body movements, blood pressure, breathing, and basal metabolic rates are reduced by as much as 30% from normal waking levels.[18] There may be some dreaming during NREM sleep, though you're unlikely to recall those dreams.[19] The majority of remembered dreaming occurs during the REM phase.

In everyone except for infants, narcoleptics, and people deprived of sleep for more than 200 hours, NREM stages precede REM. However, you may skip around from various light and deep stages or completely omit the deep sleep stages after the second or third cycle of the night. Additionally, people commonly experience a period of up to 2 hours of quiet wakefulness between 4-hour periods of regular sleep cycles. During this interval, sleepers are neither fully awake nor fully asleep, but resting and reviewing their dreams with their thoughts turned off.

Stage 1: This is the shortest phase, in which slowing alpha waves prepare you for the sleep state. As you drift in and out of wakefulness, your breathing, heart rate, metabolic rate, and body temperature begin to drop. Muscles start to relax. You may experience a sensation of falling followed by sudden muscle contractions; this is called hypnic myoclonia. You may experience hypnagogic dreams (*hypnagogic* refers to the period of drowsiness immediately preceding sleep). During stage 1, you are easily awakened by external stimuli, at which point you may only remember a few fragments of hypnagogic images and thoughts.

Stage 2: This is the longest sleep phase, marked by a light level of sleep. The brain slows down into theta waves, with intermittent surges of rapid brain waves (spindles) followed by large, slow bursts of delta waves. Breathing, heat rate, metabolic rate, and body temperature continue to decline. You may be awakened easily by sound and movement.

Stage 3: As the brain progressively slows down to large, slow delta waves, you enter a deeper stage of sleep. Muscles go limp and breathing is slow and even. You may begin to sweat. During this stage and stage 4, the body

Types of Brain Waves

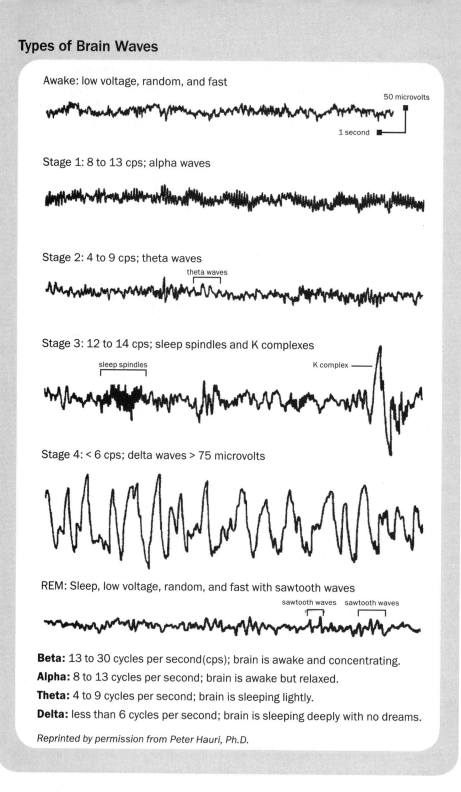

Awake: low voltage, random, and fast

50 microvolts

1 second

Stage 1: 8 to 13 cps; alpha waves

Stage 2: 4 to 9 cps; theta waves

theta waves

Stage 3: 12 to 14 cps; sleep spindles and K complexes

sleep spindles

K complex

Stage 4: < 6 cps; delta waves > 75 microvolts

REM: Sleep, low voltage, random, and fast with sawtooth waves

sawtooth waves   sawtooth waves

Beta: 13 to 30 cycles per second(cps); brain is awake and concentrating.

Alpha: 8 to 13 cycles per second; brain is awake but relaxed.

Theta: 4 to 9 cycles per second; brain is sleeping lightly.

Delta: less than 6 cycles per second; brain is sleeping deeply with no dreams.

Reprinted by permission from Peter Hauri, Ph.D.

The Five Stages of Sleep

Stage	Degree of Sleep	Duration	Level of Consciousness	Brain Wave Activity	Physiological Processes
1	"dozing," very light	30 seconds to 7 minutes	Drifting in and out of sleep; awakened easily by all stimuli	Irregular, rapid alpha waves	Muscles relax; smooth, even breathing; body temperature and heart rate begin to drop
2	light	45 to 50 minutes in first cycle, decreasing to 25 minutes in last	Awakened easily by sounds and movement	Irregular theta waves, with intermittent rapid alpha activity and bursts of delta waves	Breathing, temperature, heart rate continue to decrease; muscles further relax; eyes may roll slowly
3	moderately deep	7 to 15 minutes in first 2 or 3 cycles, then disappears	Difficult to awaken with stimuli	Brain waves slow drastically, mostly large delta waves	Breathing and heart rate continue to drop but stabilize; very relaxed; may sweat
4	very deep	12 minutes in first 2 or 3 cycles, then disappears	Very difficult to awaken with stimuli	Large, slow delta waves	Breathing and heart rate stable but slow; very relaxed; may sweat
REM	dreaming	10 minutes at first, increasing to 15 to 30 minutes as cycles continue	May be awakened more easily but difficult to adjust to reality	Smaller, more regular alpha waves resembling those of stage 1	Eyes roll back and forth; muscles freeze except for some twitching in face, toes, fingers; breathing, heart rate irregular; penile erections in men

begins to restore itself. In people under 30, during stage 3 the pituitary gland releases human growth hormone (HGH), which promotes cell division and organ growth. Awakening a person in stage 3 sleep is fairly difficult to do, and the sleeper may experience grogginess for a few seconds or minutes after awakening. After two or three sleep cycles, this stage may disappear and you may go directly from stage 2 to REM sleep.

Stage 4: This is the deepest stage of sleep. Delta waves become larger and much slower than in stage 3, and breathing, heart rate, metabolism, and temperature reach their lowest levels. Muscles continue to be inactive

In Dreams: Memory and Forgetting

Most scientists believe that dreams are the result of brain nerve cells transmitting electrical impulses into the brain's long-term memory bank, at which time electrons are released that trigger hallucinations in the cortex. But the purpose of dreams—like the purpose of sleep—has been hotly debated by both sleep researchers and psychiatrists.

A century ago, Sigmund Freud postulated that dreams allow the repressed mind a chance to act out its darkest urges. Others believe dreams impart meaningful lessons we can apply to our waking lives. While both theories may have merit, some sleep researchers believe dreaming improves the memory and capacity to learn. According to this theory, REM sleep allows the brain to transfer new material into the memory, specifically by increasing the efficiency of the left brain hemisphere, which during waking hours is active in collecting new language skills and other information.[20] Research continues into precise mechanisms of this memory consolidation process, and interesting new findings are often reported. One study links REM-induced blood flow through a part of the brain called the amygdaloid complexes to the processing of some types of memory.[21] Brain chemicals such as dopamine and epinephrine—which may be diminished by sleep deprivation—help transfer new information from the intermediate-term, high-capacity buffer in the hippocampus (a part of the brain) into long-term memory storage in the neocortex.[22]

Regardless of the mechanism, several studies confirm the correlation between REM sleep and long-term retention of learning. In one study,

scientists introduced test subjects to basic visual discrimination tasks and then allowed some of them to sleep normally overnight, while the rest were permitted to sleep during all stages of sleep except for REM sleep. The subjects who had dreamed performed significantly better on the new tasks than those who didn't dream.[23] Another study found that subjects taking a French language course reported better learning retention if their dreams contained references to the French class.[24] In a study involving learning new words and recognizing them later, sleeping and dreaming immediately after learning resulted in better long-term memory of the words than sleeping hours after learning them.[25] Other studies suggest that dreams not only help us learn better, they also help us develop new solutions or adaptations to problems.[26] Studies have shown that people deprived of REM sleep are more irritable and anxious in their waking hours—and thus are less able to cope with daily problems—than those who are allowed to dream.[27]

Although dreams have many important functions, we often forget the content of our dreams. This may be due to vasopressin, a hormone released by melatonin during sleep that acts as an amnesic agent, erasing recent memory from the hippocampus during dreams.[28] Or, as sleep expert William Dement, MD, Ph.D., hypothesizes, we may forget dreams so as to avoid confusing ourselves. "If we remembered every dream clearly," he says, "it might become difficult to sort out what really occurred and what was a dream."[29]

and the sleeper may sweat, but the body continues its restorative activities. Some sleepers may experience night terrors or sleepwalking. Toward the end of this stage, sleepers may readjust their position and may experience a muscular contraction as they enter the next stage. Rousing sleepers from this phase takes a great deal of effort. Once awakened, people feel groggy and may require several minutes to orient themselves. After two or three cycles, this stage may disappear for the rest of the night.

Stage 5: This is REM sleep, the dreaming phase, marked by small, rapid alpha waves that resemble those indicating wakefulness and sensory awareness of external stimuli. However, in this stage the brain is reacting to internally generated stimuli from dreams. Most muscles seize up to prevent the person from reacting to the action in the dreams, but the sleeper may experience some slight twitching in the face, fingers, and toes. Men experience penile erections. Breathing and heart rate speed up and slow down in reaction to dream content. A sleeper in the REM stage is difficult to rouse and, if awakened, will have a hard time adjusting to reality. This stage becomes progressively longer with each cycle, possibly lasting 60 minutes in the fifth cycle.

How Much Sleep Do You Need?

The average person sleeps 6.8 hours per night on weeknights and 7.4 hours per night on weekends[30] and completes four to five sleep cycles. A person's sleep requirements for good health vary according to age and gender, as well as level of activity during the day. Contrary to conventional wisdom, it is not necessary for all adults to get 8 hours of sleep every night to maintain good health. Some people function well with only 5 hours of sleep, while others may need 10 to feel revived in the morning. On the whole, though, most experts recommend approximately 8 hours of sleep per day. Infants require the most sleep, at 16 to 18 hours a day, and young adults generally need about 7 to 8.5 hours of shut-eye. As people age, they tend to sleep more lightly and for a shorter duration. The amount of sleep older people need has been debated over the years, but since people over age 55 spend fewer and fewer minutes in stages 3 and 4, they may actually need more than 8 hours of sleep to experience the restorative powers of deep sleep.

The modern American lifestyle can keep people from getting the sleep they need to function properly. Late nights at the office, shift work, and multiple social and family obligations eat away from the time dedicated to slumber. Many high school students are sleep deprived due to the early start times of some schools or trying to do too many activities along with homework, and this may affect their academic abilities. Such factors can run up a high sleep debt, the cumulative amount of time needed to make up for loss of sleep. If you need 8 hours of sleep but get only 6 hours two nights in a row, your total sleep debt will be 4 hours (2 nights times 2 hours). If you neglect to pay off your sleep debt, you will likely experience mood problems as well as poor cognitive function, which can be detrimental to your health and the health of those around you. According to the National Highway Traffic Safety Administration, driver fatigue (due to sleep deprivation) is responsible for an estimated 100,000 motor vehicle accidents and 1,500 deaths each year.[31]

Though there are tests that doctors use to assess whether a person is meeting their sleep requirements (see "Diagnosing Sleep Disorders," page 32), if you feel alert and emotionally stable with good memory recall and reaction times, you're probably getting enough sleep. Another clue is sleep latency, the normal length of time it takes you to fall asleep from the time you lie down. While most people can't pinpoint the actual moment they fall asleep, you can still estimate. The average sleep latency is between 15 and 20 minutes; falling asleep within 5 minutes of hitting the sack indicates sleep deprivation. Microsleep (very brief periods of sleep lasting as little as a fraction of a second) are another sign of sleep deprivation. Most people who experience microsleep aren't aware of it, but a minor lapse in attention may tip you off that this is occurring. Additionally, feeling drowsy during the day, even during tedious activities, likely means that you haven't had enough sleep.

Circadian Rhythms and the Body's Clock

As mentioned earlier, sleeping during the night likely evolved to keep animals, including the human species, out of harm's way. Supporting this theory is the fact that most of us still follow the sun's cycles, sleeping when the sun is down and waking when it's up. In fact, we possess innate cycles, called circadian rhythms, that correspond to the daily pattern of the sun. Scientists believe that these rhythms are guided partly by genes that have evolved in many species, from bacteria to humans.[32]

Circadian rhythms are regularly recurring biological changes in mental and physical behaviors over the course of the day. As indicated by the term *circadian* (Latin for "about a day"), these rhythms repeat approximately every 24 hours. Controlled by an internal clock, circadian rhythms are most commonly linked to sleep-wake patterns and account for fluctuations in alertness and drowsiness throughout the day. People with normal circadian rhythms are most alert during the morning and afternoon, tend to get drowsy toward evening, and feel the need for sleep at nighttime. Research shows that circadian rhythms occur in other physiological processes as well, including blood pressure, body temperature, hormone levels, and immune system activity.[33]

The body clock is actually part of the hypothalamus, an area of the brain just above the point where the optic nerves cross. Specifically, the clock is a cluster of hypothalamic nerve cells called the suprachiasmatic nucleus (SCN). As with other precise timepieces, researchers believe the body clock operates on the principle of oscillation. In much the same way that a grandfather clock keeps time with the evenly spaced swings of a pendulum, the body clock tells time with the slow ebb and flow of protein molecules in

Parts of the Brain Involved in the Body Clock

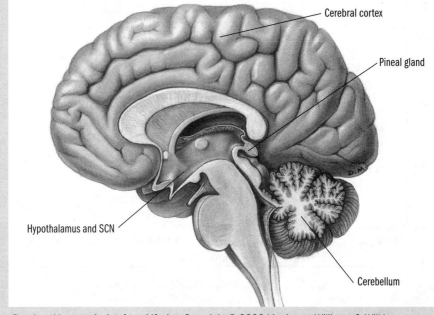

Reprinted by permission from Life Art. Copyright © 2000 Lippincott Williams & Wilkins

the SCN. In controlled conditions where test subjects are deprived of light and other time cues, a "day" by body clock standards is close to 25 hours. However, we do not exist in such a vacuum. Light, from both the sun and artificial devices, as well as environmental cues called zeitgebers (German for "time-giver"), such as alarm clocks, influence our circadian rhythms and set our body clocks to follow the 24-hour cycle of the sun.

How light manages to sway our internal timepieces also depends on the SCN nerves in the hypothalamus. The optic nerves relay information about external light levels to the SCN, which in turn sends the light signals to several regions of the brain, including the pea-sized pineal gland. The pineal gland is instrumental in sleep, because it secretes a sleep-inducing hormone, melatonin.

The Role of Melatonin

As discussed above, melatonin has been shown to have numerous health benefits, functioning as an antioxidant, stimulating the immune system, and supporting cardiovascular health. But beyond these important benefits, it is crucial in the induction of sleep and the regulation of circadian rhythms.

When it's dark, the pineal gland secretes melatonin in extremely minute amounts—blood levels of melatonin are measured in picograms, that

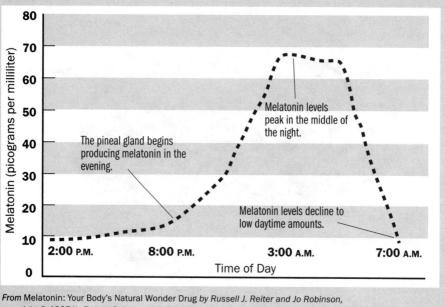

The 24-Hour Cycle of Melatonin Production

Melatonin levels peak in the middle of the night.

The pineal gland begins producing melatonin in the evening.

Melatonin levels decline to low daytime amounts.

Melatonin (picograms per milliliter)

80
70
60
50
40
30
20
10
0

2:00 P.M.   8:00 P.M.   3:00 A.M.   7:00 A.M.

Time of Day

From Melatonin: Your Body's Natural Wonder Drug *by Russell J. Reiter and Jo Robinson, copyright © 1995 by Russel Reiter and Jo Robinson. Used by permission of Bantam Books, a division of Random House, Inc.*

is, trillionths of a gram. The actual amounts depend on age and other factors, but between 5 and 10 times more melatonin is released at night than during the day.[34] Melatonin is the antithesis of another hormone, adrenaline, produced by the adrenal glands. As melatonin enters the bloodstream, it begins to slow down the waking (alpha) brain waves. Subsequently, heart rate decreases, muscles relax, blood pressure drops, and the body begins to enter the stages of sleep.

Average blood levels of melatonin throughout the day mirror typical circadian rhythms. Low amounts of melatonin correspond to periods of heightened alertness; high amounts of melatonin relate to periods of drowsiness and sleep. Between 7 A.M. and 2 P.M., melatonin is at its lowest level, below 10 picograms per milliliter (pg/ml) of blood. From 2 P.M. to about 8 P.M., melatonin levels rise slightly as the pineal gland begins production of the sleep hormone. In most people, melatonin reaches its peak (70 pg/ml) at approximately 2 A.M., then flattens for a couple of hours before beginning a dramatic drop to its lowest levels around 4 A.M.

Production of melatonin not only varies during the 24-hour cycle, it also fluctuates during our life span. Although newborns usually sleep 16 to 18 hours a day, spread out over six to seven naps, they produce very low amounts of melatonin. By the age of three months, they begin producing greater levels of the hormone; it is also during this time that babies begin to sleep through the night and become more alert during the day. Melatonin levels then surge until age of 10, when they peak at about 125 pg/ml. During this stage of life, children sleep 10 or more hours per night and undergo a dramatic growth spurt, which is aided by sleep.

When adolescents reach puberty, a time when high levels of sex hormones are being released, melatonin levels begin to decline, and this continues for the rest of the person's life. For reasons scientists are still researching, levels of other hormones, including testosterone, estrogen, growth hormone, and DHEA, also decline with age. Between the ages of 20 and 30, melatonin levels are about 40 to 60 pg/ml; by age 50, levels are below 20 pg/ml. People over 60 produce negligible amounts of melatonin, below 10 pg/ml.

The Precursors to Melatonin

The pineal gland simply doesn't make melatonin out of thin air. For melatonin to be produced, the brain needs an adequate supply of tryptophan, an amino acid that cannot be created by the body. We can only obtain this essential amino acid from dietary sources such as meat, fish, dairy products, mushrooms, spinach, and soy products. The brain is surrounded by the blood-brain barrier, so tryptophan requires the aid of a carrier, a special type of protein that transports the amino acid across the protective layer. (For dietary recommendations to facilitate tryptophan uptake by the brain, see "Eat to Boost Tryptophan Levels," page 60.)

Once tryptophan has entered the brain, a specialized enzyme helps brain cells convert it into 5-hydroxytryptophan (5-HTP). Another enzyme then helps convert 5-HTP into the neurotransmitter serotonin. Then, the enzyme N-acetyltransferase (NAT), reacts with some of the serotonin to make the chemical N-acetylserotonin (NAS). With the help of another specialized enzyme, the pineal gland is able to convert NAS into melatonin.[35]

Melatonin and the Light Paradox

Light plays a crucial—and seemingly paradoxical—role in sleep, as it both inhibits and promotes melatonin production. The enzyme NAT, necessary for melatonin synthesis, is mostly or completely inactivated by exposure to light.[36] A 100-lux light (a 100-watt bulb from a distance of 5 feet) will inhibit melatonin secretion,[37] and studies have shown that being exposed to even a fairly dim light at night can significantly reduce the synthesis of melatonin.[38]

At the same time, studies have shown that bright light also significantly boosts melatonin production.[39]

Why are these findings so contradictory? The truth is, they're not. What matters with light is when you and your nervous system—and thus your body clock—are exposed to it. During the daytime hours, when the circadian rhythm is in its more alert stages, the brain requires bright light. This promotes the increased synthesis of serotonin, which in turn means more melatonin will be produced at night. During the nighttime hours, when the circadian rhythm causes many physical functions to fall to their lowest level, the brain needs to produce melatonin to prepare the body for sleep and keep it asleep. Thus, the brain requires darkness; even a night-light a few feet from the bed or the glow from a bright digital clock can be detrimental to melatonin production.

Factors That Can Disrupt Your Body Clock

Many people with sleep disorders have disrupted circadian rhythms, often due to melatonin imbalances in which the natural sleep-wake patterns are interrupted or reversed. Many Americans spend up to 90% of their day indoors, in buildings with fluorescent lights. This lack of exposure to bright sunlight or its artificial cousin, full-spectrum light, is a major contributor to disrupted circadian rhythms and resulting reduced melatonin levels. Lack of regular exercise, structural imbalances, and chronic stress are also common factors. So, too, is a poor diet, often marked by overconsumption of stimulants such as alcohol, caffeine, spicy foods, and sugar. Over-the-counter medications can also play a role. Electromagnetic fields, both natural and artificial, may play a role in diminishing the function of the pineal gland, resulting in decreased melatonin production and an imbalanced body clock.

One of the most prevalent consequences of a disrupted circadian rhythm is an illness called seasonal affective disorder (SAD). Individuals who receive little natural light during the day often experience an imbalance in their serotonin and melatonin levels—specifically, a rise in melatonin and a corresponding decline in serotonin. When low exposure to natural light is chronic, it can lead to SAD. Often called "winter depression," SAD frequently occurs during the fall and winter months, when days grow shorter and natural light is limited. (For a thorough discussion of SAD and how to combat it, see "Beating the Winter Blues," page 123.)

two

Sleep Disorders
and Their Causes

If you're tired as you read this, you're not alone. In a 2005 survey by the National Sleep Foundation, about 30% of adults admitted to experiencing daytime sleepiness at least three days a week and driving when drowsy at least once a month.[1] Sleep deprivation is usually to blame. The average adult sleeps just under 7 hours per night during the workweek,[2] but most people function best on at least 8 hours of shut-eye. Sometimes sleep deprivation is self-imposed—you choose to stay up late working, socializing, or watching TV and still get up early to exercise or make your morning commute. But others can't get enough sleep no matter how hard they try. According to the National Institute of Neurological Disorders and Stroke, approximately 40 million Americans suffer from long-term chronic sleep disorders, while another 20 million experience occasional sleep problems.[3] But those statistics may underestimate the prevalence of slumber woes; according to the National Sleep Foundation's 2005 survey, 51% of American adults reported occasional sleep problems, and 26% said that they get a good night's sleep only a few times a month—or less.[4] In fact, it is estimated that 95% of sleep disorders are not diagnosed.[5]

Altogether Americans spend about $16 billion each year on sleep-related medical care. Unfortunately, much of this money is poorly spent, because conventional sleeping aids—potentially addictive sedatives—ultimately create more sleep disturbances than they eliminate. Conventional physicians are beginning to realize this fact, however, and are increasingly likely to suggest that their patients make lifestyle changes to remedy sleep disorders. But knowing exactly which changes to make for your particular condition can be difficult, and conventional doctors are poorly trained in recognizing the underlying causes of sleep problems.

Alternative medicine practitioners can make sure that finding the right treatment protocol doesn't turn into a nightmare. They realize that sleep disorders, including insomnia, sleep apnea, restless legs syndrome, and narcolepsy, often arise from poor diet, toxic overload, disrupted circadian rhythms, emotional stress, disruptive electromagnetic fields, and hormonal and structural imbalances. In short, the majority of sleep problems are symptoms of an unhealthy body, not diseases in and of themselves. Most people with sleep disorders will find relief by taking steps to promote overall health: improving their diet, detoxifying the body, reducing stress, balancing hormones, and correcting structural issues, among others. This chapter will introduce you to the primary underlying causes of sleep problems and provide you with an overview of alternative therapies that can help restore normality to your sleep—and your life.

Types of Sleep Disorders

Sleep disorders fall under two categories: dyssomnias and parasomnias. Dyssomnias are conditions characterized by difficulty in falling asleep or maintaining sleep or by excessive sleepiness during the day. Insomnia, sleep apnea, restless legs syndrome, periodic limb movements in sleep, narcolepsy, delayed sleep phase syndrome, advanced sleep phase syndrome, and hypersomnia are dyssomniac conditions. Parasomnias are behavioral abnormalities that occur during sleep, including sleepwalking, night terrors, and REM behavior disorder.

Sleep researchers sometimes further classify sleep disorders as primary or secondary. Primary disorders are unrelated to any existing medical conditions, whereas secondary disorders arise as the result of some other illness or hormonal change, such as menopause, pregnancy, depression, or fibromyalgia. Alternative medicine practitioners may not make such distinctions, because in their view, both the underlying medical condition and the sleep disorder arise from the same underlying causes.

Insomnia

Insomnia is a broad term casually used to describe the inability either to fall asleep or to remain asleep during the course of the night. Insomniacs usually do not feel rested the next morning and may experience excessive drowsiness, irritability, and poor cognitive function during the day.

Sleep researchers classify insomnia in terms of the time of night that it affects: sleep onset insomnia, sleep maintenance insomnia, and early-morning awakening insomnia.

- *Sleep onset insomnia:* People suffering from sleep onset insomnia take 30 or more minutes to fall asleep, after which they enjoy a relatively normal night of sleep. Of the adults who complain of having insomnia, about 22% report experiencing this type.[6] People suffering from sleep onset insomnia often exacerbate their situation by focusing on the fact that they are not sleeping; this is called psychophysiological insomnia. In this case, a person's normal presleep rituals, behavior, or sleeping environment triggers insomnia. The more the sleeper worries about falling asleep, the worse the insomnia becomes.

Types of Sleep Disorders

- Insomnia
- Sleep apnea
- Restless legs syndrome
- Periodic limb movement disorder
- Narcolepsy
- Delayed sleep phase syndrome
- Advanced sleep phase syndrome
- Hypersomnia
- Sleepwalking
- Night terrors
- REM behavior disorder
- Rhythmic movement disorder
- Bruxism (teeth-grinding)
- Bed-wetting

- *Sleep maintenance insomnia:* This type of insomnia is characterized by waking up one or more times during the course of the night and taking more than 30 minutes to fall back asleep after each awakening. This is the most common type of insomnia, accounting for around 34% of insomnia cases.[7]

- *Early-morning awakening insomnia:* If you awaken before dawn and can't get back to sleep, you have early-morning awakening insomnia. About 22% of insomniacs reportedly suffer from this type.[8] Most researchers also characterize insomnia based on frequency. Transient insomnia lasts one or several nights and is usually triggered by stress, excitement, or traveling across time zones (jet lag). Intermittent insomnia occurs sporadically over a long period of time; it, too, is generally set off by stress. Chronic insomnia occurs on most nights and lasts a month or more, and may arise from various medical conditions, including depression, anxiety disorders, arthritis, asthma, some heart and lung diseases, Alzheimer's disease, Parkinson's disease, and chronic pain.[9]

Postmenopausal women and older people tend to be more likely to suffer from some type of insomnia.

Conventional treatment for transient and intermittent insomnia is usually with over-the-counter sleeping pills or prescription benzodiazepine

The Sleepiness Scale

Sleep researchers at Stanford University in Palo Alto, California, have developed a way to document your sleep habits. Called the Stanford Sleepiness Scale, this simple questionnaire allows you and your doctor to determine if you are getting enough sleep and whether any of your sleep or daytime habits indicate a sleep disorder.[10] It is particularly useful if you also keep a sleep diary, a record of your sleep patterns that includes what time you go to bed each night (and nap during the day), how long it takes you to fall asleep, and when you get up.

To complete the Stanford scale, simply make a notation of the number that best corresponds to how you feel at different times of the day. Make notations an hour or two after you wake up in the morning (when you're usually at your peak of alertness), at around 2 P.M. (normally the sleepiest point in the day, due to circadian rhythms), and again at 7 P.M. or 8 P.M. (typically the most alert time in the evening). By comparing your responses over the course of days or even weeks, you'll be able to tell if your sleepiness and wakefulness patterns coincide with the norm or if your circadian rhythms are off track.

1. Feeling active, vital, alert, or wide awake
2. Functioning at a high level, but not at peak
3. Awake but relaxed;, responsive but not fully alert
4. A little foggy, not at peak, and feeling let down
5. Foggy, losing interest in staying awake, and slowed down
6. Sleepy; fighting sleep; would prefer to be lying down
7. Almost in a reverie; no longer fighting sleep; having dreamlike thoughts

sedatives. Chronic insomnia rarely responds well to sleeping pills.

Sleep Apnea

It's estimated that more than 12 million Americans suffer from sleep apnea, a potentially life-threatening disorder in which the sleeper experiences intermittent cessation of breathing.[11] The more common form of this condition is obstructive sleep apnea, in which the air passages become blocked, causing respiratory distress. Obstruction may be caused when the throat muscles and tongue relax during sleep, allowing the tongue and uvula (the small, fleshy tissue hanging from the back of the throat) to sag and block the airway. Excessive tissue in the airways (prevalent among overweight people) and excess swelling and mucus production in the nose (often caused by childhood allergies) can also narrow airways and substantially obstruct breathing during sleep.[12] Central sleep apnea, in which the brain fails to signal the respiratory muscles to breathe, is less common.

In an episode of sleep apnea, the sleeper involuntary stops breathing for 10 to 60 seconds, resulting in decreased blood levels of oxygen and increased amounts of carbon dioxide. This change in blood gases alerts the brain to begin breathing. To do so, the brain must awaken the body from deep sleep. The sleeper then resumes breathing, usually with a loud snort or gasp, and then quickly falls back into light sleep. People with obstructive sleep apnea usually snore heavily before and after the breathing pauses.

These apneic events can occur up to 30 times each hour, and sometimes even more frequently, although the sleeper rarely realizes this because the awakenings are so brief. However, these constant arousals prevent people from getting enough deep sleep and lead to excessive daytime sleepiness, morning headaches (from lack of oxygen), depression, irritability, sexual dysfunction, learning and memory difficulties, and falling asleep during daily activities. Sleep apnea has also been linked to irregular heartbeat and heart attack,[13] as well as high blood pressure, stroke, and sudden infant death syndrome (SIDS), so it is prudent for people who suspect that they or their children suffer from this disorder get medical care. However, it may be that a large percentage of people with sleep apnea don't realize they suffer from this serious sleep disorder; because it occurs while sleeping, they are unable to detect their problem.

Sleeping partners often observe the apnea episodes and can provide valuable information as to whether you suffer from the symptoms of sleep apnea.

Snoring and Sleep Apnea

Snoring is a common sign of sleep apnea, but it does not necessarily indicate that a person suffers from this disorder. Although 30% to 40% of adults snore, only 1% of snorers have sleep apnea.[15] So if you snore, how do you know whether it is sleep apnea or not?

In most cases, snoring does not involve obstruction of the airways. Instead, the sawing-wood sound is caused by vibrations of the soft palate and uvula during the course of breathing during sleep. If snoring is not accompanied by pauses in breathing, you can be assured that your snoring is not indicative of sleep apnea. To be sure, you may want to consult your doctor about testing for sleep apnea.

Snoring unrelated to sleep apnea has not been found to pose any health risk and doesn't cause daytime drowsiness for the sleeper (though the bed partner may be awakened by loud snoring).[16] To prevent snoring, sleep experts recommend that people sleep on their side. If you tend to roll on your back at night, sew a pocket into the back of your pajamas and put a tennis ball or golf balls inside. That will keep you on your side. Dental appliances are also sometimes used.

Doctors usually use polysomnography and/or the multiple sleep latency test (see "Diagnosing Sleep Disorders," page 32) to diagnose this problem.

People with sleep apnea should avoid alcohol and sleeping pills, as they lessen the body's ability to awaken from sleep. These sedative substances impair the body's ability to quickly awaken at night to restore breathing and could lead to suffocation in cases of severe apnea. Another downside of alcohol and sleeping pills is that either can prevent people from losing excess weight. The National Institutes of Health reports that even a little weight loss can reduce the incidence of sleep apnea.[14] Sleeping on your side and wearing a dental appliance that repositions your jaw and tongue may prove helpful in relieving mild sleep apnea.

Doctors may also prescribe the use of a continuous positive airway pressure (CPAP) device, which involves wearing a mask that forces air through the nose and keeps the throat from collapsing. In some cases, doctors recommend surgery to remove the adenoids and tonsils (most effective in young children), nasal polyps, and other tissue blocking the airway. In another surgical procedure, excess tissue in the back of the throat is removed

Treatment Guidelines for Sleep Apnea

- Use a continuous positive airway pressure (CPAP) device, a mask that forces air through the nose to keep the throat open.

- Lose weight. This reduces fat in the throat and can open up the airways.

- Sew a tennis ball into the back of the person's pajama top to prevent sleeping on the back.

- Stop smoking. Cigarettes can cause nasal and throat swelling.

- Avoid alcohol, tranquilizers, sleeping pills, and antihistamines in the evening. These can relax throat muscles to the point of collapse.

- Use nasal tape. Available over the counter, nasal strips pull the sides of the nose outward, holding the nasal passages open.

- Eliminate allergens in the home. Dust, mold, or other allergens may cause nasal congestion.

- Raise the head of the bed or add pillows. Sleeping with your head raised helps drain congestion and open your airways.

- Develop a consistent sleep schedule. Regular sleeping may help keep breathing stable and decrease snoring.

- Wash out your sinuses. A process called pulsatile nasal irrigation uses a WaterPik or similar device with a special attachment to clear out thick secretions. Ask your health-care practitioner for more information about this.

- Wear a custom dental splint. Good for people with large tongues, the dental splint holds the jaw forward so that the tongue can't fall back toward the throat and obstruct breathing.

using surgical instruments (uvulopalatopharyngoplasty) or lasers (uvulopalatoplasty). This procedure may eliminate sleeping problems but not sleep apnea itself; additionally, the long-term effects are unknown. The most drastic conventional measure is tracheostomy, in which a small hole is made in the windpipe, allowing the sleeper to breathe uninterrupted during the night. This procedure works, but it is rarely used.

Restless Legs Syndrome

Restless legs syndrome (RLS) is an unpleasant sleep disorder in which sufferers often feel creeping, crawling, prickling, burning, itching, or tugging sensations in their legs while resting or sitting for extended periods of time. Sometimes the arms may be affected as well. At night, the sensations can be so bothersome that people with RLS feel the need to move their legs and often cannot get to sleep until the discomfort subsides. The National Institute of Neurological Disorders and Stroke estimates that 80% of the 12 million Americans with RLS also experience periodic limb movement disorder (PLMD; see opposite page).[17] People with RLS often suffer from sleep onset insomnia or sleep maintenance insomnia and extreme daytime drowsiness.

Those with RLS generally find temporary relief by stretching, rubbing, or massaging their legs. Conventional doctors may prescribe dopaminergic agents (drugs that modulate or increase levels of the brain chemical dopamine), benzodiazepines (nervous system sedatives), opioids (narcotic painkillers), or anticonvulsant drugs.

Most cases of RLS are diagnosed in people between the ages of 50 and 60, but symptoms of this sleep disorder usually manifest earlier. Some children who experience "growing pains" or are labeled hyperactive because they cannot sit still may actually be suffering from RLS. According to the RLS Foundation, up to 25% of pregnant women experience RLS, usually in the third trimester; the condition often disappears within four weeks after delivery.[18] Some cases of RLS appear to be hereditary. Anemia, diabetes, kidney failure, and rheumatoid arthritis are associated with the onset or provocation of RLS. Doctors usually diagnose RLS by taking a detailed family history and sometimes polysomnography, in which increased number of brain wave spikes called K complexes, followed by bursts of alpha brain waves, indicate RLS.[19]

Treatment Options for Restless Legs Syndrome and Periodic Limb Movement Disorder

- Exercise regularly. Walking and cycling are good choices.
- Soak in a hot bath, then do 10 deep knee bends.
- Stretch your legs, particularly the calves.
- Regularly massage your legs or use a heating pad on your legs.
- Eliminate coffee, tea, and chocolate from your diet.
- Supplement with vitamins C and E, folic acid, and the minerals iron, calcium, and magnesium.
- Participate in a local support group; more than 150 exist throughout the country.

Periodic Limb Movement Disorder

Periodic limb movement disorder (PLMD) often coexists with restless legs syndrome. It is characterized by sudden, involuntary, and repetitive leg jerking that occurs at the onset of sleep as well as during the course of sleep. These movements can happen every 10 to 60 seconds, perhaps hundreds of times, usually in the first half of the night during NREM sleep. PLMD, like RLS, can cause sleep onset insomnia and sleep maintenance insomnia, and often disturbs the sleep of bed partners as well. Like those with RLS, people with PLMD often feel excessively sleepy during the day.

Conventional doctors may prescribe dopaminergic agents or opioids to treat PLMS. Some physicians may recommend 15- to 30-minute sessions of transcutaneous electric nerve stimulation (TENS); this treatment involves applying electrical charges to leg nerves before bed to alleviate nighttime leg jerking.

Narcolepsy

Narcolepsy is a chronic sleep disorder in which patients experience daytime sleepiness so extreme that they fall asleep at inappropriate times for anywhere from a few seconds to 30 minutes. These "sleep attacks" can occur repeatedly in the course of normal daily activities, such as talking, eating, working, or walking—even after a full night's sleep. Another classic symptom of narcolepsy is cataplexy, an episodic disorder marked by the sudden loss of muscle function. Cataplexy can range from slight weakness, such as limpness of the neck or knees, sagging facial muscles, or an inability to speak distinctly, to complete body collapse. Cataplexy may be triggered by sudden emotional reactions, such as anger, fear, or laughter, and can last anywhere from a few seconds to several minutes. During these events, the person remains conscious.

Narcolepsy can also cause temporary paralysis, in which the person is unable to talk or move when falling asleep or waking up, and hypnagogic hallucinations, potentially frightening dreamlike experiences that sometimes occur in stage 1 sleep. Almost everyone with narcolepsy is affected by excessive daytime sleepiness and sleep attacks, and about 70% may experience cataplexy; temporary paralysis and hallucinations are less common.[20]

Sleep researchers have discovered that people with narcolepsy experience a reversal of sleep stages. As discussed in chapter 1, the majority of people begin each sleep cycle with NREM stages and end with REM, the dream state. Narcoleptics, however, begin with REM sleep, and this abnormality extends into the waking hours as common aspects of normal REM sleep—lack of muscle tone, sleep paralysis, and vivid dreams—inappropriately occur during periods of wakefulness.

There may be a genetic component to risk for developing narcolepsy. The National Institutes of Health estimates that 10% of narcoleptics have a close relative with the disorder; however, they also suggest that genetic risk alone can't cause narcolepsy, and that other factors, such as stress, immune dysfunction, hormonal imbalance, or trauma, play a role.[21] Symptoms usually manifest in the early teen or adult years. Doctors use polysomnography as well as the multiple sleep latency test to diagnose narcolepsy.

However, since some cases of narcolepsy are infrequent and mild and others are mistaken for symptoms of depression or epilepsy or side effects of medications, this sleep disorder is underdiagnosed.

Conventional treatment involves stimulant drugs, such as Ritalin, as well as low-dose antidepressants. Doctors also advise patients to supplement their nighttime sleep with two to three short naps (lasting 10 to 15 minutes each) during the day.

Delayed Sleep Phase Syndrome

Delayed sleep phase syndrome (DSPS) is a condition in which the person chronically stays up quite late, usually until 3 a.m. to 4 a.m., and then sleeps all morning, getting up at 10 a.m. to 11 a.m. If a person with DSPS must arise earlier in the morning, they do so with great difficulty and experience daytime drowsiness and impaired performance, but still cannot go to sleep until the early morning hours. Usually teenagers or young adults are affected, and as many as 15% to 20% of college students may suffer from DSPS.[22] Eastbound travelers may experience transient DSPS as part of jet lag.

Advanced Sleep Phase Syndrome

In advanced sleep phase syndrome (ASPS), the direct opposite of DSPS, the person tends to always fall asleep very early in the evening, usually between 6 P.M. and 9 P.M., and wake up before dawn, sometimes as early as 1 A.M. People suffering from ASPS may fall asleep at dinner parties and other evening social functions. They may be able to force themselves, with great difficulty, to stay awake later in the evening; however, this can lead to sleep deprivation as they continue to arise very early in the morning. About one-third of adults over 65 tend to fall into this pattern, reports James Perl, Ph.D., author of *Sleep Right in Five Nights.*[23]

Night Owls and Early Birds: Do You Have a Sleep Phase Disorder?

We're all familiar with night owls and early birds—people who tend to prefer waking and sleeping at different hours than most other people. Owls are at their most alert during the late evening and nighttime hours and don't fall asleep until past midnight. Larks, in contrast, function best in the morning hours and fall asleep fairly early in the night. Individual variations in circadian rhythms generally determine whether you're an owl, an early bird, or less avian in your tendencies, experiencing peak performance in the normal nine-to-five schedule.

So how do you know whether your sleep personality is actually indicative of delayed or advanced sleep phase syndrome? These disorders may appear to closely resemble night owl (delayed) or early bird (advanced) characteristics; however, sleep phase syndromes are more extreme. Night owls typically have rhythms that are approximately 2 hours later than normal—not 6 to 8 hours, as is the case in DSPS. And early birds are about 2 hours ahead of everyone else, again not 6 to 8 hours off. Moreover, owls and early birds, if they get adequate sleep, generally function normally during the day. People suffering from a sleep phase disorder find it difficult to synchronize their wakeful hours with the activities of the rest of the population.

Hypersomnia

Hypersomnia describes sleep disorders in which people sleep too much, either for prolonged periods at night or during the day. Some people normally sleep longer than others—10 or more hours a day—but this does not necessarily indicate a disorder.[24] Seasonal affective disorder (SAD), described in the previous chapter and discussed at length in chapter 5, is a type of hypersomnia in which people sleep in late, among other symptoms. Other variations of hypersomnia are as follows:

● *Recurrent hypersomnia.* This disorder, which includes Kleine-Levin syndrome, lasts several weeks and can recur periodically. Some cases are marked by binge eating and hypersexuality; it usually occurs in adolescent males.

- **Idiopathic hypersomnia.** This type of hypersomnia has symptoms that may be mistaken for narcolepsy, including excessive daytime sleepiness and sleep attacks—except it does not include cataplexy.

- **Posttraumatic hypersomnia.** People who have had head injuries may develop this type of disorder, usually immediately after the injury. Other symptoms include headaches and problems with concentration and memory.

Parasomnias

Parasomnias are abnormal physical behaviors that occur during sleep. Usually these conditions involve arousal during the slow-wave stages of NREM sleep, stages 3 and 4. Parasomniacs aren't actively conscious of their actions and, upon awakening, often can't recall what happened during their nocturnal episodes. Parasomnias, which often run in families, tend to be more common in children. Research indicates that parasomniac conditions may be triggered by malfunctions in the brain mechanism that regulates the stages of sleep.[25] Conventional physicians usually treat all parasomniac disorders with medications, including benzodiazepines. Evaluation at a sleep disorder clinic is recommended if the problem is chronic or if the sleeper becomes violent during an episode.

Sleepwalking

Also known as somnambulism, sleepwalking usually occurs in stage 4, the deepest stage of sleep, during the first third of the night. As its name suggests, it typically involves walking, but sitting or other repetitive, routine motions may also occur. Each episode generally lasts between 5 and 15 minutes.[26] Sleepwalkers appear to be conscious during the episodes: their eyes are usually open with dilated pupils, and they're often able to safely navigate around obstacles, such as furniture. But they are not actively conscious of their actions and don't recall the episode upon waking. However, they are not acting out their dreams. In fact, EEGs reveal that the brain waves of sleepwalkers alternate between waking (alpha) waves and the delta waves of NREM sleep; they are literally half awake and half asleep.[27]

An estimated 4% of American adults have consulted doctors about their sleepwalking,[28] and approximately 10% to 15% of children between the ages of 5 and 12 have experienced sleepwalking.[29] Stress, fever, sleep deprivation, and even epilepsy have been shown to trigger sleepwalking. Conventional physicians sometimes prescribe sedatives or even stimulants to counter this disorder. Although it isn't harmful to awaken a sleepwalker, it may be inadvisable, as the person will usually be very difficult to arouse and may become alarmed if awakened. Instead, guide them gently back to bed and let them wake up on their own. Also, make sure sharp or fragile objects are removed from the sleepwalker's bedroom to prevent injury or property damage.

Night Terrors

Night terrors (also called sleep terrors) are frightening episodes for both sleepers and their housemates. People experiencing this parasomnia suddenly let out a piercing scream or cry and may even jump out of bed, run out of the house, or do bodily harm to themselves or others. These actions are accompanied by heavy sweating and heart palpitations. Though the sleeper may appear conscious of their acts because their eyes are open and their pupils are dilated, the person may not awaken until after the episode. Night terrors are not nightmares, because patients have no dream recall; in fact, episodes occur during the deep, NREM (nondream) stages of sleep.

As with sleepwalking and other parasomnias, young children tend to suffer from night terrors more frequently; only 3% of adults experience this disorder.[30] Night terrors are believed to be associated with a disruption in the nervous system. Stress, sleep deprivation, or sleeping in a different bed may spark night terrors. This disorder generally disappears as children mature. Some adults afflicted by night terrors may be prescribed medication; doctors may also recommend exercise and getting more sleep.

REM Behavior Disorder

REM behavior disorder is a potentially dangerous parasomnia. As indicated by its name, this disorder occurs during the REM (dream) stage of sleep. Normally, most of our muscles become paralyzed during the REM phase to prevent us from acting out our dreams. In RBD, however, it appears the brain does not properly signal the paralysis function, so sleepers physically engage in their dreams without being actively conscious of their behavior. People with RBD have been known to become violent during dreams, injuring themselves and others, and even killing people. About 75% of RBD patients repeatedly hurt themselves during RBD episodes.[31] This disorder usually affects middle-aged and older men and is often associated with some type of nerve problem or brain damage. The primary conventional drug used to treat REM-sleep disorders is a benzodiazepine called clonazepam (Klonopin).

Rhythmic Movement Disorder

Rhythmic movement disorder (RMD) involves head banging, head rolling, body rocking, body rolling, or other repetitive movements. It typically occurs immediately prior to sleep onset and is sustained into light sleep (stages 1 and 2).[32]

RMD may also last into the deep sleep stages.[33] RMD usually develops in infants at nine months of age and disappears by the age of 10 years; if it persists, it is often associated with autism and mental impairment.[34] Some adults also suffer from this disorder. Benzodiazepines, tranquilizers, and tricyclic antidepressants are usually prescribed by conventional physicians for persistent, severe forms of this sleep disorder.

Bruxism

Bruxism is characterized by grinding the teeth during sleep. Approximately 5% of adults and 15% of children experience chronic bruxism.[35] Usually this condition doesn't cause sleep deprivation or associated health and psychological problems unless it is very severe. However, any teeth-grinding can damage the teeth, bones, gums, and jaw joint.

Many people believe bruxism serves as an outlet for releasing stress experienced during the day. However, doctors contend it's the body's way of trying to correct structural problems in the mouth. Nocturnal chewing action may be an attempt to grind upper and lower teeth for a better fit. Teeth-grinding may also be the result of temporomandibular joint (TMJ) syndrome. Dentists often prescribe a mouth guard; although it doesn't eliminate the grinding instinct, it does protect the teeth from damage.

Bed-Wetting

Clinically known as sleep enuresis, bed-wetting is a common occurrence in toddlers and is only recognized as a disorder after the age of 5. It is estimated that 3% of youths between the ages of 12 and 18 suffer from chronic sleep enuresis.[36] This uncontrollable loss of bladder control during the night happens in all sleep stages and is believed to be hereditary; it seldom occurs due to emotional problems, as is commonly believed.[37] Physiological abnormalities and disorders, including a small bladder, metabolic or hormonal imbalances, allergies, bladder infections, and obstructive sleep apnea are associated with the development of this disorder.

Diagnosing Sleep Disorders

Diagnosing sleep disorders is, at best, an imprecise process; first, because scientists are still learning about the physiology of sleep, and second, because patients are unable to provide clues about problems that occur while they're sleeping. However, there are two standard tests that help doctors identify sleep disorders: polysomnography and the multiple sleep latency test (MSLT):

Polysomnography: This test monitors bodily functions during sleep, including electrical activity of the brain, eye movement, muscle activity, heart rate, airflow, and blood oxygen levels. This test is often used to diagnose sleep apnea, narcolepsy, restless legs syndrome, and periodic limb movement disorder, but may also be employed to test for other sleep disorders.

Multiple sleep latency test: The MSLT measures how long it takes a person to fall asleep at any point during the day as drowsiness occurs. Generally, people without sleep disorders fall asleep in 10 to 20 minutes; those who fall asleep in less than 5 minutes are categorized as experiencing sleep deprivation and a sleep disorder of some type. This test is typically used to diagnose sleep onset insomnia, sleep apnea, and narcolepsy.

Your doctor may also want you to undergo tests that analyze biochemical characteristics, such as a blood test called a radioimmunoassay (RIA), which can be used to measure levels of melatonin. If your physician suspects you have obstructive sleep apnea, you may undergo a breathing test while sleeping, during which technicians measure your breathing patterns, blood oxygen levels, and respiration rates.

Why Sleeping Pills Don't Work

Though the exact number is difficult to estimate, it's safe to say that millions of Americans take prescription sleeping medications, primarily benzodiazepine tranquilizers (such as Valium, Klonopin, and Xanax) and antidepressants (Elavil and Sinequan).

The number of people taking readily available over-the-counter sleeping pills (antihistamines such as Unisom, Nytol, and Tylenol PM) may be even

How Big Is Your Sleep Debt?

One clue as to whether you have a sleep disorder is a large sleep debt, the cumulative amount of sleep you've missed, whether due to choice or sleep problems. The multiple sleep latency test (MSLT) is the gold standard by which doctors measure sleep debt, but the Epworth Sleepiness Scale below will give you a good idea of how much sleep you're missing.[38] Ask yourself how likely you are to doze off or fall asleep in the scenarios below. Rate your response according to the following scale and add up your total score for an evaluation of your sleep debt. (Scale: 0 = Would never doze; 1 = Slight chance of dozing; 2 = Moderate chance of dozing; 3 = High chance of dozing)

____ Sitting and reading

____ Watching TV

____ Sitting inactive in one place (theater, meeting, etc.)

____ As a passenger in a car for 1 hour without a break

____ Lying down to rest in the afternoon when circumstances permit

____ Sitting and talking to someone

____ Sitting quietly after a lunch without alcohol

____ In a car, while stopped for a few minutes in traffic

Total Score:
0 to 5 = Slight or no sleep debt
6 to 10 = Moderate sleep debt
11 to 20 = Heavy sleep debt
21 to 25 = Extreme sleep debt

From The Promise of Sleep by William C. Dement, copyright © 1999 by William C. Dement. Used by permission of Dell Publishing, a division of Random House, Inc.

greater. While these drugs might provide a moderate amount of relief for a short period of time, they ultimately do more harm than good.

All types of sleeping medications function by sedating or depressing the brain. Benzodiazepines slow brain waves; antidepressants manipulate levels of brain chemicals; and over-the-counter drugs block histamine and other stimulating chemical reactions in the brain and body. These processes temporarily alleviate insomnia and other sleep disorders. However, most sleeping pills have a deleterious effect on the sleep cycle, increasing the time spent in light, stage 2 sleep and diminishing the time spent in deep sleep and REM sleep. As discussed in chapter 1, deep and REM sleep are required for optimal cerebral, immune, cardiovascular, and mental health. Chronic use of sedative medications impairs these functions and can open the door to illness. All of the drugs used as sleeping aids may also adversely interact with alcohol and other medications, slowing heart rate and breathing to potentially dangerous levels.

Additionally, sleeping pills, especially tranquilizers and antidepressants, can become addictive. Since the efficacy of all drugs diminishes with use, a person requires higher and higher dosages in order to feel the sedating effects, fueling the dependency on these drugs. Discontinuing these medications may cause "rebound insomnia," in which insomnia recurs, often more severely. Rebound insomnia may also disrupt REM sleep, triggering nightmares.

More recently, benzodiazepine receptor agonists (BZRAs) have been promoted as sleep aids. These hypnotic drugs are advertised to be longer lasting and less addictive. But as is the case with all medications, they may cause side effects, including dizziness and headaches. Another issue to be aware of is the wide range in duration of effect. The half-life of a drug refers to how long it typically takes the body to clear half of the substance. In BZRAs, the half-life can range from 30 minutes to two and a half days. You may experience either grogginess and memory problem as long as the drug is in your system.

A new class of drugs for promoting sleep has recently been developed; ramelteon (Rozerem) was the first to appear on the market. Called melatonin receptor agonists, these are not hypnotics; rather, they mimic the actions of melatonin. It is claimed that they offer a higher quality of sleep and have fewer side effects; however, dizziness and daytime grogginess may still occur. Because it's such a new drug, addiction and other long-term effects remain in question, but what is not open to question is that when discontinuing any sleeping pill you may still experience rebound insomnia. Your original problem may return in full force, so you might have spent a great deal of money only to wind up in the same place.

Even if used for only a short time, over-the-counter sleep aids can have many adverse side effects, including drug-induced "hangovers" or stupor. "Research that has investigated performance on mental tasks (such as learning and decision-making) and on motor tasks (such as driving a car) on days after the use of sleeping pills finds that people usually do worse after taking a pill than they do after a night of insomnia," states sleep expert Russel J. Reiter.[39] The reason this happens is that your body still retains some of the medication the next day and its sedating effects linger. Insomnia expert Peter Hauri, Ph.D., says this is particularly problematic for older adults, who tend to have more sleep disorders anyway, because they metabolize medications more slowly. Over-the-counter sleep aids can also provoke anxiety, dizziness, restlessness, confusion, amnesia, blurred vision, nausea, digestive upset, and frequent urination.[40]

Caution: People suffering from sleep apnea should not to take any sleeping medications, as they impair the body's ability to arouse itself and restore normal breathing.

If you decide you wish to approach your sleep disorder from a holistic point of view and forgo the use of drugs, there is a strong possibility that you can resolve the underlying problems that have created your sleep disorder. This is genuine healing at a deep level—and you may save some money in the process.

What Alternative Medicine Can Do for Sleep Disorders

Alternative medicine offers lasting relief from sleep disorders. While certain extreme disorders have genetic underpinnings and may require continued medical care, even cases of narcolepsy have been reversed by eliminating food allergies and by other alternative therapies. In the alternative medicine view, sleep disorders result from multiple causes, many of them with a less-than-obvious connection to the disorder or not easily detectable. As you will discover in the rest of this book, a number of underlying imbalances, with accompanying physical, mental, and environmental factors, can contribute to sleep problems.

It is essential to understand the factors that went into creating each individual's sleep disorder, because sleep disorders are rarely caused by one thing alone and no two people have exactly the same causal factors. Alternative medicine employs a battery of diagnostic tools—sleep tests, physical examination, dietary assessment, emotional evaluation, and tests for digestive, detoxification, and hormonal function—to build an individualized picture of the patient's condition. This customized approach extends beyond diagnosis to treatment. Skilled alternative practitioners take the time needed to

Sleep Problems Don't Have to Be Part of Aging

It is commonly believed that as we get older, we should expect to sleep poorly. On the contrary, how well you sleep as you age depends on your lifestyle. If you spend most of your life drinking alcohol, eating poorly, and not exercising, it is likely you will experience sleep difficulties. However, many people in their sixties, seventies, and eighties sleep soundly because they maintain healthy lifestyles.

Sleep problems are not an automatic accompaniment to aging, emphasizes H. Vafi, MD.[41] "Although uninterrupted sleep may be more difficult to achieve [with aging], insomnia may not be as much a factor in growing older as it is a by-product of a negative attitude about aging," says Dr. Vafi. While it's true that older people tend to spend less time in deep sleep, possibly due to reduced levels of melatonin, various strategies, including exercise, proper diet, melatonin supplementation, and light therapy, can help seniors—and everyone else—sleep like a baby again.

find the root causes of sleep disorders, and they also get the patient actively involved in their treatment. Alternative medicine restores health to the whole person rather than simply providing superficial symptom relief. The goal is to help each person achieve a balance among physical healing and the emotional, mental, and even spiritual aspects of their life.

Alternative medicine draws upon a wide range of therapies to help treat—and even prevent—sleep disorders. The primary keys are proper diet and nutrition, detoxification, stress reduction, and a healthy environment conducive to sleep. Diet and nutrition can have a significant impact on sleep, and special care should be taken to avoid substances that might overly stimulate the brain. Vitamins, minerals, herbs, and other natural supplements, particularly melatonin, can provide effective relief without the side effects of conventional drugs.

Removing toxins from the body has shown to be therapeutic for a wide variety of conditions, and alternative medicine offers a number of safe and effective detoxification strategies. Light therapy is especially helpful for people with disrupted circadian rhythms. Meditation, biofeedback, hypnotherapy, and other mind-body techniques can help reduce stress. Environmental imbalances can be regulated with magnet therapy and feng shui. If hormonal imbalance is a factor, addressing that imbalance can be a key strategy. Skeletal problems can be addressed through a variety of modalities, including bodywork, exercise, and yoga.

Seven Reasons Why You Can't Sleep

Sleep disorders can arise due to any of the following factors, or a combination of them: poor diet and food allergies; an accumulation of toxins in the body (from the environment, food, drugs, and other sources); emotional factors, including difficulty managing or coping with stress; electromagnetic influences; hormonal imbalances; and biomechanical stress and imbalances. All of these factors may also disrupt circadian rhythms, leading to such problems as sleep phase syndromes and insomnia.

Poor Diet and Food Allergies

Stimulants such as caffeine, sugar, and spicy foods are major contributors to sleep disorders. Caffeine, found in coffee, nonherbal teas, soft drinks, and many over-the-counter drugs, can remain in the body from 12 to 20 hours, thwarting sleep.[42] Sugar and refined carbohydrates create uneven blood sugar levels that can disrupt your sleep in the middle of the night. Another side effect of excessive sugar consumption is insulin rebound, in which the body is overwhelmed with an influx of simple sugars and as a result cannot digest food properly. This condition causes an stress reaction in the body that prevents sleep. It can also result in food addictions, a vicious cycle of bingeing on sugary foods or beverages and foods that contain caffeine, that keeps blood sugar levels and sleep patterns out of balance. Food allergies are also implicated in promoting food addictions and often are found in children with obstructive sleep apnea.

Seemingly relaxing substances, such as alcohol and nicotine, also impair the ability to sleep deeply and continuously through the night. Nicotine is actually a stimulant, similar to caffeine. Although drinking alcohol may appear to help induce sleep, it often creates shortened, lighter sleep. In addition, alcohol is a strong diuretic and may prompt you to awaken throughout the night to urinate. Sleep problems may also be caused by vitamin or mineral deficiencies, especially of B vitamins, copper, iron, and zinc.

Toxic Colon and Liver

While it may not seem readily apparent, the liver and colon play an important role in establishing and maintaining regular, restful sleep. Both the colon and the liver remove waste from the body and toxins from the air you breathe and the food and liquids you consume. If either system is not working properly, the body can become dangerously toxic, resulting in conditions such as food allergies and bacterial overgrowth, which have been shown to disturb sleep. Heavy metals, such as mercury, are particularly toxic to the body and can directly cause insomnia. Toxic load can also deplete vitamins and minerals essential to inducing a good night's sleep.

Disrupted Circadian Rhythms

Seasonal affective disorder (SAD), advanced and delayed sleep phase syndromes, and some cases of insomnia are caused by disruptions in circadian rhythms. Inadequate exposure to full-spectrum light and sunlight is a major contributor to upsetting the body's clock, but so is shift work and traveling across time zones. Poor diet, heavy use of stimulants, lack of exercise, and unmanaged stress can also upset natural sleep patterns. An often overlooked cause of circadian rhythm disruptions is extremely low frequency electromagnetic fields (EMFs), may diminish the pineal gland's ability to produce melatonin. Electrical power lines, appliances, computers and electronic devices, and commercial airplanes all generate EMFs.

Stress and Psychological Factors

Stress and pent-up emotional issues can wreak havoc on the brain, deregulating brain chemicals and also affecting organs that are instrumental in procuring a good night's rest. Unmanaged daily stress can upset your hormonal balance, deplete nutrient reserves, and create a vicious cycle of less sleep and more stress. Additionally, unresolved psychological issues, such as deep-seated internal fears or relationship conflicts, can disturb brain chemistry and hinder deep sleep.

Geopathic Stress and Environmental Toxins

Geopathic stress is defined as an abnormal energy field, often of an electromagnetic nature, created deep underground by large mineral deposits, water streams, or geological faults. Accumulated exposure to these discordant energies (usually due to the location of our homes) can create illnesses, including cancer, migraines, depression, and disrupted sleep. Most of us are also exposed to environmental assaults inside our homes that can ruin our chances for normal sleep. Toxic household chemicals, disruptive noise levels, and electromagnetic fields from power lines and appliances can impair melatonin production, nullify attempts at relaxation, and interfere with sleep.

Hormonal Imbalances

For both men and women, hormonal imbalances can disrupt sleep. While it has long been understood that women undergo hormonal shifts throughout their lives, culminating in menopause, it is now known that men undergo a similar shift, referred to as andropause or "male menopause." In both cases, levels of primary sex hormones, such as estrogen and progesterone in women and testosterone in men, decline, resulting in a host of emotional, psychological, and physical changes. Sleep is often disrupted during these transitions. As these hormonal shifts are taking place, it is common for melatonin levels to drop as well.

Structural Imbalances

Sleep can be disrupted by structural imbalances, particularly in the spine. Such conditions block the flow of nerve impulses, either causing pain that keeps a person awake at night or impinging on the nervous system's ability to send sleep signals. Lack of regular exercise can lead to sleep disorders as well, because it causes muscular tension and allows stress to build up in the body.

How This Book Can Help You Sleep Again

Alternative medicine is about getting back in balance. Only when you have addressed and resolved the imbalances in your life can you enjoy deep, restorative sleep. This book will help you understand the causes underlying your sleep problems and guide you to therapies that can get your sleep patterns and your life back on track.

Step 1: Improve diet and eliminate food allergies. In chapter 3, Improve Your Diet, you will learn how food-related problems, including hypoglycemia, insulin rebound, and food addictions, cause sleep disorders. We detail strategies for avoiding stimulants in your diet and eliminating food allergies, and also provide recommendations for integrating a whole foods diet into your life and taking appropriate nutritional supplements.

Step 2: Detoxify your colon and liver. In chapter 4, Detoxify Your Body, we detail valuable detoxification therapies for your colon and liver. You will learn the importance of detoxification diets and be introduced to organ-cleansing methods, such as enemas, colonics, and the liver flush. We also provide dietary, herbal, and supplement remedies for conditions such as candidiasis (overgrowth of the *Candida albicans* fungus) and parasites, two factors that impair the ability of the intestines to eliminate toxins, which ultimately disrupts sleep.

Step 3: Reset your body clock. The importance of balanced circadian rhythms will be emphasized in chapter 5, Reset Your Body Clock. Those of you suffering insomnia due to travel and shift work, as well those experiencing sleep phase syndromes, will learn how to reprogram your body clock to adjust to new sleep-wake schedules. Those suffering from seasonal affective disorder will learn valuable ways to improve mood during the winter months. Light therapy and melatonin supplementation will be described in detail.

Step 4: Resolve emotional issues. In chapter 6, Resolve Emotional Issues, we discuss how lingering psychological problems can adversely affect sleep. We explore different ways emotional issues can be resolved, including diet modification, cognitive therapy, hypnotherapy, and stress management techniques such as meditation. We also discuss how you can establish sleep rituals that will allow you to unwind at day's end and fall asleep easily and

Assessing Your Sleep History

As part of an examination for sleep problems, a physician will generally ask about sleep habits. These questions are also helpful for self-assessment of your own sleep problems:

■ Do you have a history of sleep problems?

■ How much sleep do you get, on average, in a 24-hour period?

■ When do you normally sleep? When do you consider the best time for sleeping?

■ What time do you go to bed and what time do you wake up?

■ How long does it normally take for you to fall asleep?

■ Is your bedroom noisy? Is it dark enough?

■ Do you frequently awaken during the night? If so, why?

■ Do you feel refreshed after a night's sleep?

■ Are you often sleepy or fatigued during the day?

■ Do you take naps during the day? If so, how often?

■ When did you last have a good night's sleep?

■ Has anyone ever told you that you snore or stop breathing during the night?

■ Have you ever been told that you walk in your sleep?

■ Have you ever been told that you exhibit jerking leg or arm movements during the night?

■ Have you ever fallen asleep suddenly while driving or at work?

■ Do you exercise regularly?

■ What types of foods do you eat and when?

■ Do you smoke or drink alcohol frequently?

■ Are you taking sleeping aids or other medications?

specific relaxation techniques that help induce sleep.

Step 5: Restore harmony to your home. Chapter 7, Protect Yourself from Environmental Factors, describes how environmental pollution and geopathic stress contribute to poor sleep and provides suggestions on minimizing these factors. You will learn how to reduce your exposure to harmful toxins and chemicals at home, and you'll also find out how magnet therapy protects you from harmful electromagnetic fields. This chapter also introduces the principles of feng shui, an ancient Chinese tradition that aims to improve health through the appropriate placement of household items. By simply rearranging some of your furniture, you can create a peaceful and sleep-promoting sanctuary in your bedroom.

Step 6: Balance your hormones. Melatonin isn't the only hormone that plays a role in sleep patterns. In chapter 8, Balance Your Hormones, you will learn how changes in sex hormones contribute to sleep disruptions. The primary focus will be on menopause and andropause, and what women and men going through these transitional times can do to improve their sleep. You will learn how to correct hormonal imbalances through traditional Chinese medicine, diet, lifestyle modifications, and stress reduction.

Step 7: Correct structural imbalances. In chapter 9, Correct Structural Imbalances, you will learn how physical disharmonies in your body can rob you

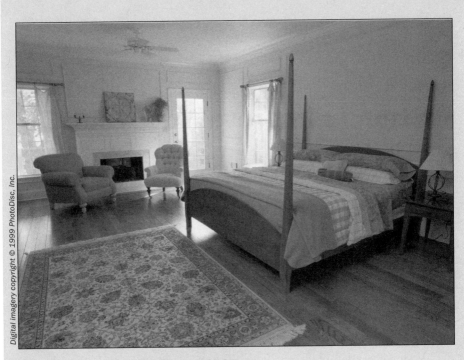

Use feng shui to restore harmony to your bedroom.

of sleep. We discuss the therapeutic effects of regular exercise and explore of how gentle forms of exercise such as qigong and yoga can be especially effective for reducing stress and restoring deep sleep. This chapter also describes how spinal and other structural misalignments can be reversed through chiropractic treatments, acupuncture, and reflexology. Additionally, we describe various forms of bodywork that may contribute to better sleep.

three

Step 1: Improve Your Diet

What you eat definitely influences the quality of your sleep. Unhealthy eating patterns, including excessive intake of stimulants such as caffeine, sugar, and alcohol, along with eating too many nutrient-depleted, processed foods, can disturb sleep. Food allergies can also cause sugar and chemical imbalances in the body that may be disrupting your sleep. Alternative medicine recognizes the importance of diet for all aspects of healthy physical functioning and has a variety of dietary recommendations for improving your sleep and your health. In this chapter, we look at the factors in your diet that may be contributing to irregular or disrupted sleep. We also recommend dietary and nutritional strategies that will help you get a good night's rest.

The Connection between Diet and Sleep

Diet is a primary consideration in sleep disorders. Many dietary factors can disrupt sleep: consumption of stimulants like caffeine and sugar, food allergies, the intake of drugs and alcohol, and poor dietary choices are the primary culprits. Fortunately, these are factors you have a great deal of control over—even though it can sometimes be hard to do. But by making some basic changes in your diet, you may be able to avoid medical treatment and other costly interventions. And your overall health will benefit, too.

Caffeine

Caffeine—present not just in coffee but also nonherbal teas, many sodas, energy drinks, chocolate, and even some foods—can have a pronounced effect on sleeping habits. Even just a few cups of coffee in the morning can have a major effect on quality and quantity of sleep at night, especially for sensitive individuals. Caffeine has been associated with insomnia, periodic limb movement disorder, and restless legs syndrome, as well as other sleep disorders.[1] If you drink coffee daily, even one or two cups, the caffeine can easily disrupt your sleep.

Dietary Recommendations for Better Sleep

- Eliminate stimulants from your diet
- Eliminate allergenic foods
- Eat more whole foods
- Take appropriate supplements

After you drink a cup of coffee, the caffeine enters your bloodstream quickly, resulting in an immediate burst of energy. Many coffee drinkers are familiar with some of the temporary stimulant effects of caffeine, including nervous jitters and irritability. This is because caffeine stimulates your central nervous system, leading to an increase in brain activity and overall energy. It also increases blood pressure, heart rate, respiration, and metabolism. More specifically, caffeine causes the adrenal glands to produce hormones that activate and energize the body, such as adrenaline, norepinephrine, and cortisol.[2] Normally, these hormones are secreted in daily cycles, peaking in the morning and having the lowest values at night. High amounts of cortisol are linked with muscle dysfunction, thyroid dysfunction, immune system depression, and sleep disorders.

Caffeine is also a diuretic, meaning that it promotes fluid loss from the body. This can lead to deficiencies in nutrients important for sound sleep, particularly the B vitamins, calcium, magnesium, zinc, and iron.[3] Some people are more sensitive to the effects of caffeine because their bodies require more time to metabolize the caffeine (clear it from the body), a function handled primarily by the liver. Caffeine can remain in the body up to 20 hours, so even caffeine ingested early in the day can inhibit your ability to get to sleep.

Coffee is not the only source of caffeine in the diet—chocolate contains caffeine as well as other stimulants. The hot chocolate that some people drink before bedtime may actually keep them awake. Tea, soft drinks, and energy drinks are other common sources of caffeine. These days you can even buy caffeinated water and prepared foods with added caffeine. In addition, many over-the-counter medications (cold and cough preparations, weight-loss drugs, pain relievers) contain caffeine or caffeine-related substances and can also increase sleep disorders.

Recently, coffee and chocolate have both been touted for their high levels of antioxidants, and in fact, caffeine itself is an antioxidant. A 2005 study found that coffee is actually the top source of antioxidants in the U.S. diet.[4] However, despite coffee's new, more healthful image, the basic fact remains:

Sugar on the Brain

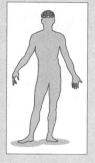

Although we generally feel satisfaction or relief after eating a sugary snack, the sensation does not come directly from the glucose that enters the bloodstream, but rather from the corresponding surge in insulin. This is because, in addition to managing glucose, insulin is used by the body to transport the amino acid tryptophan, a building block of the neurotransmitter serotonin, to the brain. (A neurotransmitter is a brain chemical that enables communications to happen between brain cells.) Serotonin is sometimes referred to as the "happiness" chemical due to its influence on mood. High levels of serotonin in the brain produce feelings of self-confidence, calm, satisfaction, and composure. However, when levels start to decline, we start to feel anxious, cannot concentrate, and become depressed.

When tryptophan is scarce, serotonin is in similarly short supply. This creates an intolerable condition for the brain, which demands immediate action, hence our cravings for sugar. Sugar causes quick satisfaction by initiating the release of insulin, which delivers tryptophan to the brain and restores serotonin levels.[5] In effect, sugar works like an antidepressant. "If serotonin levels are depressed, you're depressed," says Michael Phillips, DC, who compares sugar's action to that of the drug Prozac. "Prozac, so commonly prescribed for depression, works by elevating levels of serotonin. The emotional aspects of blood sugar imbalances are rooted in a [similar] physiological response."

caffeine consumed after noon will interfere with sleep patterns in sensitive individuals. If sleep is a problem for you, it may be best to avoid caffeine altogether. If you love the taste of coffee, consider drinking decaf, which is also high in antioxidants. Also bear in mind that antioxidant-rich fruits and vegetables contain a host of other healthful nutrients, so their overall nutritional profile is much more healthful than either chocolate or coffee.

Sugar

Much like caffeine, sugar is often consumed because it gives the body energy immediately. As effective as caffeine for providing a short burst of energy, sugar's high is also short-lived. Once the sugar is metabolized, blood sugar levels can crash or fluctuate, and this can disrupt your sleep in the middle of the night as your body demands more sugar.

Hypoglycemia, or low blood sugar (glucose), is a condition often associated with diabetes. Symptoms of hypoglycemia include anxiety, weakness, sweating, rapid heart rate, dizziness, headache, irritability, and poor or double vision Although glucose is the primary source of fuel for the brain, too much glucose in the blood can create health problems. Following a meal, glucose levels rise sharply, and the pancreas responds by releasing insulin, a substance that helps the cells absorb glucose from the blood. In healthy people, the release of insulin acts to keep blood sugar levels fairly constant; when the pancreas produces too much insulin, however, blood glucose levels drop suddenly, depriving the brain of needed fuel.

A diet high in simple sugars and refined carbohydrates can lead to nighttime hypoglycemia. Blood levels of glucose drop and the body releases adrenaline, cortisol, and other hormones to stimulate the brain and indicate that it is time to eat. This can awaken you or prevent you from entering a deep sleep state.

Food Allergies

We tend to think of allergies in terms of pollens, dust, and animal hair—the things that make us sneeze or give us a rash. However, the truth is that we can be allergic to many different types of substances, including foods, and suffer a wide variety of symptoms. Some practitioners believe that a majority of the U.S. population suffers from allergies, particularly food allergies, which frequently go undiagnosed. Allergies to foods can cause a number of reactions in the body that disturb sleep.

An allergy is the immune system's abnormal reaction to a substance that is harmless to most people. The immune system usually responds to only dangerous invaders, such as bacteria or viruses, and ignores "normal" substances such as foods. People develop allergies when the immune system has become weakened or compromised and can no longer distinguish between harmful and harmless substances. In response to these otherwise normal substances, the immune system releases chemicals, such as histamines, resulting in many of the symptoms associated with allergies—symptoms that are numerous and wide-ranging, including stomach pains, joint pain, insomnia, weight gain, mood swings, and apathy. When treating patients with sleep disorders, some alternative practitioners consider food allergies or intolerances as the first possibility. The most common culprits are yeast, wheat, corn, milk and other dairy products, egg whites, tomatoes, soy, shellfish, peanuts, chocolate, and food dyes and additives.

Herbert Rinkel, MD, was a pioneer in the issue of food sensitivities. While still a medical student, he discovered his own intolerance to eggs and began to research the field. Dr. Rinkel found that symptoms of tension and jitteriness, common to people with food sensitivities, are apt to manifest in restlessness and inattentiveness by day and insomnia by night. He concluded that insomnia, as well as tossing and turning or crying out at night, are manifestations of food intolerance. Dr. Rinkel considered fatigue to be one of the first symptoms of food intolerance and most troublesome early in the morning upon rising. This is particularly noticeable in children with food intolerances. People suffering from food allergies are often irritable during the morning hours and may need a nap in the late afternoon. They frequently suffer from insomnia as well.[6]

Intolerance to certain foods can cause release of histamine (a substance produced by the body during an allergic reaction) in the brain, which can disturb a person's biochemistry and, in some cases, lead to sleep disturbance. In the brain, histamine replaces neurotransmitters, but because it does not function like other neurotransmitters, it alters the biochemical pathways of the brain responsible for thinking, mood, and behavior. When these pathways are disrupted, the consequence is exhibited as symptoms, one of which is insomnia.

Food allergies can also disrupt blood sugar balance.[7] The mechanism is a bit complex, but here are the basics: Exposure to an allergen often cause the adrenal glands to release cortisol and adrenaline, which act as anti-inflammatory agents. Unfortunately, these hormones also causes the liver to release sugars that have been stored for later use. Faced with an influx of sugar into the bloodstream, the pancreas often responds by producing an overabundance of insulin, which can remove too much sugar from the blood-stream, causing hypoglycemia. Chronic exposure to allergens can eventually disrupt pancreatic function, leading to ongoing blood sugar imbalances and eventually to diabetes. Given that both cortisol and hypoglycemia can disrupt sleep, food allergies can potentially play major role in sleep problems. Unfortunately, the connection between sugar disorders (such as hypoglycemia) and food allergies is poorly understood and often overlooked, and thus remains undiagnosed and untreated.

Drugs, Alcohol, and Nicotine

The sleeping process can be significantly disturbed by a variety of over-the-counter and prescription drugs. Drugs that may lead to insomnia include thyroid preparations, oral contraceptives, beta-blockers, and marijuana.[8] As mentioned earlier, many over-the-counter medications also contain caffeine and can increase sleep disorders through overstimulation.

While alcohol may initially be relaxing, the end result of drinking is interrupted, less restful sleep. It may help you fall asleep, but when its effects wear off, it disrupts the deeper stages of sleep during the second half of the night.

Alcohol can reduce overall sleep time, including both REM and non-REM sleep.[9] This creates shortened, lighter, and less restful sleep, as drinkers often awaken before reaching deeper, restorative sleep (stages 3 and 4) and REM sleep. If you are deprived of these stages of sleep, you will feel fatigued the following day. In one study, 10 middle-aged men were given a moderate dose of alcohol 6 hours before a scheduled bedtime. All of the subjects experienced reduced total sleep time, sleep efficiency, and REM sleep. In the second half of the night, they showed a twofold increase in wakefulness.[10] And because alcohol is a simple sugar, it may be a factor in the development of hypoglycemia, which can disrupt sleep patterns. It can also cause decreased absorption of some nutrients essential for a good night's rest, particularly the B vitamins, magnesium, and calcium.[11] And finally, alcohol is a diuretic, so drinking may interrupt your sleep by necessitating getting up several times during the night to urinate.

Smoking also inhibits sleep. Because nicotine acts as a stimulant, many smokers have insomnia and other sleep problems.[12] In a poll conducted by the National Sleep Foundation, 46% of smokers reported experiencing insomnia a few nights a week as compared to 35% of non-smokers.[13] Nicotine is rapidly absorbed by the mucous membranes in the mouth and quickly reaches the brain, where it stimulates the release of adrenaline and norepinephrine, hormones that stimulate the body, increase heart rate, and elevate blood pressure.[14]

Poor Diet

If you eat the typical American diet, it could be making your sleeping problems worse. Highly processed foods containing large quantities of refined carbohydrates and simple sugars are empty of nutritional value and over-stimulate the body. A number of vitamin and mineral deficiencies, which may result from poor dietary choices, digestive dysfunction, or food allergies, can also affect sleep:

- L-tryptophan is a precursor to melatonin, the hormone needed for sleep. Supplementing with L-tryptophan can ameliorate the symptoms of insomnia and other sleep disorders.[15]

- The B vitamins (particularly B_6) are also important for sleep, as they regulate the body's use of L-tryptophan. In the absence of adequate vitamin B_6, the body cannot convert L-tryptophan into melatonin. Deficiencies in folic acid (also known as folacin or folate), another member of the B vitamin family, have been linked to insomnia and restless legs syndrome.[16]

- Vitamin E deficiency may be a factor in restless legs syndrome.[17]

- People suffering from insomnia may be deficient in the mineral zinc, particularly infants with frequent nighttime waking and crying.

- Deficiencies in copper and iron have been linked to greater difficulties in getting to sleep and decreased quality of sleep. Studies also indicate that low levels of iron are associated with an increased incidence of restless legs syndrome.[18]

- Calcium acts as a natural sedative in the body, producing a calming effect on the central nervous system, and deficiencies of this mineral have been linked to sleep problems. Sufficient amounts of magnesium (also a natural sedative) are necessary for the absorption of calcium.

In addition, many alternative practitioners recommend staying away from spicy and salty foods if you suffer from sleep disorders. These foods can cause indigestion or heartburn, which may interfere with sleep. Monosodium glutamate (MSG) and other artificial additives can also disturb sleep; some people who are sensitive to MSG suffer insomnia from the stimulant effects of this food additive.

Detecting a Nutritional Deficiency

Since nutrient deficiencies can be a factor in sleep disorders, one of the first steps is to determine which nutrients may be lacking in your diet so that you can design an individualized supplement program. Consult a qualified health professional trained in the intricacies of nutritional biochemistry to help you assess your needs and develop an effective, individualized dietary and nutritional supplement program. The tests described below can be used to analyze your nutrient status, pinpoint specific deficiencies, and determine the dosages of supplements that will best suit your needs.

Many mainstream physicians assess nutritional status using blood tests. These tests measure nutrient concentrations only in the blood serum (the liquid fraction of blood) and not in the blood cells (the globular or nonliquid fraction of blood). The cells are generally separated out and discarded. Unfortunately, a good deal of information about an individual's nutritional status is thrown out along with these cells.

"It's important to understand that ordinary tests on blood serum levels don't provide the correct data," says John Dommisse, MD, a nutritional medicine specialist. "What must be measured are whole blood levels." Whole blood analysis, which examines both the serum and the blood cells, is not commonly done, since most mainstream physicians are looking at blood primarily to diagnose a disease and serum testing is generally adequate for that purpose. As most mainstream physicians are oriented toward using drugs to treat symptoms, they have no interest in nutritional status and are thus not informed about or inclined to order the proper tests.

In addition to whole blood analysis, a variety of other test procedures can help assess nutrient status. These include hair analysis, the Individualized Optimum Nutrition Panel, and the Functional Intracellular Analysis.

Hair analysis: When correctly done, hair analysis measures the body's levels of various minerals, including calcium, iron, magnesium, potassium, and zinc. As the hair is a storage organ, it provides a biochemical record of nutritional status over a period of several months. This is why many health-care practitioners consider hair analysis to provide a better picture of underlying mineral imbalances than most blood or urine tests, which only provide a snapshot of nutritional status at a certain point in time. However, hair analysis cannot detect vitamin deficiencies, so other tests are needed to supplement the findings of a hair analysis.

Individualized Optimal Nutrition (ION) Profile: The ION Profile, from Metametrix Medical Laboratories (see Resources), uses blood and urine samples to measure over 100 biochemical components. Specifically, ION checks for nutritional status in categories including vitamins, minerals, amino acids, fatty and organic acids, lipid peroxides, general blood chemistries (cholesterol, thyroid hormone, glucose), and antioxidants. Each patient's nutritional level is compared with what is considered the healthy norm. In addition, ION can provide supplement recommendations based on the individual's test results. This test must be ordered by a health-care professional.

Functional Intracellular Analysis (FIA): Another accurate and comprehensive test is the Functional Intracellular Analysis, available through SpectraCell Laboratories (see Resources). It measures how micronutrients are naturally functioning within the activities of living white blood cells rather than simply measuring the micronutrient levels in the blood. This nutritional assay must also be ordered by a health-care professional, but the lab maintains a database of nutritionally oriented practitioners and will refer individuals to professionals in their area. They also provide information to consumers that they can use to educate and inform their physicians about the test.

Diagnosing a Food Allergy

Accurate diagnosis of food allergies is difficult, in part because people's reactions are often varied and inconsistent. Plus, symptoms may take several days to develop after eating an allergy-causing food. How much or how often you eat an allergenic food or how it is cooked may also be factors in whether or not you have a reaction. Or the allergy may be caused by an additive rather than the food itself.[19] In addition, more than one food may be involved in causing the reaction.

Despite the complexity surrounding the detection and diagnosis of a food allergy, mainstream medical practitioners generally take a highly simplified approach to the problem. Most rely on a procedure called the scratch test or prick-puncture test, a procedure that is only about 20% accurate in detecting food allergies.[20] In truth, this test is only useful for identifying allergens that cause immediate reactions, such as pollen or dust, and is less than effective in pinpointing food reactions. Another common test procedure is the RAST (radioallergosorbent test). This blood test is useful for diagnosing allergies to pollens, dust, molds, bee venom, and other allergens.

Do You Suffer from Food Allergies?

The following questionnaire, developed by naturopath Leon Chaitow, ND, DO, of London, England, can help you determine if you have a food allergy. If your answer is no or never to any question, give yourself a score of 0 for that particular question; the other scores are provided with each question.

- Do you suffer from unnatural fatigue? (Score 1 if occasionally, 2 if regularly—three times a week or more.)

- Do you sometimes experience weight fluctuations of 4 or more pounds in a single day, accompanied by puffiness of the face, ankles, or fingers? (Score 1 if infrequently, 2 if frequently—more than once a month.)

- Do you have hot flashes (apart from menopause) or find yourself sweating for no obvious reason? (Score 1 if infrequently, 2 if several times a week or more.)

- Does your pulse race or your heart pound strongly for no obvious reason? (Score 1 if infrequently, 2 if several times a week or more.)

- Do you have a history of food intolerance, causing any symptoms at all? (Score 2 if your answer is yes.)

- Do you crave bread, sugary foods, milk, chocolate, coffee, or tea? (Score 2 if your answer is yes.)

- Do you suffer from migraines or severe headaches, irritable bowel syndrome, eczema, depression, asthma, or muscle aches? (Score 2 if your answer is yes.)

The most anyone could score on this test would be 14. If your score is 5 or higher, there is a strong likelihood that allergies are part of your symptom picture.

Again, this test is not very accurate in testing for food allergies, and it can also be very expensive. Most alternative medicine practitioners rarely use these tests. Instead, they recommend self-testing, such as the elimination diet and the pulse test, and laboratory procedures such as the ELISA test, designed specifically to assess food allergies.

Keep in mind that no single food allergy test is a panacea; each method has its strengths and weaknesses and the key is to find one that works for you. Regardless of which test you use, it is best to consult a nutritional counselor or other health-care practitioner to help guide you through the process.

The Elimination Diet

Despite the name, this is not really a diet in the conventional sense, but a test procedure to help you identify your allergenic foods. It involves three steps:

1. Eliminating potential allergenic foods from your diet for 10 to 14 days

2. Carefully observing any changes in your symptoms

3. Testing the eliminated foods by bringing them back into your diet, one by one, and noting any return of symptoms

The foods you choose to eliminate should be those you eat every day or nearly every day, foods you crave, and foods that make you feel weak. It is important to eliminate all of the suspected foods on your list, as multiple allergies are quite common. If all allergenic foods are not eliminated, it could skew your testing results. Also, read the ingredients on any packaged foods very carefully to ensure you do not inadvertently consume whatever it is you are trying to eliminate (sugar, for example, or perhaps a flavor enhancer such as monosodium glutamate). Remember that food allergies can take as long as 72 hours to exhibit symptoms. If you experience symptoms such as irritability, fatigue, headaches, and intense cravings during the elimination period, you may be going through withdrawal, which is a sure sign that you have been suffering from an allergy.

Pulse Test

This is a relatively simple test developed by Arthur Coca, MD, a pioneer in the field of environmental medicine. Dr. Coca based his test on many years of clinical observations of patients, during which he noticed that a common symptom of many food allergies is increased heart rate. Although the pulse test can help identify food allergies, you should not conclude you are allergy free if the foods you test do not affect your pulse rate. The problem is that not all food allergens will increase heart rate. If you have no success in identifying a food allergen using the pulse test but still suspect that you are suffering from such an allergy, you should try one of the other tests.

How to Take the Pulse Test

The pulse test is easy to self-administer and involves simply recording your pulse rate before and after meals. Stephen Langer, MD, observes that "certain of my patients who use the pulse test have seen their heartbeat rise from 72 to as high as 180 after they have eaten an allergenic food."[21] To take the test, follow these simple instructions:

1. Find the pulse point on your wrist by placing the second finger of the opposite hand on the inside of your wrist.
2. Count the beats (pulses) for 6 seconds and multiply the number by 10; this is your pulse rate.
3. Record your resting pulse rate first thing in the morning before getting out of bed.
4. Record your pulse 30 minutes before each meal, then 30 minutes and 60 minutes after each meal.

If the difference between your morning pulse and either of the two after-meal rates is more than 12 to 16 beats, chances are you have a food allergy. Once you have identified a meal that triggers a rise in your pulse rate, you can begin testing individual foods eaten during that meal. However, in some cases you may find that your resting pulse is higher than your after-meal pulse or that your before-meal pulse is higher than your after-meal pulse. If you observe such a pattern, it is possible that dust or some other airborne allergen is interfering with your test.[22]

ELISA Test

The ELISA test (or enzyme-linked immunosorbent assay) is a blood test that many alternative medicine practitioners consider to be among the most sensitive and useful in detecting food allergies. Unlike other allergy blood tests, it is able to pinpoint delayed allergic reactions. It tests for a wide variety of substances, subjecting a patient's blood sample to 102 different food extracts. Blood samples can be sent by mail to any one of several laboratories that perform this test (see Resources). You can have your doctor arrange to submit a sample of your blood to the lab.

Correcting Poor Diet Results in Better Sleep

INSOMNIA CAN ARISE from a combination of poor diet and work stress. Darren, 28, complained of tiredness and depression. The fatigue, he said, was due to the fact that he had been getting only 3 to 5 hours of sleep per night for the last five months. Darren was a chemical technician, and his sleep disturbance started when his hours at work shifted from a standard daytime schedule to the swing shift, from 4 P.M. to 12:30 A.M. His body still hadn't made the adjustment to the later schedule. As a result, he stayed up until the early morning hours and then would wake a number of times once he finally got to sleep.

Darren's diet was high in sugars and fatty foods, such as cheese and peanut butter. He frequently felt bloated and gassy and estimated he was 30 pounds overweight. In addition to the insomnia, lethargy, and depression, he had suffered with hay fever since the age of 17, and also had chronic neck pain from sitting and looking down into a microscope at work.

Darren decided to get a traditional Chinese medicine (TCM) diagnosis. In TCM, the practitioner considers the flow of vital energy (qi) in a patient through close examination of the patient's pulse, tongue, body odor, voice tone and strength, and general demeanor, among other elements. Darren's tongue was flabby and slightly pale with a red tip; he also had scalloped "teeth marks" on the sides of his tongue and his pulses were "slippery." All of these signs indicated that Darren's spleen and stomach were deficient in energy, meaning he was not producing enough blood or digestive power. The deficiency was allowing a condition of "dampness" to build up in his body, causing the energy to stagnate in his liver meridian (one of the 12 principle pathways for the flow of qi through the body), which was creating heat. This dampness and heat, according to TCM, were the cause of his mental restlessness and insomnia.

Darren was given an acupuncture treatment with emphasis on points along his back to strengthen his spleen, stomach, and liver functions, as well as points on the back of his neck to ease the muscle tension. On his front side, points along the spleen, stomach, and pericardium meridians, as well as a combination of liver and large intestine points, were used to release stress and mental tension. He relaxed completely during the treatment, even dozing at times. He was also given an herbal formula called Melakava (see Resources), which contains melatonin, the sleep-inducing hormone that regulates the body's sleep-wake cycle, along with the Chinese herbs zizyphus and kava, which have sedative and antidepressant properties. (It's best to consult with a medical professional before taking kava. It can be toxic to the liver, so it is not advised for those with compromised liver function; it also may interact with some pharmaceutical drugs.)

The night of the first acupuncture treatment, Darren took two tablets of Melakava 30 minutes before bedtime. He was able to fall asleep quickly and slept without awakening repeatedly. He reported at the next treatment that he was averaging 6 hours of sleep per night and awakening refreshed for the first time in months. Darren also made significant changes to his diet, reducing his intake of dairy products, fatty foods, and sugars. He eventually eliminated cheeses completely from his diet. By the third treatment, Darren was getting an average of 8 hours of sleep per night. He was less depressed and was getting enough sleep to help him cope with stresses at work. He was also less bothered by bloating and gas and, encouraged by his improved sleep, continued to make positive lifestyle changes by getting more exercise and eating better.

Dietary Recommendations for Better Sleep

Making better food choices can have a major influence on the quality of your sleep. By eliminating stimulants, treating food allergies, switching to a whole foods diet, and taking appropriate supplements, you can help alleviate your sleep disturbances and improve your overall health as well.

Eliminate Stimulants from Your Diet

Begin by examining your diet and eliminating any foods that contain stimulating ingredients, such as caffeine, sugar, or spices, that can ruin your sleep. You might keep a food diary for about a week and write down everything you eat and drink, and also noting the times you eat and the quality of your sleep each night. According to Peter Hauri, Ph.D., author of *No*

More Sleepless Nights, insomniacs can immediately improve their chances of getting better sleep by reducing caffeine, limiting alcohol, and eliminating smoking. "No matter what other factors might be causing your poor sleep, you can do these three things immediately and have an excellent chance of improving your sleep," says Dr. Hauri.

Caffeine

Dr. Hauri advises against consuming more than 300 mg of caffeine a day—the amount in three cups of coffee.[23] Caffeine is found in many hidden forms in a variety of beverages and processed foods; read labels to avoid ingesting additional caffeine. Some medications also contain caffeine. If a person is particularly sensitive to caffeine, even drinking a single cup of coffee or tea at breakfast can affect their sleep that night. Remember that the rate at which caffeine is cleared from the body is extremely variable from person to person.

Sugar

Although pure sugar will cause the greatest insulin response, many other foods have a similar insulin-stimulating effect. To evaluate foods based on their insulin impact, a scientific rating system called the glycemic index was developed by diabetes researchers at the University of Toronto. The index offers a comparison of the insulin effect of different foods, measuring their real-life effect on blood sugar levels. Those foods with a high rating on the glycemic index cause a higher insulin response than those with a low rating. "The glycemic index ranks foods according to how fast they are absorbed into the blood as sugar," says Ann Louise Gittleman, MS, CNS, author of *Get the Sugar Out*. "A diet based on high glycemic index foods (those absorbed most quickly) usually leads to a condition of chronic low blood sugar because you have rapid rises followed by sharp dips in blood sugar levels."[24]

Richard Podell, MD, indicates that choosing foods with a low glycemic index is "the secret to keeping blood sugar stable and insulin low."[25] Dr. Podell makes the following general observations:

- Foods with a higher glycemic rating, causing a higher insulin response, include white bread and other bread products made with white flour (such as bagels and English muffins), processed and sugary cereals, instant hot cereals, low-fat frozen desserts, raisins and other dried fruits, whole milk and whole-milk cheeses, peanuts and peanut butter, hot dogs, and luncheon meats.

- Foods with a low glycemic rating, which don't cause a high insulin spike, include most fresh vegetables, leafy green vegetables, stone

A Quick Guide to Dietary Changes

Many alternative practitioners recommend a combination of nutritional adjustments to aid sleep:

■ Avoid alcohol consumption or curtail it markedly.

■ Avoid caffeine in all forms.

■ Eat a protein-rich snack at bedtime, such as yogurt. Or, for optimal uptake of tryptophan, eat a small amount of a food rich in tryptophan, along with a bit of carbohydrate (preferably in whole-grain form, not processed).

■ Eat more raw vegetables and salad greens.

■ Eat whole grains and high-fiber foods and avoid simple carbohydrates such as pastries, products made white flour, processed cereals, and foods high in sugar. Whole grains contain many B vitamins, which act as natural sedatives for calming irritability and tension that may hinder deep sleep.

■ Eat more protein in the form of moderate amounts of lean meat, seafood, eggs, nuts, brown rice, beans, and avocados. Protein is digested more slowly and doesn't cause an insulin spike, which may interfere with sleep.

■ Eat a wide variety of foods to ensure that you are getting sufficient nutrition.

■ Be aware of the fat content of foods. More important than the total fat is the kind of fat you are eating. Incorporate healthy fats such as olive oil and flaxseed oil, which contain omega-3 and omega-6 fatty acids, to be certain your metabolism is running smoothly. Cold-water fish or fish oil supplements are another good source of these fatty acids.

■ Take 1 gram of niacinamide (vitamin B_3) at bedtime. This is useful for those who fall sleep easily but awaken and cannot get back to sleep.

■ Take 500 mg of chlorella or other algae products at bedtime, as a source of tryptophan.

---

fruits and melons, 100% whole-grain breads and minimally processed whole-grain cereals, sweet potatoes and yams, skim milk, buttermilk, poultry, lean cuts of beef, pork, veal, shellfish, white-fleshed fish, most legumes, and most nuts.

● Cooked foods rank higher on the index than raw foods. Similarly, fruits and vegetables that have been juiced or pureed are higher on the index than those eaten whole.

Finding out whether a food product contains sugar requires more sleuthing today than it once did. Only a few manufacturers currently include the word *sugar* in the list of ingredients of their sugar-containing products. Instead, wanting to avoid the sugar stigma that could negatively impact sales, many food producers hide the sugars in their products behind a host of chemical synonyms. Take note that products listing any of the following ingredients really do contain sugar: corn sweetener, dextrin, dextrose, fructose, fruit juice concentrates, glucose, high-fructose corn syrup, lactose, malt, maltodextrin, maltose, mannitol, sorbitol, sorghum, sucrose, and xylitol. Although all of these are sugars, fructose does stand apart from the rest. Of all the sugars, fructose causes the least severe insulin reaction.[26]

Drugs and Alcohol

Avoiding drugs and alcohol is especially important for those with sleep apnea. Alcohol and sleeping pills slow down the respiratory drive needed during sleep and cause further relaxation of the throat muscles, which makes obstructive sleep apnea more likely to occur. Sleep laboratory tests reveal that eliminating alcohol dramatically reduces the number of sleep apnea episodes, increases the oxygen saturation levels of the blood, and leads to deeper, more restful sleep.

Eliminate Allergenic Foods

It is essential to rule out food intolerances as a cause of sleep problems. In one study of infants, sleeplessness was eliminated by removing cow's milk from the diet and then began again when cow's milk was reintroduced.[27] Once you have identified the foods you are allergic to, the next step is to eliminate them from your diet. Initially, you should completely refrain from eating all allergenic foods for 60 to 90 days. After this period, you can begin to slowly reintroduce them into your diet. You should also vary the foods that you eat on a daily basis to avoid developing new allergies. You are likely to find that as you reintroduce the foods you were once sensitive to, your old symptoms will not reappear. This is because most food allergies are temporary and can be cured through abstinence. Food allergy specialist Dr. James Braly estimates that only about 5% of delayed food allergies are permanent.

Remember that eliminating an allergenic food can cause withdrawal reactions. "The majority of people who give up foods they're allergic to go through a mild to moderate withdrawal phase, lasting one to five days, while the body detoxifies itself," says Dr. Braly. Allergic symptoms may get worse during this period and cravings can be intense. If the allergenic foods were also your comfort foods, you may experience emotional feelings of loss and distress. But as Dr. Braly explains, "Once the withdrawal phase has passed, the cravings also abate, and the allergy sufferer is free of dependence on that food, free of both the physiological and psychological desire to consume it so frequently, and in such great quantities."[28]

Dietary Recommendations

Diet can make a major difference for the person with a sleep disorder. The following recommendations can help ensure that your diet is not working

How to Stop Your Food Allergies Fast

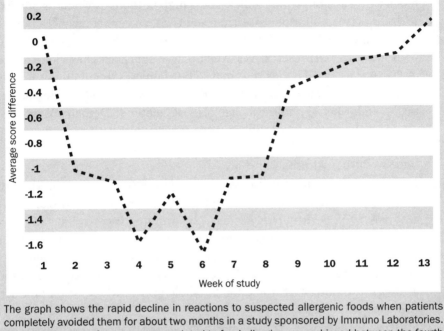

The graph shows the rapid decline in reactions to suspected allergenic foods when patients completely avoided them for about two months in a study sponsored by Immuno Laboratories. Maximum freedom from symptoms related to food allergies was achieved between the fourth and sixth weeks. Among the foods most commonly identified as allergenic are wheat, eggs, and chocolate (pictured above), as well as milk and corn.

Reprinted by permission from Immuno Laboratories

against you and your ability to sleep. All of the dietary strategies outlined below have the potential to improve your sleep and support your body as it heals. However, as you consider all of this information on diet (or any dietary advice), bear in mind the concept of biochemical individuality[29]—there is no single diet that is ideal for everyone, so remember to be sensitive to your body's response.

Eat More Whole Foods

You can't go wrong with a whole foods diet based on whole grains, vegetables and fruits, good protein sources, and healthy fats. This type of diet will provide you with the vitamins and minerals you need to reestablish regular, restorative sleep, as well as overall health and well-being.

One thing alternative and conventional medicine agree on is that Americans should consume far less animal protein, fat (especially bad fats), and processed foods, and eat more complex carbohydrates, especially whole grains rich in fiber, and at least five servings daily of fruits and vegetables. Buck Levin, Ph.D., RD, a specialist in environmental nutrition, offers a simple prescription for a healthy diet—one of natural, whole foods: "By whole foods we mean consuming a diet that is high in foods as whole as possible, with the least amount of processing, additives, and sweeteners."

Eating whole foods is always a good bet because these foods aren't laden with additives and preservatives. And because our species has a long history of use of these foods, they're suited to our bodies. Organic foods are also always a good choice because they aren't laden with residues of toxic pesticides and other agricultural chemicals. (Chapter 4, Detoxify Your Body, discusses the interrelationship between toxicity and sleep.)

Choose Carbohydrates Carefully

Earlier in this chapter, we discussed how excessive intake of sugar (the basic unit of carbohydrates) can cause hypoglycemia, which can disrupt sleep. One way to prevent hypoglycemia is by avoiding excessive sugar intake. However, glucose is the body's primary fuel, so how can you provide that fuel in a form that won't cause unhealthy fluctuations in blood sugar levels? The easy answer ties in with the previous recommendation: eat carbohydrates in the form of whole foods: whole grains, whole-grain products, vegetables, and fruits.

To understand why choosing the right carbohydrates can help keep blood sugar levels more even, let's take a step back and look at carbohydrates as a whole. There are two different types of carbohydrates. Simple carbohydrates are made up of single sugar molecules or two sugar molecules joined together. Complex carbohydrates are also made up of sugars, but the sugar molecules are strung together to form longer, more complex chains. Complex carbohydrates include starches and fiber, and they are abundant in most plant foods, especially grains, legumes, and vegetables.

In the body, complex carbohydrates are ultimately broken into down into usable energy units (glucose molecules), but the conversion happens slowly, sending a steady stream of glucose into the blood. Unfortunately, once complex carbohydrates are refined—stripped of fiber and other essential nutrients during milling and other processes—the body breaks them down into sugars much more rapidly, and as a result, they have effects similar to simple carbohydrates. For balanced blood sugar levels, improved sleep, and, ultimately, for optimum health, it's best to eat whole grains and products made from whole grains. It should be fairly easy to increase your consumption of familiar grains like brown rice, oats, barley, and bulgur, but consider making it an adventure. Experiment with some of the interesting alternatives now more commonly available, such as amaranth, quinoa, and millet.

In truth, processing also plays an important role where simple carbohydrates are concerned. For example, fruits are fairly high in simple

Guidelines for Healthy Eating

Avoid These Foods	Use These Foods Instead
Refined sugar in all its forms: white sugar (sucrose), fructose, corn syrup, sorbitol, mannitol, and many others. Synthetic sugars: aspartame, saccharin, and others.	Natural sweeteners: fruit juice, raw honey, organic maple syrup, molasses, barley malt syrup, dehydrated organic sugarcane juice. Avoid even these if you're diabetic or sugar intolerant.
Refined flours: white, bleached, unbleached, and enriched flour and products containing these flours.	Organic whole grains: heirloom varieties, which aren't genetically altered, are best—such as Kamut, quinoa, amaranth, and spelt. People with gluten intolerance or celiac disease may tolerate these better.
Synthetic fats: margarine, hydrogenated or partially hydrogenated oils, vegetable shortening, and olestra and other fat substitutes. High levels of saturated fats.	When cooking or baking: moderate amounts of healthy monounsaturated fats (olive oil or canola oil) and saturated fats (organic butter or coconut oil). If not heated: unsaturated oils (corn, safflower, soy, and flaxseed oil). Always use cold-pressed oils that are fresh; rancid oils can be harmful.
Commercial nuts and seeds with added oil, sugar, or salt. Also beware of peanuts. They often are contaminated by a mold that produces aflatoxin, a toxic, carcinogenic compound.	Organic dairy products, especially cultured milk products (kefir, yogurt, buttermilk), goat's milk, and unprocessed cheeses. Use dairy products in moderation if you are lactose intolerant.
Commercial dairy products, especially homogenized, pasteurized, or nonfat milk and processed cheese.	Organic nuts and seeds soaked for 6 hours or blanched or roasted to destroy enzyme inhibitors in their skins.
All commercial meat, poultry, and eggs.	Organic meats, free-range poultry, and eggs, in moderation. Seafood is fine if it is not from polluted waters, and cold-water fish is an excellent source of both high-quality protein and EFAs.
Junk food and canned, precooked, microwaved, or processed fast foods.	Buy fresh, organic foods first, fresh nonorganic second, and frozen third. Only use canned if that is the only option available.
Commercial, sugared fruit juices, juice drinks, and soft drinks (both diet and regular).	Fresh juices, preferably raw and organic, and natural spritzers containing only fruit juice and carbonated water.

carbohydrates, yet they are a healthful food. Why? Because in their whole form, they come packaged with complex carbohydrates, vitamins, minerals, enzymes, phytochemicals, and more—a veritable cornucopia of healthy nutrients. Plus, the fiber that they contain helps moderate the release of sugars into the bloodstream. These days, most of us are aware that fiber has many health benefits, from promoting good digestive function to helping reduce risk of certain diseases, including heart disease and cancer. In later chapters, we'll look at how dietary fiber can benefit sleep by aiding in detoxification (chapter 4) and promoting hormonal balance (chapter 8).

Eat to Boost Tryptophan Levels

You might try altering your diet to help your brain get more tryptophan, a precursor of melatonin. Tryptophan is one of the eight essential amino acids; in typical diets, it's also the least plentiful of all the amino acids. Because it's an amino acid, you might be tempted to think that eating more protein would boost your body's stores of nutrients, but it doesn't work that way. To make its way into the brain, where it's converted into serotonin and, ultimately, melatonin, tryptophan must be transported across the blood-brain barrier by a carrier molecule, and it has to compete with other amino acids for a carrier. Since it's the least abundant amino acid, it has the lowest chances of winning that competition. Eating more protein just introduces more competitors.

Interestingly, the best way to get more tryptophan into the brain is to eat an evening meal that consists primarily of carbohydrates (complex carbohydrates from whole foods, of course). This stimulates the production of insulin, which has functions other than regulating blood sugar. One of those other functions is to direct amino acids to various body tissues where they're needed. Tryptophan is more resistant to this action, so it keeps circulating in the blood longer; eventually, it exists in higher concentrations in the blood than other amino acids, facilitating its access to transport across the blood-brain barrier.[30] Another strategy is to eat an evening or bedtime snack consisting primarily of carbohydrates, but with a small amount of a food rich in tryptophan. Foods with a relative abundance of tryptophan include turkey, chicken, eggs, dairy products, nuts and seeds, soy products, oatmeal, and bananas.

Eating a meal high in protein actually has the opposite effect. In most foods, the amino acid tyrosine is more abundant than tryptophan. Tyrosine is a precursor of the stimulating neurotransmitters adrenaline, noradrenaline, and dopamine. If supplies of these neurotransmitters are low, your body will use the tyrosine to create more, which can have a stimulating effect. (At this juncture, you may find yourself wondering why that high-tryptophan

Thanksgiving meal featuring turkey induces sleepiness. The answer isn't tryptophan—it's overeating, which directs more blood to your digestive tract, making less blood available to your brain.)

Be Aware of the Timing of Meals

As discussed above, hypoglycemia can disrupt sleep. Fluctuating blood sugar levels are influenced not just by the foods you eat, but also by when and how much you eat, as well as skipping meals and snacking habits. Stress and exercise can also play a role. If you skip meals, your blood sugar level can get too low. Your body will respond by releasing sugars (stored in the liver in the form of the starch glycogen) into the bloodstream. This is one reason it's important to eat a good breakfast. After sleeping—and fasting—all night, your body needs to be refueled.

Insomnia expert Peter Hauri recommends a "triangle" plan—a large breakfast to start the day, a lighter lunch, and an even lighter meal for dinner—to ensure that your body isn't working on

Foods to Avoid before Bedtime

As mentioned in the discussion of boosting tryptophan levels, tyrosine can have a stimulating effect, so you might want to avoid high-protein meals at the end of the day. In addition to concentrated protein sources (animal products, and also soybeans and other legumes), other foods high in tyrosine include green beans, oats, peas, seaweed, and wheat. You wouldn't want to try to avoid tyrosine in your diet, because the neurotransmitters made from this amino acid are critical for healthy functioning of the body. But you might experiment with avoiding these foods in the evening.

Another dietary rule of thumb is to avoid foods that contain tyramine, a breakdown product of the amino acid tyrosine. Many people can metabolize tyramine just fine, but in some people, tyramine makes its way into the bloodstream, where it increases the release of the stress hormone norepinephrine, which acts as a stimulant. Tyramine can also trigger migraine headaches. Foods that contain tyramine include aged cheeses, sauerkraut, bacon, ham, sausage, other aged and processed meats, yeast concentrates, soybeans, fava beans, eggplant, potatoes, spinach, tomatoes, and overripe avocados and other overripe fruits. Certain alcoholic beverages contain tyramine, especially Chianti, port, sherry, and vermouth; wine and beer may also contain tyramine.[31]

digesting a large meal when you go to bed. In addition, foods eaten later in the day should be lower in fat, because fats take longer to digest.

Although it's important not to go to bed too full, it's also important not to go to bed hungry. Like any other discomfort, this can make it harder to get to sleep or awaken you during the night. If you find you're hungry at bedtime, have a small, low-calorie snack. This is be especially important if you have issues with low blood sugar (or if you have a fast metabolism). To prevent nighttime hypoglycemia, avoid foods high in sugar and refined carbohydrates for bedtime or evening snacks; complex carbohydrates are a good bet, but some practitioners recommend a protein-rich snack, and some people do benefit from this approach. Experiment to find what works best for you. Eating well-balanced meals at regular times during the day (4 to 5 hours apart) will also help stabilize your blood sugar.

Heartburn and gastroesophageal reflux disorder (GERD) can both interfere with sleep, not only due to the inherent discomfort, but also because both are exacerbated by lying down. If you suffer from either, be sure to avoid foods that may be triggers late in the day. Common culprits include spicy food, fried foods, tomatoes, citrus fruits, chocolate, garlic, onions, mint, and anything with caffeine (which you should be avoiding in the evening anyway!).

If gas is a problem for you, avoid foods that cause this problem before bedtime. Although this varies from person to person, common offenders are beans, soy foods, peanuts, and cruciferous vegetables, such as broccoli, cauliflower, and cabbage. If you're trying to consume more of these healthful foods with unfortunate side effects, start with small amounts and increase how much of them you eat slowly. This may allow your body to adjust. Other causes of gas include fried foods, fatty meats, dairy products, many starches, carbonated beverages, and excessive amounts of fruits and vegetables. As you can see, the list is potential causes is long. You'll need to identify which are a problem for you.

Though it may sound obvious, it can't hurt to mention that those who are frequently awakened by a need to urinate may want to consume fewer liquids late in the day. Drinking enough water is important for overall health and good sleep, so don't cut back on the amount you're drinking, just adjust when you drink. It's particularly important to avoid diuretic beverages, such as coffee, alcohol, sodas, and tea (even some herbal teas) in the evening hours. If you do have to get up during the night, use the dimmest light possible to move around safely, to avoid disrupting your sleep-wake cycle.

Eat Lower on the Food Chain

Because toxins become more concentrated higher up in the food chain (a concept known as bioaccumulation), animal products generally are more burdened with toxins. If you choose to eat meat, poultry, eggs, and dairy products, protect your health—and your sleep—by eating organic products. In addition, the hormones—both supplemental and natural—in animal products can disrupt hormonal balance, which can have negative impact on sleep (more on that topic in chapter 8, Balance Your Hormones). Cold-water fish, such as salmon, cod, and mackerel, can be especially beneficial. In addition to being a great source of lean, high-quality protein, they are rich in essential fatty acids, which play an important role in many physiological functions, including balancing hormones.

Take Appropriate Supplements

Aside from making certain that you are consuming a balanced whole foods diet, you may want to consider supplementing with vitamins, minerals, and herbs that have been shown to help improve and restore sleep. The following information highlights specific nutritional supplements known to aid sleep.

Vitamins

Good nutritional status is essential for good health, and any serious deficiencies are likely ultimately have some impact on your sleep. However, a few specific vitamins are more directly involved in sleep, particularly B vitamins and vitamin E. Let's take a look at B vitamins in general before getting into the specific B vitamins recommended for sleep. The B vitamins (collectively known as B complex) nutritionally support the brain, eyes, intestines, liver, muscles, and skin. They act as a team to help maintain healthy energy metabolism and are important for sleep. The B vitamins are known to have a sedative effect on the nerves and regulate the body's use of L-tryptophan. Stress levels, diet, and lifestyle can cause the body to use B vitamins relatively quickly. And because they are water-soluble, they aren't stored in the body; therefore, it's important to get enough B vitamins daily, either through diet or supplementation.

Vitamin B_1 (thiamin) and vitamin B_2

Vitamin B_1 (thiamin) and vitamin B_2 (riboflavin) primarily serve in the maintenance of mucous membranes, formation of red blood cells, and metabolism of carbohydrates. Deficiencies of vitamin B_1 may lead to blood sugar imbalances.

Food sources: Brewer's yeast is an excellent source of both of these vitamins.

Supplements: B_1 and B_2 are commonly found in B complex supplements.

Typical therapeutic dose: 25 to 100 mg daily.

Vitamin B_3 (niacin)

Vitamin B_3 (niacin) is necessary for oxygen transport in the blood and formation of fatty acids and nucleic acids. Also known as niacinamide, this vitamin has been shown to prolong REM sleep and is helpful to people with sleep maintenance insomnia, who wake up in the middle of the night and can't fall back to sleep. Low levels of B_3 can cause muscle weakness, fatigue, irritability, and depression. Eating a diet high in refined sugar as well as prolonged use of antibiotics will deplete B_3 reserves in the body.

Food sources: Meat, chicken, fish, peanuts, wheat germ, brewer's yeast, and whole grains, particularly rice.

Supplements: Niacin, the natural form of vitamin B_3, is available in supplement form. When taken in dosages of over 100 mg, niacin can cause a very distinctive flushing, tingling, and redness that begins in the lower part of the body and moves up to the face, hands, and head. Niacinamide causes no flushing and is the form found in many modern supplements.

Typical therapeutic dose: 50 to 100 mg daily.

Precautions: Liver enzymes may be affected when taking high doses of B_3 or niacinamide. Inositol hexaniacinate, another form of vitamin B_3, has shown no toxicity and may be the best choice for this supplement.

Vitamin B₅ (pantothenic acid)

Vitamin B_5 (pantothenic acid) is vital for synthesis of hormones and support of the adrenal glands. Pantothenic acid deficiency can cause fatigue, insomnia, and depression.[32]

Food sources: Liver, meat, chicken, whole grains, and legumes. Eating a variety of foods can ensure adequate levels of vitamin B_5.

Supplements: Pantothenic acid is the most common form of vitamin B_5 in supplements, but sometimes pantothine is used.

Typical therapeutic dose: 10 to 2,000 mg daily.

Vitamin B₆ (pyridoxine)

Vitamin B_6 (pyridoxine) strongly influences the immune and nervous systems. The body requires vitamin B_6 to convert the amino acid tryptophan into the neurotransmitter serotonin, which helps control sleep. Deficiencies occur as a result of eating a diet high in fats and low in fruits and vegetables.

Food sources: Brewer's yeast, whole grains, legumes, nuts, and seeds.

Supplements: There are two forms of B_6, pyridoxine hydrochloride and pyridoxal-5-phosphate (the most active form). For efficient absorption of pyridoxine by the body, sufficient levels of riboflavin and magnesium should be present.[33]

Typical therapeutic dose: 50 to 100 mg daily can help prevent insomnia.

Precautions: High levels of pyridoxine can cause toxic side effects.[34]

Vitamin B₁₂ (cobalamin)

Vitamin B_{12} (cobalamin) is virtually absent in vegetable food sources, which means vegetarians are at risk of deficiency in this vitamin. B12 is essential for normal formation of red blood cells and the maintenance of the nervous system.

Food sources: Meat, most fish (especially trout, mackerel, and herring), egg yolks, and yogurt.

Supplements: B_{12} can be given in injectable form or as an oral supplement.

Typical therapeutic dose: 25 micrograms (mcg) daily.

Folic acid (folacin, folate)

Folic acid (folacin, folate), also a member of the B vitamin family, is important for red blood cell formation, breakdown and utilization of proteins, and proper cell division. It is also useful for fighting anemia, atherosclerosis, fatigue, immune weakness, infection, and osteoporosis.

Food sources: Asparagus, broccoli, lima beans, green peas, sweet potatoes, bean sprouts, whole wheat, cantaloupe, strawberries, brewer's yeast, and leafy green vegetables, such as spinach and kale.

Supplements: The folic acid content in foods can be depleted by cooking, so supplementation may be necessary.

Typical therapeutic dose: 400 mcg daily.

Vitamin E (alpha-tocopherol)

Vitamin E (alpha-tocopherol) has been proven effective in treating restless legs syndrome, which may be caused by decreased circulation to the legs. In one study concerning vitamin E and restless legs syndrome, a 78-year-old female with a history of restless and jumpy legs was cured after supplementing with 300 IU of vitamin E daily for two months.[35] In another study, a 37-year-old female with a 10-year history of severe nightly restless legs experienced complete relief after taking 300 IU of vitamin E daily for six weeks and 200 IU daily for the following four weeks.[36]

Food sources: Cold-pressed polyunsaturated vegetable oils (such as sunflower and safflower), leafy green vegetables, avocados, nuts, seeds, and whole grains.

Supplements: Vitamin E is actually a group of compounds called tocopherols. When purchasing supplements of vitamin E, avoid products that contain vitamin E in the DL-alpha-tocopherol acetate form. This means that it is a petroleum-based synthetic form of the vitamin. The natural form of vitamin E will be designated with the letter "D."

Typical therapeutic dose: 30 IU daily. Those suffering from restless legs syndrome should take 800 to 1,200 IU per day.

Minerals

The minerals the human body requires can be divided into two categories: macrominerals and trace minerals. Macrominerals are those we need large quantities of, often because they are incorporated into important body structures, such as bones, teeth, hair, and skin. Trace minerals often play a role in facilitating metabolic processes. Calcium and magnesium are the macrominerals that most directly play a role in sleep. Key trace minerals involved in getting good sleep are chromium, copper, iron, and zinc.

Calcium

Calcium and magnesium nourish the nervous system and act as natural relaxants. Many people have systems that are too acidic and benefit from taking these mineral supplements, which are both alkaline and also have sedative qualities. Low levels of calcium and magnesium have been associated with muscle cramping, which can disrupt sleep.[37] Calcium absorption can be compromised by whole grains and cereals, spinach, the tannins in tea, antacids that contain aluminum, or a diet high in protein, refined sugar, and commercial sodas.[38]

Food sources: Almonds, hazelnuts, oats, lentils, beans, figs, currants, raisins, broccoli, cabbage, brussels sprouts, cauliflower, kelp, and leafy green vegetables, especially kale, which is very high in an easily absorbed form of calcium.[39]

Supplements: Bone meal, dolomite, and oyster shell calcium supplements have been found to have the highest levels of lead and should not be used as a supplement.[40] Calcium citrate and calcium gluconate have a much better absorption level.[41] One of the best forms of absorbable calcium is microcrystalline hydroxyapatite.

Typical therapeutic dose: 600 mg of liquid calcium can have a relaxing effect (take calcium in a 2-to-1 ratio to magnesium).

Precautions: Excessive intake of calcium oxalate may cause the formation of kidney stones, but this risk can be decreased by using the calcium citrate and calcium gluconate forms. High calcium intake can interfere with iron absorption and cause chronic constipation, and may also increase blood pressure.[42]

Magnesium

Magnesium is second only to potassium as the most concentrated mineral within the cells. Magnesium helps form bones, relax muscle spasms, and decreases the pain involved in arthritis. It activates cellular enzymes, plays a large role in nerve and muscle function, and helps regulate the body's acid-alkaline balance.[43] Magnesium deficiency can cause anxiety, muscle tremors, confusion, irritability, and pain. Processed food or foods cooked at high temperatures can be depleted of their magnesium content.

Food sources: Tofu, nuts, seeds, sea vegetables, and leafy green vegetables, especially kale.

Supplements: Oral supplements of magnesium are absorbed well and will increase the measurable levels of this mineral inside red and white blood cells.[44] The forms best absorbed are magnesium glycinate, magnesium fumerate, and magnesium citrate, which also have less of a laxative effect.[45] Epsom salts (magnesium sulfate), an old-fashioned remedy, is an excellent addition to a bath, but it has a strong laxative effect if taken as an oral supplement.

Typical therapeutic dose: 250 mg daily.

Precautions: Very high doses of magnesium may be dangerous for those with kidney disease.

Chromium

Chromium is essential for regulating the production of the hormone insulin, which is responsible for stabilizing blood sugar levels. Although the body requires only small amounts of this important mineral, Americans are more likely to be deficient in chromium than any other micronutrient. Chromium is found in the outer bran portions of grains, but much of it is lost in the milling and processing of white flour, the primary ingredient in most refined bread and pasta products. The chromium that we do obtain from food sources can be depleted in the body by various factors, including a high-carbohydrate diet, infections, and physical and emotional stress. Urinary excretion of chromium can increase as much as fiftyfold under stress.[46] A high intake of refined sugar also tends to deplete the body of chromium, as the mineral is used up in removing sugars from the blood.[47]

Food sources: Brewer's yeast is an excellent source of chromium; other good sources include wheat germ, beef, chicken, liver, whole grains, potatoes, eggs, apples, bananas, and spinach.

Supplements: Chromium and other minerals are better absorbed in the body when chelated, meaning they are bound in a "transporter" molecule. In this form, minerals are better protected from damage in the digestive system. Chromium chelated with glucose tolerance factor (GTF chromium) tends to be a more bioavailable form than chromium salts, such as chromium chloride.[48] Chromium polynicotinate, another chelated variety, is chemically bound to vitamin B_3. According to some researchers, this form of chromium is superior to either chromium chloride or chromium picolinate.

Typical therapeutic dose: 250 to 500 mcg twice a day.

Copper

Copper is important for normal functioning of the central nervous system. Deficiencies in copper have been linked to greater difficulties in getting to sleep and decreased quality of sleep. This mineral may also help alleviate allergic reactions, particularly elevated levels of histamine. The body's absorption of copper is blocked by a diet high in refined foods or high levels of zinc, iron, and vitamin C.[49]

Food sources: Beans, lentils, shellfish (especially oysters), liver, nuts, and leafy green vegetables.

Supplements: There are various forms of supplemental copper, such as copper sulfate, copper gluconate, copper picolinate, and others.

Typical therapeutic dose: 2 to 5 mg daily.

Precautions: Copper toxicity is seen more often than is copper deficiency. Use only after a copper deficiency has been clearly established through hair or urine analysis.

Iron

Iron is essential to red blood cell synthesis, oxygen transport, and energy production. A diet low in iron is one cause of anemia and can also cause hypothyroidism.[50] Supplementing with iron has produced significant relief of symptoms in restless legs syndrome.[51]

Food sources: Kelp, organ meats, egg yolk, blackstrap molasses, lecithin, certain nuts and seeds, millet, and parsley.

Supplements: The heme form of iron, found in desiccated liver or a liquid liver extract, is most easily absorbed and has fewer side effects. Of the nonheme forms of iron, ferrous fumerate and ferrous succinate are recommended.

Typical therapeutic dose: 30 mg daily between meals.

Precautions: Overdose in infants can be serious or even fatal, so be sure that your iron supplements are out of the reach of children. Ferrous sulfate, commonly used in conventional supplements, can cause the production of free radicals and should not be used. Elevated levels of iron in the blood are associated with an increased risk for heart attacks and other cardiovascular problems, as well as low immunity.[52] Women who are menopausal and those who experience a heavy menstrual flow should consult their physicians about supplementing with iron.

Zinc

Zinc may be deficient in people suffering from insomnia, particularly infants. Vegetarians may be more likely to have a zinc deficiency because beans, legumes, and grains—often the staples of a vegetarian diet—are high phytates, substances that inhibit absorption of zinc (and other minerals).[53]

Food sources: Zinc is commonly added to animal feed, making meat one of the best sources of this mineral. Oysters, shellfish, nuts and seeds are also good sources. In spite of reduced absorption due to phytates, whole grains are also a fairly good source.

Supplements: Zinc sulfate, found in many multivitamin-multimineral preparations, is not easily absorbed by the body. Other forms of zinc that are more readily absorbed are zinc picolinate, zinc citrate, and zinc monomethionine.

Typical therapeutic dose: 25 mg of zinc daily, along with 3 mg of copper (zinc tends to deplete copper reserves).

Precautions: With medical supervision, the dosage of zinc could be increased if necessary. However, dosages should be increased with caution, as too much zinc can interfere with the functioning of the immune system. Toxicity of zinc is rarely reported; however, prolonged use of over 150 mg a day can cause anemia.

Amino Acids and Other Supplements

Amino acids are the building blocks of proteins, and proteins are, in turn, the building blocks of the body. Of the 22 amino acids vital to the body's growth, development, and maintenance, some can be manufactured in the body while others, called essential amino acids, must be obtained from the diet or nutritional supplements. Semi-essential amino acids can be made by the body in amounts that are adequate to maintain basic protein requirements; however, additional dietary sources are required during times of growth or stress. Although often undetected, amino acid deficiencies may be an underlying factor in many sleep disorders. It's commonly thought that vegetarians and vegans (vegetarians who eat no eggs or dairy products) will have difficulty meeting their protein requirements. However, most foods contain a variety of amino acids, and as long as the diet is varied, obtaining all the amino acids the body needs for manufacturing proteins isn't an issue. In fact, it isn't necessary to combine various foods, such as rice and beans,

A Guide to Taking Supplements

In addition to knowing what supplements to take, it is also important to know how to take them. Jeffrey Bland, Ph.D., and Lindsey Berkson, DC, offer the following recommendations and precautions:

- Nutritional supplements should be taken with meals to promote increased absorption. Fat-soluble vitamins (such as vitamins A and E, beta-carotene, and the essential fatty acids linoleic and alpha-linolenic acid) should be taken during the day with the meal that contains the most fat.

- Amino acid supplements should be taken on an empty stomach at least 1 hour before or after a meal, and taken with fruit juice to help promote absorption. When taking an increased dosage of an isolated amino acid, be sure to supplement with an amino acid blend as well, to avoid an imbalance.

- If you become nauseated when you take supplements in pill form, consider taking a liquid form, diluted in a beverage.

- If you become nauseated or ill within 1 hour after taking nutritional supplements, consider the need for a bowel cleanse or detoxification program prior to beginning a course of nutritional supplementation.

- If you are taking high doses of a nutrient, don't take the entire amount at one time; divide it into smaller doses throughout the day.

- Do not take mineral supplements with high-fiber meals, as fiber can decrease mineral absorption.

- When taking an increased dosage of an isolated B vitamin, be sure to supplement with B complex.

- When taking supplements, be sure to drink adequate amounts of liquid to mix with digestive juices and prevent side effects

Reprinted by permission from Jeffrey Bland

to eat "complete protein" at any given meal. The body can utilize amino acids consumed at different meals to make proteins. That said, vegetarians who eat a poor diet or only a limited variety of foods should take an amino acid complex supplement.

L-tryptophan is considered the most important amino acid for sleeping problems. L-tryptophan is a precursor to serotonin, which is then converted into melatonin. Adequate levels of melatonin allow the body to drop off into slumber. Tryptophan occurs naturally in certain foods, most notably turkey, and also other meats, milk, cheese, and soybeans and other legumes. Other tryptophan-containing foods include cashews, mushrooms, spinach, bananas, figs, dates, yogurt, tuna, and whole grains. Research shows that tryptophan helps about half of the people who suffer from insomnia.[54]

During the 1980s, L-tryptophan got a bad reputation when several batches from one specific manufacturer made more than 1,000 people ill; 37 people died. While high-quality L-tryptophan supplements should be perfectly safe, if you have concerns, there is an alternative: 5-HTP, or 5-hydroxytryptophan, which is a form of tryptophan that is a step closer in the conversion process to serotonin. In the brain, tryptophan is usually converted into 5-HTP, which is then turned into serotonin. 5-HTP has been shown to be effective in treating depression, fibromyalgia, headaches, and insomnia.[55] A Norwegian study on animals showed that 5-HTP had an effect on sleep patterns by increasing levels of serotonin.[56] The typical recommended dosage of 5-HTP is 25 to 50 mg daily. Higher dosages (over 100 mg) could cause some side effects, including mild nausea. Vitamin B_6 should be taken on the same day as 5-HTP, because it is necessary for converting 5-HTP into serotonin.

Other amino acids may play a role in sleep disorders, depending on the person and their nutritional status. Jonathan Wright, MD, a pioneer in nutritional medicine, has had success in treating insomnia using supplements of essential amino acids. He reports the case of a man who had been suffering from insomnia most of his adult life. Over the previous 18 years, doctors had prescribed 14 different drugs, starting with sleeping pills and progressing to antidepressants. The sleeping pills left the patient feeling groggy, while the antidepressants resulted in nightmares and, in the case of two drugs, heart trouble. He had also tried L-tryptophan supplements, but his insomnia did not improve. A blood test determined that the patient was deficient in five of the eight essential amino acids (his tryptophan levels were normal). Dr. Wright prescribed an amino acid blend to be taken (stirred into applesauce) twice a day. After three weeks, the patient's condition had improved markedly and, within three months, his insomnia had cleared up completely.

The best amino acid supplements are labeled USP pharmaceutical grade, free-form, L-crystalline amino acids. The term *USP* means that the product meets the standards of purity and potency set by the United States Pharmacopeia. The term *free-form* refers to the highest level of purity of the amino acid. The *L* refers to one of the two forms in which most amino acids come, designated D- and L- (as in D-lysine or L-lysine). L-form amino acids are appropriate for human biochemistry, as proteins in the human body are made from this form.

Generally, it is not advisable to take individual amino acids for extended or indefinite periods, as this can create an imbalance among the body's amino acids and possibly cause other health conditions. If individual amino acids are taken for specific health conditions, follow this course of treatment with a complex of free-form amino acids to ensure balanced amino acid nutrition. Please consult a qualified health-care professional before beginning such therapies. Individual amino acids often come with warnings or precautions for women who are pregnant or for people with certain health conditions.

One final nutrient also bears discussion: phosphatidylserine. Classified as a phospholipid, it isn't, strictly speaking, an amino acid, but it does contain the amino acid serine. Phosphatidylserine plays a critical role in the normal functioning of the cell membranes of neurons. It also helps the hypothalamus regulate the amount of cortisol produced by the adrenals. This makes it a useful supplement for those who cannot sleep because of high cortisol levels, usually caused by stress. Cortisol is usually at high levels in the morning, for wakefulness, but in stressed individuals it may be high at night and prevent sleeping.

four

Step 2: Detoxify Your Body

Alternative physicians working with sleep disorders know that removing toxins from the body is an essential phase in restoring patients to health and vitality. Each year, people are exposed to thousands of toxic chemicals and pollutants in air, water, food, and soil. People carry within their bodies a chemical cocktail of industrial chemicals, pesticides, food additives, heavy metals, and the residues of conventional pharmaceutical drugs, as well as legal drugs like alcohol, tobacco, and caffeine and illegal drugs such as marijuana, amphetamines, cocaine, and heroin.

Today people are exposed to chemicals in far greater concentrations than previous generations were. For example, over 158 million Americans live in areas that exceed smog standards.[1] It's estimated that 20% of the U.S. populations drinks water that violates safety standards;[2] even worse, EPA safety standards only exist for about 120 pollutants in drinking water, but studies have shown that at least 260 contaminants occur in tap water.[3] Some 3,000 chemicals are added to the food supply, and as many as 10,000 chemicals in the form of solvents, emulsifiers, and preservatives are used in food processing and storage. Many of these toxins can remain in the body for years.[4]

To make matters worse, there's no way food and product labels can list every possible contaminant. When you consume many foods—especially seafood, meat, poultry, and dairy products—you're ingesting all the chemicals and pesticides that have accumulated as contaminants in the food chain.

Some of these pollutants are stored in the body, loading it up with poisons, and this can manifest in a variety of symptoms, including decreased immune function, damage to nerve cells, hormonal dysfunction, psychological disturbances, and sleep disorders.

Alternative Medicine Approach to Detoxification

- Colon cleansing programs
- Liver cleansing programs
- Eliminating yeast
- Eliminating parasites

The Loading Theory of Toxicity

The loading theory of toxicity, according to its formulator, Serafina Corsello, MD, founder of the Corsello Centers for Complementary and Alternative Medicine, states that no single factor causes a disease. Rather, the cumulative load of multiple poisons creates an illness like insomnia.

This is compounded by layers of toxicity, malnutrition, and dysfunction. Dr. Corsello explains that people don't *get* a disease—they develop it. Over time, multiple factors weigh down the immune system and eventually throw it out of balance. Among the typical stressors are toxic metals (mercury leaching from fillings, aluminum), petrochemical residues (from pesticides and fertilizers), chemical pollutants (in the water and air), electromagnetic pollution (from power lines), undiagnosed food allergies, nutritional deficiencies, biochemical imbalances, insufficient exercise, and emotional stress. All these factors impinge on the immune system's natural ability to resist the downhill slide into illness.

Increasingly, toxicity is being identified as the predisposing factor in a long list of acute and chronic illnesses, including sleep disorders, environmental illness, chronic fatigue, degenerative diseases, and cancer.[5] "The current level of chemicals in the food and water supply and the indoor and outdoor environment has lowered our threshold of resistance to disease and has altered our body's metabolism, causing enzyme dysfunction, nutritional deficiencies, and hormonal imbalances," says Marshall Mandell, MD, a pioneer in environmental medicine.

Detoxification can play an important role in both preventing and healing many of these conditions. It's an important component in promoting healthy immune function and addressing other factors that may be contributing to your sleep disorder. As our environment and food become increasingly saturated with chemicals, the body's mechanisms for elimination of toxins cannot keep up with the chemical deluge. The constant circulation of toxins in the body taxes the immune system, which must continually strive to destroy them. It is advisable to take measures to remove the toxins stored in the body.

Detoxification Defense System

The detoxification system has two lines of defense: specific organs that prevent toxins from entering the body, and others that neutralize and excrete the poisonous compounds that get through this initial line of defense. When functioning properly, the body's defenses protect healthy tissues from damage by circulating toxins and harmful free radicals. Key components of the detoxification system include:

- The gastrointestinal barrier, including the walls of the intestines
- Liver
- Lymphatic system, which transports waste products from the cells to the major organs of detoxification
- Kidneys, bladder, and other components of the urinary system
- Skin, including sweat glands and sebaceous glands
- Lungs

The gastrointestinal system is typically the first line of defense against toxins and, when compromised, the first place to harbor seeds of disease. "The digestive system is one of the first screening systems against the daily load of contact with bacteria, viruses, and parasites, that, if left unchecked, would constitute a grave threat to our entire immune system," says Dr. Corsello. A healthy intestine is immunologically vigilant against undesirable pathogens and toxins. One that is overburdened and compromised fails to perform its defensive role and may start contributing to the emergence of chronic disease. The intestines consist of a complex and delicately balanced population of mixed microflora in which the friendly, beneficial bacterial should outnumber the harmful ones. But this ecology is easily upset, leading to a condition of imbalance called dysbiosis.

Within the intricately convoluted lining of the 25 feet of the intestines, there are many hiding places for disease-causing agents. If these pathogens aren't neutralized by the immune system in the gut, they can break through the intestinal membrane and gain access to the bloodstream. This is one facet of how sleep disorders begin—once the bowel is toxic, the entire body soon follows. If the intestines are letting toxins through, then the liver, lymph, kidneys, skin, and other organs involved in detoxification become overwhelmed.

The liver bears most of the burden for eliminating toxins. Located beneath the right lower part of the rib cage, the liver is the largest internal organ. It's also one of the most complicated organs in the body, rivaled only by the brain. The liver collects and removes foreign particles and chemicals from the blood and detoxifies these poisons through three systems:

1. The Kupffer cells

2. Phase I and phase II systems, involving over 75 enzymes

3. The production of bile

Each system feeds into the others, and all three need to be operating at full efficiency for proper detoxification.

Approximately 1.6 quarts of blood pass through the liver each minute for filtering. The major players in this filtering project are the Kupffer cells, a type of white blood cell that engulfs foreign matter in the blood before it passes through the rest of the liver. When the liver is damaged, toxic, congested, or sluggish, the filtration system breaks down, allowing increased levels of antigens, foreign proteins, bowel microorganisms, and dietary waste products to pass through the liver and enter the general circulatory system.

When a toxic chemical like alcohol

The Digestive System

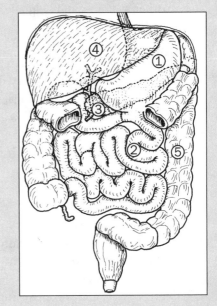

Digestion begins in the mouth, then food travels to the stomach (1), where it is further broken down by gastric juices. Next, the partially digested food goes to the small intestine (2) where enzymes from the pancreas (3) and bile produced by the liver (4) act upon the food to extract nutrients for absorption into blood and lymph cells. The unusable food materials are sent to the large intestine (5) for evacuation from the body.

enters the liver, the phase I and phase II reactions begin, which attempt to break down these chemicals into harmless substances. Phase I is the oxidation phase, in which enzymes oxidize toxins, reacting with them to form intermediate substances. Phase II enzymes work to combine these intermediate substances with other molecules (such as sulfur, glutathione, and glycine) to make them more water soluble and easier for the body to excrete.[6] These wastes are excreted via bile, a fluid that's stored in the gallbladder and then pumped into the small intestine as needed to make intestinal contents less acidic and prevent them from putrefying.

Other toxins are eliminated through the lymphatic system, kidneys, skin (by sweating), and respiratory system. When imbalances occur in any part of the body's detoxification system, the result can be poor digestion, constipation, bloating and gas, immune dysfunction, reduced liver function, sleep disorders, and a host of degenerative diseases. Detoxification can reduce or eliminate the body's toxic load, restore proper functioning of the immune and other systems, and help alleviate your sleep problems.

Sources of Toxins

We are exposed to toxins every day of our lives, in air and water pollution, chemical and pesticide residues, mercury amalgam dental fillings, biological contaminants such as pollen and parasites, and genetically altered foods, among other sources. Even our own bodies can produce toxins, called endotoxins, which can be harmful if their numbers become excessive or if they aren't adequately neutralized.

Environmental Pollution

Toxins emanate from a variety of sources, but chiefly from environmental pollution. Unavoidably, many of us carry around an internal chemical cocktail of toxins we've absorbed: industrial by-products (coal tar or fuel exhaust), pesticides, herbicides, household contaminants (found in cleaners, paints, plastics, and solvents), and biological contaminants (pollens, molds, dust mites, and parasites). We are also exposed to toxins from processed or genetically altered foods, alcohol, tap water (which usually contains heavy metals), and even newspapers (from the inks used in printing).

In the 1980s, physicians began using the term *sick building syndrome* (SBS) to refer to a host of symptoms produced by low-grade toxic environmental conditions found in living or office spaces—especially those with inadequate ventilation. SBS symptoms include headaches, memory loss, fatigue, lethargy, temporary weight loss, infections, irritability, impaired balance, and diseases of the respiratory system, eyes, and skin. All of these suppress the immune system, rendering the individual susceptible to long-term chronic illness.

Environmental estrogens, or xenoestrogens, are a particularly insidious toxin. These foreign compounds that mimic the effects of estrogen in the body have been linked to disruption of the endocrine system and severe breakdown of the integrity of the digestive system. Many different types of synthetic chemicals can have estrogenic effects, particularly herbicides, pesticides, and industrial by-products from the manufacture of plastics and paper, as well as from the incineration of hazardous wastes.

Each year an estimated 2,000 new synthetic chemicals enter the world market, swelling the planetary total to well over 100,000. All of these are completely foreign and potentially harmful to the function of the digestive system and endocrine glands. The endocrine glands, including the testicles, ovaries, pancreas, adrenals, thyroid, parathyroid, and pituitary, are central to the regulation and normalization of all the body's complex, interconnected systems, from metabolism and heat production to reproduction. Evidence is accumulating that environmental estrogens, even at very low concentrations and limited exposure, cause hormone havoc—resulting in autoimmune diseases, clinical depression, and reproductive system disorders, among others.

Though we tend to think of inhaling or ingesting toxins, they can also enter the body in other ways—in particular, through the skin's pores. (Those same pores, of course, also facilitate the elimination of toxic chemicals). Tap water in the United States often contains chlorine, aluminum, pesticides, lead, copper, and other toxic substances. Approximately 70% of the toxins from tap water enter the body through the skin; the remaining 30% of the toxins enter via ingestion.[7]

Chemicals found in dry-cleaning fluids (trichloroethylene), paint solvents (toluene), municipal water supplies (phenol and chlorine), carpets and flooring (formaldehyde), and some imported produce (pesticide residues) are also potentially harmful, depending on your level of susceptibility. Studies have proven that these chemicals can interfere with proper nerve and muscle function, cause skeletal and muscular changes, and alter mental functioning.[8]

Harmful Metals and Chemicals

Conventional dental amalgams or "silver" fillings are actually made of tin, copper, silver, nickel, zinc, and the toxic metal mercury. These fillings disintegrate over time, and in some instances, have been shown to release these metals into the body, affecting the bones and the central nervous system and brain. Evidence now shows that mercury amalgam fillings are the major source of mercury exposure for the general public, at rates six times higher than those found in fish and seafood.[9] One of the symptoms of mercury toxicity is disturbed sleep.

Copper-lined pipes in plumbing systems can be another source of toxicity. A greenish brown ring in the tub, sink, or toilet can indicate that your water is contaminated with copper, which is toxic at high levels. According to Paul C. Eck, Ph.D., and Larry Wilson, MS, of the Eck Institute of Applied Nutrition and Bioenergetics, many of the most prevalent metabolic dysfunctions of our time are in some way related to a copper imbalance and/ or copper toxicity. Copper toxicity can cause liver problems, adrenal fatigue, allergies, and osteoarthritis.[10] Other sources of copper include birth control pills, intrauterine devices, fungicides, and pesticides, all of which contain copper as a main ingredient. A thorough analysis from a health-care practitioner, including assessment for nutritional status and heavy toxicity, can determine whether copper detoxification or supplementation is needed.

Symptom Analysis of Patients Who Eliminated Mercury-Containing Dental Fillings

The following represents a summary of 1,569 patients in six different studies evaluating the health effects of replacing mercury-containing dental fillings with nonmercury fillings. The data was derived from 762 Patient Adverse Reaction Reports submitted to the Food and Drug Administration by patients and 807 patient reports from Sweden, Denmark, Canada, and the United States.[11]

% of Total Reporting	Symptom	Number Reporting	Number Improved or Cured	% Cured or Improved
14	Allergy	221	196	89
5	Anxiety	86	80	93
5	Bad temper	81	68	84
6	Bloating	88	70	80
6	Blood pressure problems	99	53	54
5	Chest pains	79	69	87
22	Depression	347	315	91
22	Dizziness	343	301	88
45	Fatigue	705	603	86
8	Gum problems	129	121	94
34	Headaches	531	460	87
12	Insomnia	187	146	78
15	Intestinal problems	231	192	83
10	Irregular heartbeat	159	139	87
8	Irritability	132	119	90
17	Lack of concentration	270	216	80
6	Lack of energy	91	88	97
17	Memory loss	265	193	73
17	Metallic taste	260	247	95
7	Multiple	113	86	76
8	Muscle tremor	126	104	82

Inner Toxins

Environmental toxins are only one layer of the toxic load that our bodies must process. Endotoxins—toxins produced within the body—are also present and are potentially dangerous if not efficiently eliminated. Endotoxins include uric and lactic acid, homocysteine, nitric oxide, intestinal toxins, and cellular debris from dead microorganisms. These are normal by-products of metabolic processes that are typically broken down by the liver and excreted from the body. But in someone with a compromised immune system, they tend to accumulate in the blood, where they burden the detoxification pathways or initiate an allergic reaction.

The Yeast Connection

Yeast is a type of single-celled fungus found throughout nature—in the soil, on vegetables and fruits, and in the human body. *Candida albicans*, commonly referred to as candida, is a very common variety of yeast frequently present in small quantities in the intestines and in a woman's vagina. It is not harmful under normal conditions (that is, when its numbers are few), but it can cause considerable damage when its colonies grow and multiply. Candida then becomes pathogenic, taking on an aggressive filamentous form. This potential for transforming from a benign organism to a pathogenic one is why William Crook, MD, describes candida as a kind of microbiological "Dr. Jekyll and Mr. Hyde." Candidiasis causes a lengthy and diverse list of allergic reactions, which makes it particularly difficult to diagnose. The symptoms can range from sleep disturbances, fatigue, and digestive difficulties to joint pains, food cravings, and emotional problems.[13] According to James Braly, MD, candida can cause a person to develop food allergies by burrowing into and damaging the intestinal lining.[14] This may cause breaches in the lining, allowing food particles to seep out of the intestines and into the bloodstream, a condition known as leaky gut syndrome.

Toxins That Can Poison the Liver

- Pesticides, herbicides, and fungicides
- Antibiotics and growth hormones used in agriculture
- Vaccinations
- Food additives and preservatives
- Prescription drugs
- Auto exhaust
- Fluoride
- Household cleaning fluids
- Mercury amalgam fillings
- Recreational drugs
- Electromagnetic fields
- X-rays
- Alcohol
- Tobacco
- Coffee
- Hydrogenated fats
- Fried foods
- Cosmetics[12]

The Parasite Connection

Parasite infections are often overlooked because they can cause a wide variety of health problems that mimic other diseases. Among the conditions that can be caused by parasites are fatigue, hypoglycemia, skin problems, sleep disorders, depression, upper respiratory tract infections, environmental illness, PMS, and gastrointestinal problems. According to Hermann Bueno, MD, an international authority on parasitic disease, parasites can neutralize the action of hormones. They do so by blocking the receptor sites where hormones attach to the cells of the target organ. This blocking at the cellular level prevents hormones from stimulating the body's organs, which, in turn, can cause a myriad of illnesses. Several of these illnesses, such as hypoglycemia (low blood sugar) and hypothyroidism (an underactive thyroid), are known to cause sleep disorders. The parasites themselves may also invade the bloodstream, causing the immune system to channel much of its energy and resources to subduing them. Such an immune response can cause widespread, allergy-like symptoms that contribute to sleep disturbances.

Toxic Overload and Its Impact on Sleep

When our bodies become overloaded with toxins and our detoxification pathways are overwhelmed, one result is disturbed sleep. While it may not seem readily apparent, the detoxifying roles of the liver and colon are important for establishing and maintaining regular, restful sleep. If either system is not working properly, the body can become dangerously toxic. One of the main causes of sleeplessness—especially sleep maintenance insomnia, in which people wake up in the middle of the night—is trouble in the liver and the gastrointestinal tract.

We treated a woman named Laurie, a professional hair colorist. She came to our clinic in desperation because of her insomnia. Laurie would wake up after 2 hours of sleep and rarely be able to fall asleep again. She also suffered from sinus infections and several skin conditions. Conventional medicine hadn't helped her insomnia, and antibiotics actually made her sinus infections and skin conditions even worse. We suspected that the coloring chemicals she worked with and the antibiotics had made her liver toxic. A functional liver detoxification profile (described below) confirmed our diagnosis. At our suggestion, Laurie took a month off from work and followed a liver detoxification program we designed for her. In addition, we taught her breathing techniques, self-hypnosis, and acupressure as stress reduction tools to help her sleep. After three weeks on this program, Laurie began to sleep through the night, and she continues to do well. She was not able to change her profession, so every month she repeats the liver detoxification. That, along with the adjustments she's made in her lifestyle, keeps her sleeping soundly.

Let's take a look at some of the main ways that toxic conditions in the body can interfere with sleep.

Heavy metal–induced reactions: Poisoning from toxic metals such as mercury, lead, copper, thallium, and arsenic can lead to insomnia, fatigue, and lethargy. Mercury (often from amalgam fillings) in particular causes a number of reactions that can disturb sleep. It interferes with the transmission of nerve impulses from the brain to the rest of the body, producing tremors, tingling sensations, and numbness. Mercury also interferes with hormone function and can deactivate minerals such as calcium and magnesium, which are important for sound sleep.[15] A recent study found that patients with dental amalgams had a significantly higher incidence of insomnia (as well as anger, depression, and anxiety) than those without amalgams, because of mercury's effects on neurotransmitters in the brain.[16]

Candida: Candida infection can directly alter sleep patterns, according to a study with animals.[17] Yeast infections can also cause food allergies to develop.

Allergies and chemical sensitivity: Overproduction of insulin, the hormone that controls blood sugar levels, is one potential effect of food allergies, and the resulting blood sugar imbalance (hypoglycemia) can potentially result in sleep problems. Chloride and fluoride in water, along with pesticides that leach out of the soil and into our food and water supply, are among the toxic chemicals people are most commonly exposed to. People who are sensitive to these chemicals can have allergic responses that include insomnia. In those who are environmentally sensitive, breathing car fumes and other toxic substances can trigger a cascade of internal biochemical events that disturb sleep.

Blood sugar imbalances: Parasites can cause hypoglycemia or low blood sugar. Nighttime hypoglycemia releases adrenaline, cortisol, and other hormones to stimulate the brain and indicate that it is time to eat. This can awaken you or prevent you from entering a deep sleep state.

Slow metabolism: If the liver is toxic, it will not be able to adequately process toxins out of the body. This may mean that caffeine, medications, and other stimulants remain the body and disrupt your sleep.

Nutrient deficiencies: It is also important to remember that exposure to environmental toxins depletes certain vitamins and minerals from the body and can lower the immune system's ability to fight off infections. "When nutrients such as the B vitamins, iron, antioxidants and specific trace minerals are depleted in the diet, the liver's ability to function effectively as a detoxification organ is impaired. This impairment causes the individual to become more vulnerable to the environment," according to nutritional medicine specialist Dr. Jeffrey Bland.[18] These nutrients are also critical for the formation of neurotransmitters and hormones necessary for sleep.

Testing Your Detoxification Capabilities

Determining how efficiently the body can detoxify itself is especially useful for those with sleep disorders. Two laboratory tests that can help are the functional liver detoxification profile and the oxidative stress profile.

Functional liver detoxification profile: If your liver is unable to adequately detoxify your body's store of toxins and waste products, this situation may contribute significantly to the emergence and continuation of a sleep disorder. Excess free radicals and by-products of incomplete metabolism resulting from poor detoxification can interfere with the movement of substances across cell membranes. The functional liver detoxification profile determines whether the enzymes needed for phase I and phase II are present and the rate at which the two phases are operating.

Oxidative stress profile: When your ability to detoxify is impaired or you are deficient in antioxidants, free radicals run unchallenged throughout your body, damaging cells. They tend to affect the immune, endocrine, and nervous systems, interrupting communication among cells and depleting key nutrients and antioxidants. This is called oxidative stress. The oxidative stress profile assesses the degree of free radical damage in the body and measures the body's levels of glutathione, an amino acid complex central to detoxification.

Diagnosing Candidiasis

Candidiasis causes systemic illnesses that produce a wide variety of symptoms. This makes candidiasis difficult to accurately diagnose, since it shares symptoms with so many other conditions. One clue that candidiasis may be an issue is if symptoms are chronic rather than acute or sudden. If specific symptoms have been previously treated without success, this is another clue suggesting candidiasis. Some physicians rely on laboratory test results to diagnose the condition. While these tests are helpful, it is important not to depend on them exclusively. For example, blood tests can be used to pinpoint candida antibodies. But since most people normally have candida organisms in their systems, the tests may show antibodies even if the person is not suffering from candidiasis. The truth is, there is no single diagnostic test for yeast overgrowth. Stephen Langer, MD, indicates that "the clincher to any diagnosis is not so much what is happening in the laboratory as what is happening in the patient."[19] The combination of an individual's complete medical history and examination, their response to treatment, and information culled from laboratory tests is the key to a correct diagnosis.

Leon Chaitow, ND, DO, describes the likely candidate for candida overgrowth as someone whose medical history includes steroid hormone medications (cortisone or corticosteroids, often prescribed for skin conditions such as rashes, eczema, or psoriasis), prolonged or repeated use of antibiotics, medications for ulcers, or oral contraceptives. Certain illnesses, such as diabetes, cancer, and AIDS, can also increase susceptibility to candida overgrowth.

"All too often more than one influence is operating," says Dr. Chaitow. "Over a few years, a patient may have had antibiotics for a variety of conditions, while using steroids as well, perhaps in the form of the contraceptive pill. If the patient also happens to be living on a diet rich in sugars, then the candida is very likely to have spread beyond its usual borders into new territory."[20]

A qualified practitioner should take a complete medical history to determine if you have a candida infection, but here are a few questions to ask yourself to see if you are at risk (the more questions that you answer yes to, the greater your risk):

- Have you taken repeated courses of antibiotics or steroids?

- Have you used birth-control pills?

- Have you had repeated fungal infections (athlete's foot, ringworm, jock itch, etc.)?

- Do you regularly have any of these symptoms: bloating, headaches, depression, fatigue, memory problems, impotence or lack of interest in sex, muscle aches with no apparent cause, or mental fogginess?

- Do you experience symptoms of premenstrual syndrome?

- Do you have cravings for sweets, products containing white flour, or alcoholic beverages?

- Do you repeatedly experience any of these health difficulties: inappropriate drowsiness, mood swings, rashes, bad breath, dry mouth, postnasal drip or nasal congestion, heartburn, urinary frequency or urgency?[21]

If you suspect you may have candidiasis, several tests can help confirm the diagnosis whether this is the case. Because some amount of candida is normal, these tests aren't always definitive, but they may shed light on your situation.

Blood tests: Blood tests can look for candida antibodies. (An antibody is a protein molecule made by white blood cells in the lymph tissue and activated by the immune system against specific foreign substances, or antigens. Antibodies, also referred to as immunoglobulins, bind to antigens as a first step in destroying it.) When candida assumes its filamentous form and spreads beyond its usual confines, the immune system responds by producing special antibodies to fight off the infection. Consequently, if a large concentration of these antibodies is found in the blood, you may be experiencing a candida outbreak. Dr. Langer notes that "if the yeast antibodies are elevated and the test is positive, the yeast infection is active and threatening."[22] However, the antibody test may be misleading, because most people normally have candida organisms in their bodies. The Anti-Candida Antibody profile, from Genova Diagnostics (see Resources) is a blood test measures the levels of antibodies (specifically, the immunoglobulins IgG and IgM) against candida. IgG levels indicate both past and ongoing infection, while IgM level may be a truer reflection of present infection.

Darkfield microscopy: The blood can also be examined visually using a darkfield microscope to detect the presence of the candida fungus. Darkfield microscopy is a way of studying living whole blood cells under a specially adapted microscope that projects the image (magnified 1,400 times) onto a video screen. A skilled physician can detect early signs of illness in the form of abnormalities in the blood known to be associated with disease. Specifically, darkfield microscopy reveals distortions of red blood cells (which indicates nutritional status), possible undesirable bacterial or fungal life-forms (like candida), and other blood ecology patterns indicative of health or illness.[23]

Stool analysis: Another test used to diagnose candidiasis is a stool analysis, which can help assess digestive function through laboratory examination of a stool sample. The Genova Diagnostics Comprehensive Digestive Stool Analysis (CDSA) can measure how much yeast is actually present in the intestines. If the stool contains abnormally large amounts of candida, this may indicate candidiasis. The CDSA can also look at levels of beneficial bacteria in the intestines as well as other digestive markers for determining candida levels.

Diagnosing a Parasite Infection

Symptoms and personal history are the first two things a physician should check with diagnosing a possible parasite infection. "I always begin with a detailed picture of the symptoms and then gather a complete history that will indicate if exposure to parasites should be factored in," says Leo Galland, MD, author of *The Four Pillars of Healing.* "Red flags are things like a recent trip out of the country, extensive use of antibiotics which weaken the immune system, or having a child in day care, where it's estimated 30% of staff are infected."

After determining whether a parasite infection may exist from a patient's symptoms and history, physicians generally confirm the diagnosis with various testing procedures. Different

Assessing Parasite Exposure

A medical history assessing the person's potential exposure to parasites is crucial to getting an accurate diagnosis. Alternative medicine practitioners typically ask patients questions along these lines to assess the likelihood of a parasite exposure:

- What is your travel history (inside and outside the United States)?
- What is the source of your drinking water? Have you ever drunk untreated water while camping?
- Do you have pets in your household, or are you in close contact with animals?
- Do you frequently eat out, particularly at ethnic restaurants, sushi bars, or salad bars?
- Do you eat raw fruits and vegetables?
- Do you eat raw or undercooked meat or fish?
- Do you work in a hospital, day care center, sanitation department, or garden, or around animals?
- Do you engage in oral or anal sex?
- Do you have some or all of these symptoms: dark circles under your eyes, distended abdomen, bluish lips, allergies, diarrhea or constipation, anemia, skin eruptions, anal itching, chronic fatigue, loss of appetite, insomnia, depression, or sugar cravings?[24]

parasites require different formulations to kill them, so an accurate diagnosis is an important step in any treatment program. A number of diagnostic tools can be useful in determining if you have parasites, including a purged stool test and mucus and blood tests.

Purged stool test: Ann Louise Gittleman, MS, recommends using a purged stool test for parasites. This method differs from standard stool analysis; the patient ingests 1½ ounces of a high-sodium solution on an empty stomach to encourage more frequent and powerful bowel movements. These induced stool samples have higher levels of mucus, which provides higher numbers of organisms. Parasites generally begin to appear after the fourth bowel movement, but sometimes it may take as many as a dozen bowel movements to dislodge them. The purged stool test may be more accurate than conventional stool analysis for diagnosing a parasite infection. The problem with a random stool sample is that parasites cling to the wall of the intestines, so they may not be present in the feces.[25]

Uni Key Health Systems (see Resources), makes a do-it-yourself purged stool test kit endorsed by Gittleman. You can do this test at home and send the sample to a parasitology laboratory for analysis. The test can detect 15 types of worms, more than a dozen types of protozoa, and yeasts like *Candida albicans*. The test results are sent to Gittleman's office and she will offer advice on treatment options.

Caution: A purged stool test is not recommended for individuals with high blood pressure, as the high-sodium solution may exacerbate their blood pressure problems. Pregnant women and those suffering from an intestinal obstruction or appendicitis also shouldn't take this test.

Blood tests: Blood tests may be useful for diagnosing some parasitic infections. Elevated levels of eosinophils, a type of white blood cell, may indicate a parasite infection. Blood tests can also measure levels of antibodies to some parasites. In addition, abnormal blood levels of some nutrients may indicate parasites. For example, low levels of iron, folic acid, and calcium may indicate the presence of giardia.[26]

success story

Correcting Candida Cures Insomnia

"IF ONLY I COULD SLEEP, I know I would be better," said Sally, a schoolteacher in her thirties who had a candida infection and chronic fatigue syndrome. She had been unable to work for the past year because of her severe tiredness. She often spent the day in bed, but barely slept at all. In addition, she suffered from bloating after eating, chronic constipation, and emotional swings. Sometimes she would force herself to exercise, but the next day she would feel worse.

During her initial visit to an alternative practitioner, Sally said that she had suffered from teenage acne. In order to cure the acne, she underwent a year of antibiotic therapy. In addition, she had a series of upper respiratory infections in her early twenties, for which she was given more antibiotics. Heavy doses of antibiotics can destroy healthy bacteria in the intestines, resulting in digestive problems and also setting the ground for candida to develop. The results of a stool test showed that had indeed occurred: Sally suffered from malabsorption of nutrients and dysbiosis, a condition in which unfriendly bacteria in the intestines predominate and produce toxic by-products that interfere with the normal elimination cycle. She also had problems with liver toxicity, and as a result, her liver was sluggish and inefficient in eliminating toxins.

Sally was placed on a yeast-free diet and given garlic and grapefruit seed extract to detoxify and rehabilitate her intestinal tract and liver. She also received various physical treatments, including acupuncture, applied kinesiology, and craniosacral work. (Applied kinesiology and craniosacral therapy are discussed in chapter 9.) After one month on the program, Sally began to sleep through the night. As her energy and strength began to return, she started on a very minimal exercise program to tone her muscles. She also received hypnotherapy for attitudinal changes, relaxation exercises to do at home, and recipes for herbal baths to help her relax before bed. After three months on the program, Sally was not only sleeping well, she was also refreshed and able to return to her teaching job.

Alternative Medicine Approach to Detoxification

A detoxification program should be tailored to the individual's specific condition, including disease state, toxic burden, and the functional capacity of their major detoxifying organs (the intestines, liver, and lymphatic system, among others). The process must progress at a rate that the body can handle without causing greater injury. During detoxification, many people experience a healing crisis, or brief worsening of symptoms, immediately followed by significant improvement. Although a healing crisis is uncomfortable, it usually indicates that toxins are being effectively removed from the body. However, a health-care professional should be alerted when symptoms worsen during detoxification to avoid complications or unintended injury. It's important to increase consumption or supplementation of antioxidants prior to any detoxification program; this can help avert or diminish a healing crisis.

Caution: Any detoxification effort should always be planned and executed under professional supervision. Alcoholics, diabetics, people with eating disorders, people recovering from substance abuse, and those who are underweight, physically weak, or have an underactive thyroid or hypoglycemic condition are urged not to detoxify without consulting a licensed healthcare professional.

In the following pages, we outline a number of detoxification strategies for cleansing the colon and liver and for eliminating parasites and yeast infections.

Colon Cleansing Programs

There are two basic approaches to colon cleansing: taking herbs and supplements and internally bathing the colon via enemas or colonic irrigation. Colon cleansing supplements can work quite well, but those with a more toxic colon might benefit from combining the two approaches.

Colon Cleansing Formulas

Increased interest in colon health has led to a surge in the development of colon cleansing formulas and supplement programs. Most of these programs utilize a cleansing supplement in addition to recommending a basic dietary program. The supplements generally contain a combination of herbs, nutrients, enzymes, and toxin absorbers designed to help remove the buildup mucoid plaque from the colon and enhance digestion and absorption of food. Many of these supplements include ingredients that also cleanse the liver, gallbladder, and lymph. It's important to note that cleansing supplements should not be confused with laxatives. The latter are not considered to be a healthy alternative. Laxatives can cause dehydration, and they only stimulate the muscular movement of the colon but do nothing to loosen and remove mucoid plaque. Laxatives may also weaken the colon by irritating and overstimulating it.

Note: It is common to have physical reactions to the colon cleansing process. These reactions may include headaches, vomiting, diarrhea, fatigue, or dizziness. For all the discomfort, this is actually a sign that the process is working and that you are eliminating toxins from your body. If these symptoms occur, you may need to temporarily cut back on your cleansing procedure.

Such a wide variety of different cleansing formulas and products are available that it can be difficult to sort out the wheat from the chaff. We list a few recommended products below, because products are always changing and improved formulas will become available, you might wish to consult with your health-care practitioner or someone knowledgeable in this field.

Ultimate Cleanse: This cleansing program from Nature's Secret (see Resources) includes two formulas: Multi-Herb and Multi-Fiber. The formulas include cleansing herbs, amino acids, antioxidants, digestive enzymes, vitamins, minerals, and five kinds of fiber. Both formulas are taken in the morning and evening, in gradually increasing dosages, for several weeks. These formulas target not only the bowel, but also the liver, lungs, skin, and lymph. At the end of the program, a person should be having two to three bowel movements every day.

Whole Body and Colon Program: Made by the Pure Body Institute (see Resources) this program uses a combination of two formulas; each uses a blend of herbs chosen for their ability to flush toxins out of the organs and old fecal matter from the intestines. The program is designed to last about 30 days. First-time users may find that three courses of the program are required for complete inner cleansing and detoxification.

Cleanse 28: Available from Arise and Shine Herbal products (see Resources), this 28-day program cleanses the entire alimentary canal, from the tongue to the stomach and all the way down to the colon. The program usually begins with the mildest phase in the first week and progresses to the most demanding level in the fourth week, but the schedule should be adjusted to the individual. All of the details are covered in a helpful guide that comes with the kit, which includes everything needed for the cleanse: an herbal laxative formula, an herbal formula for nutritional support, bentonite and psyllium for use in cleansing shakes, and a probiotic supplement to help restore healthy intestinal bacteria.

Enemas and Colonic Irrigation

Some health-care practitioners recommend using either an enema or colonic irrigation to augment a colon cleansing program. Using either of these therapies at the very beginning of any colon cleansing program may help achieve better results more quickly. An enema involves injecting water into the colon via a small plastic tube inserted into the rectum. The tube is attached to an enema bag, which is basically just a compressible sack. About 1 cup to 1 quart of warm water is generally used. The water flushes out the lower portion of the colon. Because of the body's natural evacuation reflex, the fluids injected can't remain there very long—the bowel demands to be emptied promptly.

A colonic irrigation, also called a colonic or a high enema, follows a similar procedure; however, it goes further and accomplishes more. A colonic irrigation moves water slowly through the entire length of the colon, so that the waste matter lining the walls of the intestine will soften and detach. The patient usually lies on a treatment table, and a specially designed funnel, called a speculum, is inserted into the rectum. Several gallons of water flow in and out of the colon through the speculum and the attached tubing during the irrigation. The therapist monitors the temperature and pressure of the water and also massages the abdomen. The colonic machine is self-sanitizing, featuring a built-in check valve that prevents waste water from contaminating the water source. All instruments used in the treatment are sterile and disposable, preventing any possible contamination of the patient. A single treatment can take anywhere from 20 to 45 minutes.

The number and frequency of colonics or enemas needed will vary depending on the condition of the colon and the nature of the overall cleansing program. It's not unusual to require anywhere from 6 to 18 treatments, which can be given daily or weekly. Your colon therapist should be a trained, licensed professional, though need not be a doctor.

Caution: Colonics are contraindicated for those with ulcerative colitis, diverticulitis, Crohn's disease (in the acute inflammatory stage), severe hemorrhoids, spasms of the muscles surrounding the prostate, and intestinal or rectal tumors. People in a generally weakened condition should only undergo colonics under the supervision of a medical professional.

Dietary Support for Your Colon

The foundation of any colon cleansing program must begin with a healthy diet and adequate intake of fiber and water. During a colon cleanse, your diet should be very high in fiber and fresh raw vegetables and fruits, and low in acid-forming foods that stimulate the intestines to secrete mucus (most animal products, grains, and legumes). During the cleansing period, it is preferable to completely stop eating sugar, all milk products, and all refined white flour products, such as pastas, breads, and baked goods. You should also reduce your intake of eggs, meat, chicken, most fish, nuts, seeds, and unsprouted beans and grains.

Fiber acts like a sponge, absorbing water as it goes through the stomach and the small intestine and arriving in the colon full of moisture. Diets low in fiber cause fecal material to become dry and hard to expel, whereas a diet high in fiber will greatly reduce transit time. Fiber consists of the cell walls of plants and certain indigestible food residues. There are two basic types of fiber: soluble and insoluble. Insoluble fiber is found in wheat and corn bran, whole grains, nuts, legumes, and some vegetables; it increases fecal size and weight and promotes regular bowel movements. However, insoluble fiber can also irritate the bowel, especially if it is already sensitive or inflamed. Soluble fiber, which isn't irritating to the bowel, is found in fruits and vegetables, oat bran, barley, beans, and peas. Ingesting foods containing soluble fiber stimulates bowel movements, decreases appetite, and leads to weight loss. One excellent source of soluble fiber is powdered psyllium husk. It is often used for intestinal cleansing because of its superior ability to absorb moisture, lubricate the intestines, and mop up contaminants. Other good sources of soluble fiber are flaxseed, guar gum, and apple pectin.

Caution: Increasing your intake of dietary fiber too rapidly can cause unpleasant side effects, such as gas, bloating, and even diarrhea. To avoid these unwanted side effects, increase fiber consumption gradually.

Soluble fiber requires copious amounts of water to carry it to the colon. Adults need at least 8 to 10 cups of water daily (2 to 2½ quarts), but few people drink that much. Other liquids, such as milk, coffee, tea, juice, and soda, are not substitutes for pure water. Even if you drink plenty of these other liquids, you need to consume 8 to 10 cups of purified water daily.

Liver Cleansing Program

Appropriate cleansing treatments for the liver vary depending on the extent of the toxic overload. In general, mild toxicity can be corrected by consuming ample quantities of fresh fruit, vegetables, whole grains, and a limited amount of high-quality proteins. It is important to stop eating and drinking harmful substances, such as alcohol, caffeine, and unsaturated fats. Periodic liver cleansing treatments can also help prevent an excess buildup of liver toxins. One of the hallmarks of natural medicine is attention to the condition of the internal organs, especially the liver and gallbladder. It is surprisingly easy to use herbs and nutrients to safely and effectively cleanse these organs. Many holistic practitioners, in fact, recommend such an organ cleansing on a yearly basis as a strategy for disease prevention and health maintenance.

Flushing the Liver

"Liver flushes are used to stimulate the elimination of wastes from the body, to open and cool the liver, to increase bile flow, and to improve overall liver function," says Christopher Hobbs, L.Ac., herbalist and author of *Foundations of Health*. Here are his instructions for preparing and administering a liver flush:

1. Squeeze enough fresh lemons or limes to produce 1 cup of juice. Dilute with a small amount of distilled or spring water, if desired, but the more sour, the better it will perform as a liver cleanser. Orange or

How to Administer a Coffee Enema

Here is the procedure for administering a coffee enema:

1. Add 3 tablespoons of ground organic coffee (not instant or decaffeinated) to 2 pints of distilled water. Boil for 5 minutes (uncovered) to burn off the oils; then cover, lower the heat, and simmer for an additional 15 minutes.

2. Strain and cool to body temperature. Lubricate the rectal enema tube with K-Y Jelly or another lubricant. Hang the enema bag above you but not more than 2 feet from your body; the best level is approximately 6 inches above the intestines. Lying on your right side, draw both legs close to your abdomen.

3. Insert the tube several inches into your rectum. Open the stopcock and allow fluid to run in very slowly to avoid cramping. Breathe deeply and try to relax.

Retain the solution for 12 to 15 minutes. If you have trouble retaining or taking the full amount, lower the bag; if you feel spasms, lower the bag to the floor to relieve the pressure. After about 20 seconds, slowly start raising the bag toward the original level. You can also pinch the tube to control the flow.

4. If experiencing symptoms of toxicity, such as headaches, fever, nausea, intestinal spasms, and drowsiness, you may increase the frequency of enemas. Take in 1 to 2 pints each time for these conditions.

5. Upon waking the next morning, if you experience headaches and drowsiness an additional enema is recommended that night. Eat a piece of fruit before the first coffee enema of the day to activate the upper digestive tract. Sanitize all equipment after each use.

grapefruit juice may also be used, provided they are blended with some lemon or lime juice.

2. Add the juice of 1 to 2 cloves of garlic and a small amount of ginger juice. To make ginger juice, shred a piece of raw ginger using a grater, then press the shreds with a garlic press to get juice. Alternatively, you can put a 1- to 2-inch piece of ginger root through a juicer.

3. Add 1 tablespoon of high quality, organic, extra-virgin olive oil to the juice. Blend or shake until all of the ingredients are thoroughly combined.

4. Take the drink in the morning and do not eat any food for 1 hour afterward.

5. After 1 hour has elapsed, drink 1 pint of an herbal blend that Dr. Hobbs calls "Polari Tea." To prepare Polari Tea combine the following dry herbs: fennel (1 part), flax (1 part), burdock (¼ part), fenugreek (1 part), and licorice (¼ part). Simmer 3½ tablespoons of this blend in 2½ cups water for 20 minutes, then add 1 tablespoon dried peppermint and steep for an additional 10 minutes. For convenience, several quarts of Polari Tea may be prepared in advance and refrigerated.

6. Do the flush for 10 days, discontinue for 3 days, then resume for 10 days—this is one cycle. Repeat for another cycle. Dr. Hobbs suggests during the liver flush (two full cycles) twice yearly.[27]

Coffee Enema

This therapy, easily done at home, helps to purge the liver of accumulated toxins, dead cells, and waste products. The enema is prepared by brewing organic caffeinated coffee, letting it cool to body temperature, and delivering it via an enema bag. Coffee contains chloretics, substances that increase the flow of bile from the gallbladder.[28] Early research by Max Gerson, MD, founder of the Gerson Institute and originator of Gerson Diet Therapy, established that a coffee enema is effective in stimulating the complex system of liver detoxification.[29]

Castor Oil Packs

Castor oil comes from the bean of the castor plant (*Oleum ricini*). The plant itself is quite poisonous, but the oil pressed out of the bean is safe to use, since the toxic constituents remain in the seeds. The ancient Egyptians used castor oil as a laxative and as a scalp rub to make hair grow and shine. Castor oil packs have been used for many conditions, including liver problems, constipation, and other ailments involving elimination, as well as nonmalignant ovarian fibroid cysts and headaches.[30] The oil helps to draw out toxins, release tension, and improve blood circulation, especially in the lower abdomen.

Nutritional Support for Liver Detoxification

Certain dietary recommendations will help support the liver during the detoxification process. Try to avoid fats from animal sources (meat, eggs, and dairy) and limit the overall amount of animal foods you eat. Incorporate more chlorophyll-rich foods (particularly dark leafy greens) and raw vegetables into your diet. Artichokes, asparagus, celery, radishes, and beets are all considered to have liver cleansing properties. When the liver becomes toxic,

Castor Oil Pack Instructions

1. Fold a flannel sheet into three sections to fit over your whole abdomen.

2. Cut a piece of plastic 1 to 2 inches larger than the folded flannel sheet.

3. Soak the flannel sheet in gently heated castor oil. Fold it over and squeeze until some of the liquid oozes out. Unfold.

4. Prepare the surface where you will be lying. Place a large plastic sheet and an old towel over the surface to prevent staining.

5. Lie down on the towel and place the oil-soaked flannel sheet over your abdomen. Place the fitted plastic piece over the flannel sheet. Apply a hot water bottle over the area.

6. Wrap a towel under and around your torso.

7. Rest for 1 to 2 hours.

8. Wash your body with a solution of 3 tablespoons baking soda to 1 quart water to rinse off the oil.

9. Repeat as instructed by a physician.

more water is required to help flush impurities from the liver out through the kidneys. You should drink eight large glasses of pure water daily (at least 2 quarts) to bring your liver back to health.

Certain herbs have a mild detoxifying effect on the liver. Taken regularly, these herbs can be used to prevent liver disease and maintain the health of this vital organ. Milk thistle (*Silybum marianum*) is native to Europe, where it is often prescribed to treat and protect the liver. As far back as the seventeenth century, this herb was known as "a friend to liver and blood." The active ingredient in milk thistle is silymarin, a substance that prevents inflammation and protects against the harmful effects of free radicals. It also stimulates liver cell growth and the production of bile. Milk thistle seeds can be used to make a tea or powdered seeds can be taken in capsule form. To make a tea, steep 1 teaspoon of seeds in ½ cup of water; drink 1 to 1½ cups of tea daily. For the powdered form of milk thistle, take one capsule (approximately 1 teaspoon) with water five times per day.

"Dandelion root (*Taraxacum officinale*) is regarded as one of the finest liver remedies, both as food and as medicine," according to naturopaths Michael Murray, ND, and Joseph Pizzorno, Jr., ND, authors of *A Textbook of Natural Medicine*. It has been used for centuries both for the liver and as a weight-loss aid. Its ability to stimulate the production and secretion of bile was first noted by researchers in 1875. Dandelion is also a potent diuretic, meaning it promotes the excretion of urine, which helps flush toxins from the body. A typical dose is 4 grams of dried root (available in capsule form) or 4 to 8 milliliters (ml) of dandelion extract, three times daily.

Oregon grape root (*Berberis aquifolium*) is considered a gentle stimulant for the liver and gallbladder. It helps improve the overall functioning of the liver as well as its detoxification processes. Because of its bitter taste, Oregon grape root is generally taken as a tea: mix 1 part Oregon grape root with 1 part dandelion root and ¼ part fennel seeds.

Chlorophyll is an excellent liver remedy. Chlorella (a food algae) is one of the best sources of chlorophyll. It can heal liver toxicity and supply needed minerals to this hardworking organ. It can also soothe bowel tissue, stimulate bowel function, and reduce candida overgrowth. A typical dose is 100 mg of chlorella daily. Other sources of chlorophyll are barley juice, wheatgrass juice, and spirulina (available at most health food stores).

Eliminating Yeast

As noted above, chlorophyll can be effective against candida. Several other nutritional supplements have also been shown to be effective in treating candidiasis. In addition, probiotic supplements can help resolve yeast overgrowth and prevent it from occurring in the future, and Ayurvedic medicine is also quite effective.

Anti-Candida Supplements

Garlic, a well-known folk remedy, is now formulated as an odorless extract. Allicin, the active ingredient in garlic, has been found to be more potent than many other antifungal agents; a typical recommended dose is 4 mg daily (equal to about one clove of fresh garlic). As an alternative to garlic extract, you can also take either liquid garlic (available at health food stores) or fresh garlic cloves.

Caprylic acid, a naturally occurring fatty acid found in coconut oil, has been shown to be an effective antifungal agent. In one study, patients taking 3.6 grams of caprylic acid daily for two weeks completely eliminated their candida overgrowth. A typical dose is 1 to 2 grams daily, taken with meals. Since caprylic acid is readily absorbed into the system, it should be taken in an enteric-coated or sustained-release form so that it is absorbed in the small intestine rather than the stomach. Other fatty acids, derived from olives (oleic acid) and castor beans, have also been found useful for treating candidiasis.

Herbs are often used by alternative medicine practitioners to kill harmful yeasts and enhance immune function. They can be taken in teas, dried in capsules or tablets, or in suppository form. Herbs effective against candida include oregano, thyme, peppermint, and rosemary. Barberry (*Berberis vulgaris*) and Oregon grape (*Berberis aquifolium*) can also be helpful. These herbs contain berberine, a natural antibiotic that acts against candida overgrowth, normalizes intestinal flora, helps digestive problems, has antidiarrheal properties, and stimulates the immune system by increasing blood supply to the spleen. They may be taken three times daily as a tea (2 to 4 grams), tincture (6 to 12 ml), fluid extract (2 to 4 ml), or powdered solid (250 to 500 mg).

Caution: Berberine-containing plants are generally nontoxic at recommended dosages, but high doses can interfere with the metabolism of B vitamins. They are not recommended for use by pregnant women.

Goldenseal (*Hydrastis canadensis*) is also effective. The preferred form is an extract of the root standardized to 5% or more of its active ingredient (hydrastine), at a dose of 250 mg twice daily. Pau d'arco, another herb that has long been used to treat infections and intestinal complaints, is reportedly also an analgesic, antiviral, diuretic, and fungicide. This South American

Beneficial Flora

Friendly bacteria refers to beneficial microbes inhabiting the human gastrointestinal tract, where they are essential for proper nutrient assimilation. The human body contains an estimated several trillion beneficial bacteria comprising over 400 species, all necessary for health. Among the more well-known of these are *Lactobacillus acidophilus* and *Bifidobacterium bifidum*. Overly acidic bodily conditions, chronic constipation or diarrhea, dietary imbalances, consumption of highly processed foods, and the excessive use of antibiotics or hormonal drugs can interfere with the function of these helpful microbes and even reduce their numbers, setting up conditions for illness.

herb, also known as taheebo, is often prepared as a tea. Other antifungal and antibacterial herbs used to treat candidiasis include German chamomile, ginger, cinnamon, gentian, and licorice. (Because certain compounds in licorice can be toxic at high doses, it's best to take deglycyrrhizinated licorice supplements).

Probiotics

A healthy growth of "friendly" bacteria in the intestines—particularly *Lactobacillus acidophilus* and *Bifidobacterium bifidum*—is the best defense against yeast infections. Cabbage is one of the best food sources of friendly bacteria; eat it raw or juice it daily. Other foods that can help revitalize the colon and encourage the growth of normal bacteria include rice, chicory, onions, garlic, asparagus, and bananas. Cultured products such as yogurt and kefir (a fermented milk drink) are excellent sources of probiotics. Another way to repopulate the intestines with friendly bacteria is to take a probiotic supplement, particularly one containing *L. acidophilus* and *B. bifidum*.

Ayurvedic Medicine

In this ancient healing tradition, which originated in India, candidiasis is considered to be a condition caused by *ama*, the improper digestion of foods, according to Ayurvedic practitioner Virender Sodhi, MD, ND. As do other alternative physicians, Dr. Sodhi attributes this malfunction, and thus candidiasis, to environmental stress, society's addiction to sugar in the diet, and widespread use of antibiotics, birth-control pills, and hormones. "Ayurvedic medicine believes that these stresses on the system cause carbohydrates to be digested improperly," he says. "Furthermore, the immune system in the gut becomes worn down."

To address the candida overgrowth and bolster immunity, Dr. Sodhi uses grapefruit seed oil and tannic acid, which act as antifungals and antibiotics, along with *L. acidophilus* to help restore the balance of friendly bacteria in the intestines. Long pepper, ginger, cayenne, and the Ayurvedic herbs trikatu and neem are taken 30 minutes before meals to increase immune and digestive functions. Dr. Sodhi further recommends that patients cleanse toxins from their systems using the *panchakarma* program, which involves herbs and dietary modification (see "Ayurvedic Detoxification," opposite page). With Dr. Sodhi's approach, candidiasis can usually be eliminated in four to six months.

Eradicating Parasites

Like other toxins, parasites can make it harder for the liver, kidneys, and intestines to detoxify and eliminate wastes from the body. If testing reveals that you have a parasitic infection, you may want to consider taking the following practical steps to rid your system of parasites.

Caution: Before beginning any parasite elimination program, consult a qualified health-care professional. This is especially important if you are pregnant.

1. *Cleanse the intestines.* Parasites tend to embed themselves in the intestinal wall, but over the course of several weeks you can flush them out by using some of these natural substances (preferably in combination): psyllium husks, agar, citrus pectin, papaya extract, pumpkin seeds, flaxseeds, comfrey root, beet root, and bentonite clay (take bentonite only in combination with another substance, such as psyllium). You might also take extra vitamin C (at least 2 grams daily, but higher amounts up to individual bowel tolerance are more useful) to help flush out your intestines. Note, however, that vitamin C taken at the same time as wormwood (below) renders wormwood ineffective.

2. *Do an enema.* Use up to 2 quarts of water, to which you may add black walnut tincture or extract (4 teaspoons per quart), vinegar (2 tablespoons per quart of water), or blackstrap molasses (1 tablespoon per quart of water), or use coffee brewed from organically grown beans (2 tablespoons of grounds per quart of water). For a garlic enema, simmer 3 cloves of crushed garlic in 2 quarts of water). Use filtered or distilled water for the enema; further sterilize it by boiling or ozonating it for 10 to 15 minutes before use, including before using it to prepare the coffee.

3. *Prepare your system.* It is prudent to give your gallbladder and liver a week to prepare for the parasite program. To flush the gallbladder of its toxins, take lime juice in warm water or Swedish Bitters before each

Ayurvedic Detoxification

Practiced in India for the past 5,000 years, Ayurvedic medicine is a comprehensive system of medicine that combines natural therapies with a highly personalized approach to maintaining health. Ayurveda describes three metabolic, constitutional, and body types (*doshas*) based on combinations of the five basic elements of nature in combination. These are *vata* (air and ether, rooted in intestines), *pitta* (fire and water, rooted in the stomach), and *kapha* (water and earth, rooted in the lungs).

An Ayurvedic procedure called *panchakarma* can be used for sleeping disorders where the body is in a toxic state and in need of cleaning. *Panchakarma* is often very effective in pacifying and calming the body because it assists in cleansing the intestines, and, by transference, the mind, leading to restful sleep.

Panchakarma actually is a series of treatments that includes massage with medicated herbs (*abhyanga*) and *shirodhara*, a treatment involving dripping oil on the forehead. *Panchakarma* can be done five to seven days in a row, 2 or more hours a day, or every other day. In addition to the massage and warm oil drip, it can include the following: *nasya*, a nasal administration of herbs in which drops of medicated oils are placed in the sinuses; *basti*, herbalized oil enemas that are injected into the colon with a catheter and syringe; *swedna*, a steam treatment with herbs designed to open up and detoxify the body through sweating; and *virechana*, a purgation.

meal. Eliminate all sugars—both refined and natural, meat, and dairy products during the parasite program; even better, start cutting back on them during this preparatory week. Take barberry bark capsules, dandelion root, or other herbs to help cleanse the liver. The amount depends on your state of health and the strength or composition of the specific product used.

4. **Use an herbal cleanout formula.** Naturopathic physician Hulda Regehr Clark, ND, Ph.D., recommends using a blend of three herbs to flush the parasites out of your system: black walnut hull tincture, worm-wood capsules, and freshly ground cloves (to kill the parasites' eggs). (Her protocol is very specific; see Resources.)

Antiparasite Dietary and Herbal Support

If you suspect a parasitic infection, you should eliminate all uncooked foods from your diet and cook all meats until well-done. Also, soak all vegetables—both organic and inorganic—in salted water (1 tablespoon per 5 cups) for a minimum of 30 minutes before cooking. It is also advisable to eliminate coffee, all sugars including fruits and honey, and all milk and dairy products with the possible exception of raw goat's milk. Raw goat's milk contains IgA and IgG immunoglobulins, types of antibodies that help strengthen the immune system, and which may be helpful in the treatment of parasites.

Gittleman says that the best diet for a parasite infection is one that "supports the host and starves the parasite." Specifically, she recommends against eating any sugar, white flour, or processed foods (such as prepack-aged snack foods). Once inside the body, these foods provide ideal condi-tions for parasites to breed. She has found that a diet composed of 25% fat, 25% protein, and 50% complex carbohydrates is best for people with par-asite infections. Gittleman also advises limiting your intake of raw fruits and vegetables; instead, cook both fruits and vegetables. Sufficient levels of vitamin A are particularly important for preventing parasites, as this vita-min seems to increase resistance to penetration by larvae. Good dietary sources of vitamin A include salad greens and properly cooked carrots, sweet potatoes, and squash. A combination formula of digestive enzymes, taken between meals, may also be helpful for eliminating parasite larvae or eggs in the intestines.

Certain foods are antiparasitic, according to Gittleman, and you should incorporate more of these foods into your diet. These include pineapple and papaya, either as fresh juice or in supplement form, eaten in combination with pepsin (a stomach enzyme) and betaine hydrochloric acid (a supple-ment form of stomach acid). Avoid all meats and dairy products for at least one week at the beginning of therapy. You can also use pomegranate juice (four 8-ounce glasses daily), papaya seeds, fresh figs, finely ground pumpkin seeds (¼ cup to ½ cup daily), or two cloves of raw garlic daily. Because pomegranate juice can irritate the intestines, you should not drink it for more than four to five days at a time. Other antiparasitic foods include onions, kelp, blackberries, raw cabbage, and ground almonds.[31]

Herbal remedies have been used effectively for centuries for the treatment of parasitic infections. These remedies can also help prevent a parasitic infection when water or food conditions are questionable. Some practitioners advise continuing any treatment regimen until at least two parasite tests, performed one month apart on purged stool specimens, are negative. Here are a few of the most effective antiparasitic herbs:

- **Citrus seed extract.** Citrus seed extract is highly active against protozoa, bacteria, and yeast, and has long been used in the treatment of parasitic infections. It is not absorbed into the body's tissues, is nontoxic and generally hypoallergenic, and can be administered for up to several months, a length of time which may be required to eliminate giardia and the candidiasis that often accompanies it.

- **Artemisia annua.** This is an herbal remedy of Chinese origin. Its antiprotozoal activity is especially effective against giardia, but some caution is advisable—it can initially cause a worsening of symptoms, allergic reactions, and some intestinal irritation. *Artemisia annua* is sometimes prescribed along with citrus seed extract. It may also be used with other herbs known for to have antiparasitic activity and can also be used in conjunction with conventional drug therapy.

- **Artemisia absinthium.** This herb, which is similar to *Artemisia annua*, is one of the oldest European medicinal plants. Known as wormwood, it was highly prized by Hippocrates. When taken alone, it can be toxic, though, and therefore should be used in combination with other herbs to nullify its toxicity.

Caution: Before using any of the herbal remedies listed here, it is important that you first consult with a health-care professional who has been properly trained in their use. *Artemisia annua* should not be used during pregnancy. Garlic, if taken in too high a dose, may cause intestinal irritation.

Traditional Chinese Medicine
In traditional Chinese medicine, herbs are the primary treatment for parasites; the type used depends on the location of the parasites in the body, according to Maoshing Ni, DOM, Ph.D., L.Ac., cofounder of the Yo San University

How Chinese Medicine Views Insomnia

In conventional Western medicine, two insomniacs who come to a physician with the same complaint—restless sleep—in all likelihood would leave the physician's office with the same prescription for the same sleeping pills. In traditional Chinese medicine, however, the practitioner might look at one person and determine the restless sleep to be caused by a deficiency of heart yin energy, for example. For that person, the practitioner would prescribe heart- and yin-strengthening herbs and acupuncture treatment of heart- and yin-tonifying points, as well as lifestyle changes such as improved diet, exercises, and meditation. For the other person, the practitioner might see the restless sleep as being caused by an excess in liver yang energy, and thus would prescribe herbs and acupuncture treatments to calm the liver, as well as lifestyle changes tailored to reduce stress.

While that type of customized diagnosis may be complex, the basic premise of Chinese medicine is very simple. The underlying cause of an illness or condition is always the same: an imbalance in the person's energy field. It's the practitioner's job to determine what part of the energy field is out of balance and which organ systems are affected. The concept of the human being as an energy field is essential to an understanding of how Chinese medicine works.

Once a Chinese medicine practitioner has determined where a person's energy is out of balance, they can suggest acupuncture treatments. Along with herbal therapies, acupuncture is one of the primary tools Chinese medicine practitioners have been using for more than 5,000 years. The procedure involves the insertion of slender, sterilized, solid needles into the body at specific points on 12 different energy pathways called meridians or channels. The channels are associated with organ systems of the body, such as the kidney channel, liver channel, or stomach channel. Chinese scientists have found that acupuncture can affect blood sugar and cholesterol levels, gastrointestinal function, and immune system activity, and American researchers have found evidence that acupuncture releases the body's own anti-inflammatory agents, as well as sending pain-blocking signals to the spinal cord.

Specific treatments for insomnia will vary greatly, depending on both the patient and the practitioner. The acupuncturist will want to know, for example, if you have trouble falling asleep or staying asleep. People who can't fall asleep may be deficient in blood energy, whereas those who wake up during the night could be deficient in yin energy. Another common question is what time you wake up during the night. Chinese medicine recognizes an organ time clock—2-hour time periods in which certain organ systems are more active. If you always wake up at 1:30 A.M., for example, you're in liver time (1 A.M. to 3 A.M.), which could mean you have an imbalance in your liver channel.

Acupuncturist Giovanni Maciocia, a noted author of several textbooks on Chinese medicine, says there are at least four main excess, or full, patterns of insomnia and at least five main deficient, or empty, patterns. In the excess patterns, one of the body's energy systems, such as liver fire (fire is a yang energy) or heart fire, is overactive. In the deficient patterns, one or more of the energy systems, such as spleen, blood, kidney, heart, or liver yin, is weak and not doing its job. Each of those nine main patterns requires a different set of acupuncture points and a different herbal formula.[32]

Acupuncturist Dr. Roger Jahnke, author of The Healer Within, tends to look at insomnia as mainly a deficiency of yin—whether in the kidneys, the liver, or the heart. Most of the insomnia cases Dr. Jahnke sees are from yin deficiencies, although he does see some people with insomnia caused by digestive problems.

of Traditional Chinese Medicine. For intestinal parasites, purgative herbs are usually used. Pumpkin and quisqualis seeds are two common remedies. The pumpkin seeds are eaten raw, while the quisqualis seeds are usually roasted. Both are taken every morning on an empty stomach, approximately 10 to 12 seeds of each, for about two weeks. "Quisqualis and pumpkin seeds are mild and safe enough for adults and children to take daily as a preventative measure as well," says Dr. Ni.

Meliae seeds are much stronger than either pumpkin or quisqualis and should only be taken in more severe cases. The meliae seeds paralyze the parasites for approximately 8 hours, allowing the body to eliminate them through the bowels. Betel nut is another tropical treatment for intestinal parasites. The nut is chewed raw like chewing tobacco. "It can give a certain sense of euphoria, too, because it is slightly toxic," says Dr. Ni. "This is negligible, but some people might get diarrhea." Depending on the type of parasite, they may be able to get through the intestinal walls and into the bloodstream. "In situations like this you have to use some very strong antibiotic-like herbs," says Dr. Ni, "such as goldenseal and coptidis which are antiparasitic as well." While eliminating the parasites with herbs, Dr. Ni also strengthens the immune system in order to get at the underlying cause of the parasitic infestation. He reports that nutrition and herbs such as ginseng, ligustri berries, and schisandra berries can accomplish this. He has good success with his three-month treatment program addressing both components.

five

Step 3: Reset Your Body Clock

The body clock and circadian rhythms primarily determine our sleep-wake patterns. When these functions are thrown off course—by factors both in and out of our control—sleep problems ensue. Sleep onset insomnia, advanced and delayed sleep phase syndromes, and even REM behavior disorder can be caused by disrupted circadian rhythms and melatonin imbalances. While not a sleep problem per se, seasonal affective disorder (SAD), or the "winter blues," is also an outgrowth of a confused body clock.

Trappings of our modern lives generally cause sleep-wake rhythm disruptions. Both shift work and traveling across time zones set up the body for sleep problems. Other factors, including inadequate exposure to light, improper diet, pharmaceutical drugs, electromagnetic fields, and stress, can impair the pineal gland's ability to produce the sleep-inducing hormone melatonin, drastically altering sleep patterns.

Sleep problems due to disrupted circadian rhythms are reversible if you take steps to reset your body clock to follow a new schedule. Light therapy, chronotherapy, and magnet therapy are proven alternative therapies for disruption of circadian rhythms. Melatonin supplements, dietary changes, exercise, stress management, and good sleep hygiene can also alleviate many sleep disorders. While avoidance of factors that disturb the body clock is the best way to prevent ongoing sleep problems, even shift workers and frequent flyers can use these therapies to their advantage.

Free-Running and Entrained Circadian Rhythms

Alternative Therapies to Reset Your Body Clock

- Lifestyle modifications
- Light therapy
- Chronotherapy
- Magnet therapy
- Melatonin supplementation

To comprehend how disruptions in circadian rhythms can cause sleep disorders, it's important to understand how the body clock keeps time. As described in chapter 1, a bundle of nerves in the hypothalamus called the suprachiasmatic nucleus (SCN) measures the passage of time. The SCN also transmits light signals from the optic nerves to various organs of the nervous system, including the pineal gland. Light signals suppress the pineal gland's secretion of the sleep-inducing hormone melatonin into the bloodstream; darkness activates the process. Melatonin receptors have been found on SCN cells, leading researchers to speculate that the SCN's functions are to some degree regulated by melatonin. Together, melatonin and the SCN appear to guide our circadian rhythms, natural cycles governing fluctuations in body temperature, hormone release, and sleep-wake patterns (see "The Circadian Rhythms of the Body," page 104).

Circadian means "around a day," and human circadian rhythms do indeed repeat approximately every 24 hours. But our body clocks do not naturally follow the sun's 24-hour day. Several experiments have been conducted to test the innate length of circadian rhythms. In these tests, the lab environments (ranging from caves in the Swiss Alps to a hospital in the Bronx) were strictly controlled to eradicate all time cues (zeitgebers, meaning "time-givers" in German): the sun's rising and setting, clocks, TVs and radios, the male five o'clock shadow, and, in some studies, electromagnetic fields. Researchers discovered that when freed from the constraints of 24-hour time cues, the human biological clock runs according to a 25-hour day. At the beginning of the Bronx test, subjects were sent to bed at 11 P.M. and awakened around 8 A.M. for 20 days. At the end of this time, the subjects were allowed to decide their own sleeping schedules. At first the subjects voluntarily went to sleep at 11 P.M. and arose at 8 A.M., but as the days progressed, they started sleeping 1 hour later each subsequent night, awakening 1 hour later each morning (midnight and 9 A.M.; 1 A.M. and 10 A.M., and so on). Weeks into the test, subjects were falling asleep at 4 P.M. and waking up at midnight, ready for breakfast.[1]

These findings proved that the free-running biological clock, without time cues, measures 25-hour days and that the sleep-wake circadian rhythms likewise follow 25-hour cycles. A gene discovered in 1997, popularly called the "clock gene," may be responsible for the free-running instinct.

The Circadian Rhythms of the Body

Sleep-wake patterns are not the only type of bodily function recurring according to circadian rhythms. Body temperature and hormone levels also fluctuate throughout the day and, for the most part, correspond directly or indirectly to sleep-wake patterns. For instance, during the daytime wakeful period, blood levels of the hormone melatonin are low while body temperature is high; during sleep phases, melatonin is high—spiking at around 3 A.M. then declining rapidly—and body temperature is low, down approximately 1.5°F from daytime peak levels. Human growth hormone levels are very low during the waking hours, but rise during sleep, usually spiking in the first 2 hours. It's important to note that reducing body temperature will not induce secretion of melatonin or sleep.[2] On the contrary, raising the body temperature is correlated with an increase in melatonin and may provide therapeutic benefits for people with sleep problems (see "Take a Hot Bath for a Good Night's Sleep," page 115).

Cortisol, a naturally occurring adrenal hormone, has a different cycle (it's also produced during the stress response). Levels of this hormone start off very high in the morning waking hours and decline over the course of the day, reaching a low midway through sleep; the level then spikes around 5 A.M. or approximately 1 hour before awakening. When stress disrupts cortisol's circadian rhythms, especially at night, cortisol levels become elevated when they are normally low. This shift can have profound effects on sleep-wake patterns and potentially cause sleep disturbances.

It's believed that this genetic predisposition makes us more adaptable to seasonal changes (although some of us do suffer from physiological and psychological problems during seasonal changes—see "Beating the Winter Blues," page 123).

These and other studies elucidate the power and function of zeitgebers, showing how we use light and other environmental cues to live and sleep by the sun's 24-hour cycle. At the same time, our circadian adaptability makes us extremely susceptible to zeitgebers. Normally time and light cues reset, or entrain, our body clocks to run by the sun's 24-hour cycle. In fact, our body clocks and circadian rhythms can easily adjust within a 4-hour range, allowing us to perform normally on 23-hour or 27-hour schedules.

However, when we change work schedules drastically, travel across time zones, or are chronically exposed to electromagnetic fields, inadequate light, and other disruptions, our normal temporal cues vanish or become erratic, confusing the body clock. Called internal desynchronization, this situation ultimately disrupts the timing and duration of melatonin secretion, leading to sleep-wake rhythm disturbances such as insomnia, advanced or delayed sleep phase syndromes, and REM behavior disorders, as well as seasonal affective disorder.

Factors That Disrupt Sleep-Wake Rhythms

As discussed above, traveling across time zones and shift work can disrupt circadian sleep-wake rhythms, but so can other factors that alter levels of melatonin. Abnormal exposure to light—whether too little in the day or too much at night—is a predominant cause of melatonin imbalances. Extremely low frequency electromagnetic fields, emotional stress, some medications, and poor diet can also impair melatonin secretion.

Traveling across Time Zones

If you've ever traveled by plane across time zones—for instance, from San Francisco to New York or from New York to Paris—more than likely you've experienced jet lag. This condition is characterized by fatigue, irritability, difficulty in concentration, and an inability to sleep at the local bedtime. Flying across time zones can drastically disorient your circadian rhythms because the temporal cues (light and dark) of the destination are different from those you're synchronized with.

Jet lag only occurs following airplane travel, and only when traveling east-west or west-east. Were you to walk or even drive from San Francisco to New York, the transit time would be slow enough for you to gradually adjust to new time zones and zeitgebers. And should you fly from New York to Lima, Peru, you may be uncomfortable or restless during the long flight, but your sleep rhythms would be unaffected because you'd remain in the same time zone.

West-east travel affects sleep more adversely than east-west, and the more time zones you cross traveling to the east, the more difficult it will be to adjust to the local time and sleep patterns. Suppose you leave San Francisco at 7 A.M. on a nonstop flight bound for New York. If the flight takes approximately 5 hours, you'll land at noon San Francisco time, which is 3 P.M. in New York. During the course of the day, you will likely feel more alert than New Yorkers, but by bedtime, say 10 P.M., your body clock will think it's 7 P.M. Try as you may, you will likely have a difficult time falling asleep this early in your sleep-wake cycle—even though darkness has fallen and other environmental cues indicate it's bedtime. You will probably also have trouble awakening the next morning at your usual time, say 7 A.M., even though it's light outside, as it will feel like 4 A.M.—the time when your circadian rhythms are at their deepest sleep phase.

Research shows that, without intervention, it takes a little less than a day for each time zone crossed to entrain your body clock to the new time schedule.[3] Therefore, it will take approximately two days to adapt to New York time. Flying from New York to Paris, a 10-hour flight, will entail crossing five time zones. Thus, your circadian rhythms will act as if it's 5 P.M. when it's 10 P.M. local time, and it will take about four days before you feel comfortable with the Parisian time and sleep patterns. Meanwhile, your mental function will be impaired due to sleep deprivation. As you can imagine, safety is a special concern for airline pilots and others adversely affected by jet lag.

East-west travel usually presents fewer disruptions to sleep-wake patterns. If you leave from New York at 7 A.M. local time on a 5-hour nonstop flight, you'll arrive at San Francisco at noon New York time, which is 9 A.M. in San Francisco. You may feel more tired that night and go to bed earlier than your San Francisco counterparts, and awaken earlier the next morning, but in general your sleep will be only minimally and briefly affected because synchronizing to the new time and light cues won't require advancing your circadian rhythms. As the human internal clock is genetically predisposed to 25-hour days, a delayed phase shift is easier to accommodate than an abbreviation.

Shift Work

Approximately 25 million Americans work regular or rotating hours outside the nine-to-five daytime schedule.[4] These include hospital employees, industrial plant workers, and security personnel. As our society demands more around-the-clock services, businesses such as financial institutions, photocopy shops, supermarkets, and communications companies have also established around-the-clock shifts. Sleep researchers, ironically, also are among this population. While nonstop work increases productivity and provides convenience for the rest of us, shift work is a burden for circadian rhythms. Studies indicate that shift workers are about three times more likely to suffer from sleep-wake disturbances than daytime workers are.[5] Sleep deprivation can have numerous detrimental consequences to personal health and safety, including tension, fatigue, emotional problems, and poor mental performance; one result is that about 20% of shift workers report having an auto accident or a near miss each year. Shift work is associated with increases in gastrointestinal problems, cardiovascular disease, and infertility, as well as a higher incidence of smoking and overuse of other stimulants.[6]

In the 1880s, the invention of the lightbulb allowed factories to operate 24 hours a day, seven days a week. Until that time, the duration of daylight determined work schedules: approximately 14 hours during the summer and 11 during the winter. But with the advent of artificial light, industrial plants imposed shift work, in which two or three sets of workers rotate around the clock, keeping production at a consistent pace. Today, three shifts are common: day (8 A.M. to 5 P.M.), swing (4 P.M. to 1 A.M.), and graveyard (midnight to 9 A.M.). Some shift workers maintain a regular schedule, while others may rotate, alternating, for example, between several days or weeks of day shift to a period of evening shift then a period of graveyard shift, with days off interspersed.

The fundamental problem with shift work is that it requires the individual to disregard circadian rhythms and temporal cues. Whereas in cases of jet lag, travelers can ultimately reset their body clocks to synchronize with the local sunrise and sunset, night- and rotating-shift workers are expected to function contrary to natural cycles. For instance, millions of Americans are at work between 3 A.M. and 5 A.M. This is the sleepiest time for most people, when melatonin levels are high, muscles are relaxed, and body temperature is low. This is also the time of night when many accidents occur on the job.

When night workers go home in the morning, sunlight suppresses melatonin production and the circadian rhythms enter the alert phase. Daytime sleep is therefore often lighter and less restorative than nighttime sleep, and as a result, many night-shift workers suffer from sleep onset and sleep maintenance insomnia. And of course there's more activity and noise in the daytime, which can further disrupt sleep. In fact, most night workers get 2 to 3 less hours of sleep than the average person—and the average person is already sleep deprived![7]

Rotating-shift workers may experience even more frequent and severe disruption of sleep and associated health problems. The most debilitating rotation schedules are those that run counterclockwise; for example, night then evening then day, with days off in between. These schedules require the person to constantly advance their sleep-wake phases. Since we innately run on a longer, 25-hour time schedule, advancing phases by up to 8 hours during any given week causes serious circadian disturbances. Animal studies have found that weekly drastic (12-hour) changes in light-dark patterns (the equivalent of weekly rotating day and night shifts) reduces life span by 11%.[8] Human studies indicate that counterclockwise shift rotation increases the likelihood of coronary heart disease. Less disruptive rotation schedules are those that run clockwise (day then evening then night).

All of these problems are further exacerbated by the fact that on weekends or days off, shift workers tend to resynchronize their sleep-wake rhythms with zeitgebers, sleeping at night and rising in the morning. Resuming shift schedules often intensifies the sleep-wake disturbances.

Light—Too Little or Too Much

As we've seen in the case of night-shift workers, light plays a crucial role in determining our sleep-wake patterns. This is due to the interplay between ambient light and the pineal gland. In chapter 1, we described how the suprachiasmatic nucleus—the circadian pacemaker in the hypothalamus—sends outside light signals to the pineal gland, the primary producer of the hormone melatonin (the gastrointestinal system also secretes some melatonin). The pineal gland needs darkness to produce melatonin, because light deactivates certain enzymes necessary for converting serotonin into melatonin.[9] Several studies have shown that melatonin production significantly drops or is completely inhibited by inadequate exposure to natural bright light during

Testing for Melatonin Levels

In diagnosing and reviewing your sleep problems, your doctor may test for melatonin levels at different times of the day. This is usually done by analyzing urine or blood samples with a radioimmunoassay (RIA). This test measures the minute amounts of melatonin excreted in the urine or circulating in the blood. Melatonin is present in the body in picograms, or trillionths of a gram. Since each person's levels of melatonin vary, it's difficult to assess "normal" values. However, if your melatonin levels are significantly lower than expected during sleep, this can indicate that various lifestyle or dietary factors may be impairing the pineal gland's ability to produce melatonin. In this case, your doctor may recommend melatonin supplementation or other therapies.

the day and also by excessive exposure to artificial bright light at night. Both factors can cause sleep onset insomnia as well as seasonal affective disorder.

Americans spend the vast majority of their time indoors, usually in windowless cubicles and energy-efficient homes under low-intensity artificial lights. A 1994 study found that middle-class, middle-aged adults in San Diego, California, spent 4% of their time outdoors—most of that time in their cars.[10] It's likely that people who live in less sunny climates spend more time indoors. Night-shift workers are worse off, spending only 2.6% of their time outdoors.[11] It's estimated that the majority of people are exposed to light levels of less than 100 lux (a measurement of light intensity) for much of the day[12] (100 lux is the amount of light that would enter your eyes if you were looking at a 100-watt bulb from a distance of 5 feet in an otherwise dark room). Ordinary fluorescent lights may emit 400 lux, while a room lit by sunlight can be up to 3,000 lux. On a clear summer day, the light outside can be up to 100,000 lux, and even on gloomy, stormy days, outdoor light is rarely below 500 lux.[13]

The lack of exposure to bright sunlight—or at least high-intensity artificial (full-spectrum) light—is associated with diminished nocturnal melatonin production. This may be due to reduced daytime levels of serotonin. Studies indicate that people subject to typical amounts of indoor light have lower serotonin levels than those exposed to bright sunlight.[14] It appears that the enzymatic process of converting the amino acid tryptophan into serotonin requires light, just as the conversion from serotonin into melatonin requires darkness. Less serotonin produced during the day means less melatonin made at night, and this correlates with sleep onset insomnia. In one study, night-shift workers who were not exposed to sunlight or full-spectrum light between 600 and 900 lux experienced lower melatonin levels and took longer to fall asleep than those who were exposed to bright light.[15] Interestingly, 90% of blind people frequently suffer from insomnia, probably due to their inability to receive light signals.[16]

Conversely, exposure to light at night—even for 5 minutes—is detrimental to melatonin production.[17] In one study, six men exposed to bright artificial light (greater than 3,000 lux) from sunset to 2 A.M. on one night experienced delayed pineal secretion of melatonin during the light exposure. The subsequent night, when the subjects resumed normal exposure to light and darkness, melatonin secretion was still delayed, this time by 1 hour.[18] Even nighttime exposure to as little as 100 lux can inhibit nocturnal production of melatonin in some people.[19] The effect of nighttime light on sleepers varies greatly; 500 lux of light has been shown to impair melatonin production by 8% in some people, but by 98% in others,[20] and delay sleep onset for 30 minutes.[21] Common practices such as leaving bright lights on before going to bed or even sleeping with a night-light on can negatively impact your melatonin production and lead to sleep disturbances.

Magnetic and Electromagnetic Fields

Light—whether natural or artificial—isn't the only environmental phenomenon proven to affect and potentially impair the pineal gland's ability to secrete melatonin. Numerous studies have indicated that electromagnetic fields (EMFs)—both natural and artificial—can also cause sleep-wake disturbances by inhibiting melatonin production. Electromagnetic fields are defined by two properties: electrical current (measured in units of hertz, or cycles per second) and magnetic strength (measured in units of gauss). The best way to comprehend gauss is to consider that the earth's magnetic field is 0.5 gauss, and a refrigerator magnet is approximately 10 gauss. The intensity of electromagnetic devices such as computer monitors and electric ranges are often described in terms of milligauss (thousandths of a gauss) and sometimes hertz. Studies have shown that EMFs of less than 300 hertz and more than 2 milligauss can disrupt melatonin production.

The pineal gland is sensitive not only to light, but also to magnetic fields. This makes sense when you consider that visible light is actually a very high frequency electromagnetic field, oscillating at 1,015 hertz (Hz), or 1 trillion

Light, Melatonin, and the Elderly

For reasons still being researched, the elderly produce very low levels of melatonin and suffer a corresponding increase in insomnia, advanced sleep phase syndrome, and other sleep disorders. Some sleep researchers speculate that this is caused by neurochemical alterations of the suprachiasmatic nucleus (SCN) that occur during the aging process.[22] Other researchers believe calcification of the pineal gland or a more sedentary lifestyle leads to disruptions in sleep-wake patterns.

However, other studies suggest that a deficiency of sunlight contributes to depleted melatonin levels in older people. One study compared melatonin levels of elderly subjects who lived independently and were exposed to more bright sunlight to melatonin levels of elderly patients who lived in nursing homes and were less likely to have outdoor activity. The results of this study indicated that a lack of exposure to bright light may lead to reduction of melatonin secretion in old age.[23] In another study, researchers concluded that sunlight deprivation is a significant factor in disturbed sleep patterns in institutionalized elderly patients. They recommend that older people with sleep problems be exposed to sunlight for at least 2 hours each day to boost nighttime melatonin production.[24]

times per second. In comparison, human brain waves in deep sleep oscillate at about 2 to 4 Hz.

In studies on migratory birds, scientists discovered that the pineal gland, in conjunction with the hormone melatonin, functions as the brain's navigating system. This "master gland" is able to detect variations of the earth's magnetic field and use that information to locate geographical directions (north, south, east, west) and determine seasonal cues (the earth's magnetic fields changes daily and seasonally).[25] In one study, researchers removed the pineal glands of pied flycatchers, a type of migratory bird. A subset of the birds received melatonin supplementation while the other birds did not. The researchers observed that the birds lacking pineal glands and melatonin supplementation did not migrate during the expected season (autumn) and were unable to orient themselves to the migratory pattern. Birds that received melatonin supplementation, however, chose the correct season and direction in which to migrate.[26]

Other studies have found that the pineal glands of several animal species have magnetically sensitive cells.[27] While there is no conclusive evidence that human pineal gland cells are likewise receptive to magnetic fields, human studies confirm that drops in the earth's magnetic field—which occur during various solar and lunar events—cause a significant decline in melatonin levels.[28] (For more about electromagnetic fields, see chapter 7, Protect Yourself from Environmental Factors.)

Geomagnetic fields are obviously not the only magnetic phenomena in our lives. Indeed, we're exposed to numerous artificial magnetic and electromagnetic fields every day, in varying frequencies: from radios, artificial lights, microwaves, refrigerators, TVs, computer monitors, and many other common appliances. Several animal and human studies indicate that chronic exposure to extremely low frequency EMFs (less than 300 Hz) may suppresses nighttime melatonin secretion.[29] In one study, 12 men were exposed to extremely low frequency EMFs (29 milligauss, 40 Hz) for three weeks, either in the morning or in the afternoon. All test subjects showed significant drops in nocturnal melatonin secretion regardless of when they were exposed to the EMFs.[30] Another study showed that work-related exposure to 16.7-hertz magnetic fields ranging from 10 milligauss to 200 milligauss significantly decreased nighttime melatonin levels; levels rebounded on the test subjects' days off.[31] The nighttime use of electric blankets, which have extremely low frequency EMFs, is also linked to suppressed melatonin secretion.[32] Because they also can pose a fire risk, the best advice is not to use an electric blanket.

It's also worth noting that extremely low frequency EMFs have been linked to the development of breast cancer, although more research needs to be done before the connection is certain. There are thousands of melatonin receptor sites in a woman's reproductive system. Melatonin enhances intercellular communications and lower levels may cause a less efficient reproductive physiology and a greater vulnerability to breast cancer. Extremely low frequency EMFs may not only suppress melatonin secretion—they may also impair the body's ability to fight cancer cells. The proliferation of electronic devices in our lives parallels the increase in the incidence of breast cancer over the same years.

Physical and Emotional Stress

Stress can have a detrimental effect on nocturnal melatonin production, often causing insomnia and other sleep-wake rhythm disturbances. For the purposes of this chapter, we'll define stress by the presence of high blood levels of cortisol, a hormone secreted by the adrenal glands, which are located atop the kidneys. Secretion of cortisol (as well as other adrenal hormones such as DHEA, adrenaline, and aldosterone) occurs in daily cycles, peaking in the morning and having the lowest values at night. Cortisol promotes protein building, regulates insulin and glucose metabolism, and helps produce prostaglandins, fatty acids with hormonelike functions. Under conditions of stress, high amounts of cortisol are released; chronic excess secretion is associated with obesity and suppressed thyroid function. Cortisol imbalances are also linked with low energy, muscle dysfunction, impaired bone repair, thyroid dysfunction, immune system depression, sleep disorders, poor skin regeneration, and decreased growth hormone uptake. In addition to obvious stressors such as traumatic events and emotional problems, intense physical exercise can also trigger the stress response, resulting in a large release of cortisol.

As with melatonin, cortisol release is regulated by circadian rhythms, with levels the highest in the dawn hours—the same time that melatonin levels begin to dramatically decline. Research indicates that cortisol helps the body make the transition from deep sleep (which is prompted by melatonin) to light sleep and wakefulness.[33] Scientists believe that cortisol is able to reverse deep sleep by reducing the brain's uptake of serotonin, thereby suppressing production of melatonin.[34]

When large amounts of cortisol are released at night, whether due to physical exercise or emotional upset, people will likely experience difficulty falling asleep or staying asleep. In one study, nighttime exercise and the associated high cortisol levels produced a 1- to 2-hour phase delay of nocturnal melatonin release in men.[35] These findings prompted the study's researchers to claim that stress may act similarly to light in shifting human circadian rhythms—in other words, causing sleep-wake pattern disturbances.

Medications

Several commonly used medications can suppress melatonin production, leading to sleep-wake disturbances. Short-term use of over-the-counter pain relievers, heart medications, antianxiety drugs, and even sleeping pills has been shown to interfere with nocturnal secretion of melatonin. Although avoiding these medications is the only definite way to reverse or avoid their effects on melatonin, taking these drugs earlier in the day may minimize their impacts on sleep. Statistics regarding sleep deprivation in older people rarely take into account the use of multiple medications and their effects on sleep patterns.

Nonsteroidal anti-inflammatory drugs (NSAIDS), which include the widely used over-the-counter painkilling drugs ibuprofen, aspirin, and indomethacin, greatly reduce melatonin secretion at night and even disturb the amount of restorative deep sleep. This is due to their inhibitory effect on the synthesis of prostaglandins, which are necessary in the production of melatonin.[36] In one study, subjects administered standard dosages of aspirin or ibuprofen twice in one day suffered significantly higher rates of delayed sleep onset and repeated nighttime awakenings than did the control subjects. Additionally, subjects who took ibuprofen also experienced delayed onset of the deep stages of sleep.[37] In another study, one standard dosage of indomethacin given at 6 p.m. completely suppressed normal nocturnal secretion of melatonin.[38] Acetaminophen, a non-NSAID painkiller, does not appear to significantly interfere with melatonin production, but research indicates that it does have a slight adverse effect on sleep.[39]

Two commonly prescribed types of heart drugs—beta-blockers and calcium-channel blockers—also impair melatonin production. Beta-blockers are often used to treat heart problems such as high blood pressure, angina, and arrhythmias (abnormal heart rhythms). They function by interfering with specific cell receptors called beta-adrenergic receptors, which results in relaxed heart rate and lowered blood pressure, but also suspension of normal nighttime melatonin production. The beta-blockers propranolol and atenolol are particularly damaging to melatonin levels. Calcium-channel blockers also seriously impair nighttime melatonin levels. As their name suggests, these drugs impede the flow of calcium to cardiovascular cells, thus relaxing the arteries and reducing the amount of oxygen needed by the heart. But they can also suppress the flow of calcium to pineal cells, which need calcium to make melatonin.[40]

Benzodiazepines are tranquilizing drugs frequently prescribed for anxiety and insomnia. However, several studies show that benzodiazepines, including diazepam, alprazolam, and flunitrazepam, may impair the central nervous system's ability to relay light information to the pineal gland.[41]

In one test, six healthy subjects were given diazepam and their nocturnal melatonin levels were then measured. In all subjects, melatonin levels were suppressed throughout the night.[42] Other studies have found that another benzodiazepine, alprazolam, also diminished nighttime melatonin levels, resulting in less time spent in deep sleep stages.[43] Benzodiazepines may also lead to melatonin rebound during the day, in which melatonin production nearly reaches regular nighttime levels during the day, causing excessive daytime sleepiness.[44]

Poor Diet

Caffeine and alcohol, the usual suspects in sleep problems, have been shown to impair melatonin production. One study showed that 200 mg of caffeine (the amount found in two cups of brewed coffee) significantly reduced nighttime melatonin levels.[45] Alcohol has been found to depress nocturnal melatonin secretion due to its inhibitory effect on the adrenal hormone norepinephrine, which promotes production of melatonin by pineal cells.[46]

Imbalances of certain vitamins and minerals may also affect melatonin levels. In several studies, vitamin B_{12} deficiencies have been shown to suppress melatonin production.[47] For this reason, B_{12}, in conjunction with light therapy, is effective for sleep phase syndromes. Deficiencies of magnesium and vitamins B_1 and B_6 may also reduce melatonin levels, since these nutrients are essential in activating the enzymes that facilitate production of serotonin and melatonin.[48]

Alternative Therapies to Reset Your Body Clock

Alternative medicine offers a broad range of therapies to reset your body clock and resolve sleep-wake rhythm disturbances. Some are simple, no-cost steps: avoid caffeine and alcohol, exercise, and spend more time outdoors. Other therapies require special purchases, such as light boxes or magnets, and are best administered under the guidance of a health-care practitioner. Melatonin supplements are effective and widely available. However, most alternative medicine practitioners recommend integrating lifestyle changes (such as dietary changes and light therapy) before turning to melatonin supplementation; with proper nourishment and light-dark cycles, the body can naturally produce sufficient amounts of this hormone.

Lifestyle Modifications

Making a few adjustments to your daily routine can get you snoozing again. One of the most important steps to improving your sleep is avoiding caffeine and alcohol. If you decide to continue consuming caffeine-containing beverages and foods, do so earlier in the day. Drink coffee no later than 10 A.M.

Alcohol consumption should be discontinued completely. Also, steer clear of NSAIDs and other melatonin-suppressing drugs at night. You might try taking them earlier in the day, but make sure you talk to your physician about altering your dosage schedule for prescription medications.

Next, eat foods that will boost your body's natural melatonin production. Though research on this front is just beginning, we now know that many foods contain melatonin, including walnuts, oats, corn, rice, tomatoes, and bananas. Eating these shortly before bedtime will promote higher nocturnal melatonin secretion. Tryptophan is a precursor of melatonin, so increasing levels of tryptophan in your brain may also be helpful. For information on dietary strategies to help accomplish this, see "Eat to Boost Tryptophan Levels," page 60. Russel J. Reiter, Ph.D., author of *Melatonin: Your Body's Wonder Drug*, recommends supplementing with calcium (1,000 mg), magnesium (500 mg), and niacinamide (100 mg) before bed, since these minerals are essential in converting tryptophan into serotonin and then melatonin.[49]

Starting to exercise is an important way to manage stress, which can interfere with sleep. Additionally, it can elevate your body temperature; the following drop in body temperature 4 to 6 hours later, may facilitate sleep.[50] However, proper timing is crucial. The best time to exercise to improve your sleep is during the late afternoon (5 P.M. or earlier). As discussed above, physical exertion at night can incite a stress response, resulting in overstimulation due to high levels of cortisol.

Light Therapy

Light therapy relies on the body's natural ability to reset its sleep-wake rhythms according to the zeitgeber of light. As discussed earlier, the presence of external light inhibits melatonin secretion; darkness promotes it. The premise behind light therapy is simple: get more light exposure during the day and less at night. Dimming the lights at night probably won't be a hardship, but making sure that you receive adequate amounts of bright light during the day can be difficult.

One way you can increase exposure to bright light is by going outdoors more often—for 1 hour or more each day. Make it a habit to get outdoors first thing in the morning to exposure yourself to natural sunlight. Alternately, you can sit by a large, east-facing window while you eat breakfast or spend your lunch break outdoors. Unfortunately, the sun's ultraviolet rays can damage the skin and eyes, leading to various health problems, so be sure to wear UV-protective sunglasses (with minimal tint so the light can enter your retinas) and sunscreen.

Many things may prevent you from spending prolonged periods outdoors: cold weather, illness, work, and other obligations. To enjoy the benefits of natural sunlight indoors, install full-spectrum lightbulbs in your home and office. Full-spectrum lightbulbs provide a balanced blend of all colors in the visible spectrum, closely resembling natural sunlight, whereas conventional incandescent lightbulbs illuminate more intensely in the yellow part of the color spectrum. Lee Hartley, Ed.D., a researcher on light therapy, suggests mounting a row of four to six full-spectrum bulbs in a vanity fixture over your bathroom sink. "This is an excellent method for maximum impact," she says, "because the body receives the same effect as natural sunlight in the morning. You wake up quicker and with less morning shock."

Additionally, you may consider using a light box; these specially designed devices use full-spectrum fluorescent lights to simulate early-morning sunlight. Light boxes typically cost $100 to $450 and are widely available in various sizes and styles, from wall units to desk lamps to visors. They usually come in values of 5,000 to 10,000 lux. Most standard therapy protocols recommend 10,000 lux for at least 30 minutes daily or 2,500 lux for at least 2 hours; because lux values are affected by distance from the light source, it's important to clearly understand the specifications of any unit you use. Ideally, light therapy would take place first thing in the morning. Sit before the light box with your eyes open but not staring directly into the light, either at home or at work (assuming you work at a desk or in some manner of stationary pursuit). Interestingly, research has found that external light is sensed by organs other than the eyes. In fact, one study found that exposing the back of the knees to light suppressed melatonin production. (The therapeutic applications of these findings are not assessed at this time.) Recently, some manufacturers and practitioners have advocated using blue light. However, the safety and effectiveness of blue light have yet to be established, and there are credible concerns that blue light may be more damaging to the eyes.

Some doctors may also recommend vitamin B_{12} supplements in conjunction with light therapy, as this vitamin appears to enhance a person's

Take a Hot Bath for a Good Night's Sleep

A hot bath isn't just a relaxing experience, it's also a natural sleep aid. In the National Sleep Foundation's 1999 sleep survey, 65% of adults reported that they fell asleep more quickly and slept better than usual after soaking in a hot bath, and research substantiates these claims.[51] In one study, researchers found that after taking a hot bath, subjects' body temperature rose about 2°F and melatonin levels also increased.[52] Apparently, the pineal gland responds to a sudden rise in body temperature by producing melatonin, which lowers and normalizes body temperature. A pleasant side effect is that you are lulled to sleep.

To enhance these relaxing effects, consider adding ¼ to ½ cup Epsom salts or baking soda to the bath. For aromatherapy benefits, add a few drops of relaxing essential oils, such as lavender, chamomile, pine, eucalyptus, orange blossom, or ylang-ylang. Alternatively, infuse herbal essences into the water using a muslin bag or tea ball; beneficial herbs include chamomile, linden flowers, and lavender.

photosensitivity. Researchers have found that 3 hours of light therapy (2,500 to 3,000 lux) accompanied by intravenous vitamin B_{12} (5 to 6 mg daily) reset the circadian rhythms of melatonin secretion and was effective in resolving delayed sleep phase syndromes and other sleep-wake disturbances.[53]

Generally, it takes about 14 days of light therapy to see if you're getting benefits. Never stare into the light during therapy and be careful to choose light sources that screen out ultraviolet rays. People with eye problems such as diabetic retinopathy or macular degeneration should not use light therapy without their doctor's consent.

Chronotherapy

The majority of people suffering from sleep-wake rhythm disturbances will find relief through increased daytime exposure to sunlight or a light box. However, for those who experience extreme delayed sleep phase syndrome, chronotherapy (which literally means "time therapy") may be appropriate. Chronotherapy is based on the theory that by delaying bedtime for several days, it is possible to move the person's sleep time to a more conventional time frame, such as 10 P.M. to 6 A.M. Here's an example of how it works: If you don't get to sleep until 2 A.M. and rise at 10 A.M., you can begin by delaying your bedtime until 5 A.M. the first night. Each successive day, add another 3-hour delay until you have moved around the clock. In this example, the second day you go to bed at 8 A.M. and rise at 4 P.M. This method is best done during a vacation or at a time when you aren't committed to a regular work schedule or other obligations.

Magnet Therapy

Magnetic fields exist everywhere, emanating from the earth, from changes in the weather, and even from the human body. The use of magnetic devices to generate controlled magnetic fields has proven to be an effective therapy for rheumatoid disease, inflammation, cancer, circulatory problems, and other illnesses. Magnet therapy can influence the flow of varying electrical currents (normally present in all organisms) that govern the nervous system and other biological systems. Controlled use of magnetic fields can benefit those who suffer from sleep disorders by reversing the detrimental effects of extremely low frequency electromagnetic fields on the pineal gland.

For sleep disorders arising out of disruptions in melatonin production, alternative medicine doctors recommend therapy with negative-polarity magnets. Magnet therapy may offer permanent relief to those with various sleep-wake disturbances, including insomnia and even sleep apnea. Though the use of magnets has been shown to improve cases of multiple sclerosis and Parkinson's disease, very few studies have tested their effectiveness against sleep disorders. However, one study did show that three weeks of magnet therapy permanently eliminated a chronic case of sleep paralysis in a multiple sclerosis patient. This report suggests that magnet therapy promoted melatonin secretion, since REM sleep disorders such as sleep paralysis have been linked to melatonin deficiency.[54]

In treating sleep disorders, magnets are used in various placements: on the abdomen (some amount of melatonin is secreted by the intestines), on the eyes, and in specially designed mattress pads. Commercially available, negative-polarity mattress pads are the easiest way to use magnet therapy for sleep disorders. You simply place the pad on top of the mattress (for maximum strength) or between the mattress and box spring. However, mattress pads can be costly, and your doctor may determine that magnets placed on your eyes or abdomen will be more effective for your condition. In most cases, you can discontinue magnet therapy once your condition has improved, or you can continue to use magnets as a preventive measure.

As an alternative to a magnetized mattress pads, you might use a 5 by 6-inch flexible multiple-magnet mat. This type of mat is composed of strips of plastiform magnets placed sufficiently close together to make a solid field, but far enough apart for flexibility. Before going to bed, place four ceramic magnets measuring 4 by 6 by 1 inch at the headboard. Once you get into bed, place the mat across your forehead and down to the tip of your nose to cover your eyes, sinuses, and nose. Directly on top of this mat and over your eyes, place two neodymium disk magnets measuring 1 by ½ inch, which will magnetically adhere to the mat. Sleep with these magnets in place throughout the night. Be sure to keep your bedroom dark, too. To increase the depth of sleep, place a flexible multimagnet mat measuring 5 by 12 inches across your abdomen before going to sleep. (Alternatively, you can use a plastiform magnet strip measuring 4 by 12 by ⅛ inch.) For additional magnetic reinforcement, center a ceramic magnet measuring 4 by 6 by ½ inch on the mat, positioned lengthwise on the body.

Cautions: There are conflicting methods of naming the magnetic poles. To be effective, magnets need to be marked correctly, so be sure to use magnets marked according to the Davis-Rawls system (developed by Dr. Albert Roy Davis in 1936). Avoid touching the sides of thick therapeutic magnets and never use magnets with holes in the middle. Keep magnets 1 to 2 feet away from your computer, audiotapes, videotapes, computer disks, and other magnetic storage media, credit cards, and the like. People with cancer or any infection (including candida, viruses, and bacteria) should avoid exposure to bipolar magnets. Don't use magnets on your chest if you have a pacemaker. A pregnant woman should not use magnets on her abdomen. Do not use magnetic beds for longer than 8 to 10 hours a day. For long-term

A Quick Review of Magnetic Basics

All magnets have two poles: positive (or S for south, usually marked in red) and negative (or N for north, usually marked in green). If you are using magnets for therapeutic purposes, only use magnets specifically designed for this purpose. Do not substitute refrigerator or other magnets. Negative magnetic energy normalizes and calms human physiological systems, while positive magnetic energy overstimulates or disrupts these systems. For this reason, negative poles are most frequently directed toward the body. Do not apply positive magnetic poles directly to the body unless under medical supervision.

The strength of a magnet is measured in gauss units (which measure the intensity of magnetic flux). Every magnetic device has a manufacturer's gauss rating; however, the actual strength of the magnet at the skin surface is often much less than this number. For example, a 4,000-gauss magnet transmits about 1,200 gauss to the body. Magnets placed in pillows or mattress pads will render even lower amounts of field strength at the skin surface, because a magnet's strength quickly decreases with the distance. The strength of the magnet also depends on its size and thickness. Therapeutic magnets use from 200 gauss to 1,500 gauss (only a fraction of what an MRI machine emits), while a common refrigerator magnet emits 120 gauss.[55]

The most common types of magnets used in magnetic therapy are ceramic and neodymium (a rare-earth element). These substances are mixed with iron to increase the magnet's strength or the duration of magnetic charge. Neodymium magnets are more powerful (and expensive), while ceramic magnets are less expensive but still keep their charge for many years. These magnetic materials are incorporated into various types of products that are widely available: wrist and back supports; seat pads; strips worn inside shoes, and plastiform strips that attach to the skin by an elastic adhesive. Magnetic blankets, mattress pads, other bedding products, and even beds are also available for promoting sleep and reducing stress.

results, use magnets at night and supplement with magnet treatments during the day as is convenient. It is best to use magnets under the supervision of a health-care professional. Don't combine melatonin supplementation with magnet therapy without first consulting your doctor.

Melatonin Supplementation

Melatonin is popularly regarded as a wonder drug for its immune-boosting, age-defying, and, of course, sleep-enhancing properties—and rightly so. Research repeatedly confirms the benefits of melatonin supplementation for various sleep-wake rhythm disturbances. Further studies have found that melatonin supplements are nontoxic and very safe for short-term use, with only mild side effects such as headaches and abdominal cramps in test subjects who received extremely large doses (3 to 6.6 grams).

Melatonin effectively relieves insomnia (including cases associated with jet lag and shift work), sleep phase syndromes, and REM behavior disorders in all age groups. It has been shown to decrease sleep onset latency in stages 1 and 2 (light sleep), a helpful boost for those suffering from sleep onset insomnia.[56] Melatonin has also been found to significantly increase deep sleep, REM sleep, and sleep efficiency (time spent in sound asleep), all without the "hangover" or stupor effects common with other over-the-counter and prescription sleeping aids. In addition, it has been shown to dramatically improve the sleep-wake cycle in blind people, who often suffer from problems with free-running circadian rhythms due to their inability to detect light.[57] Melatonin pills work quickly; people usually fall asleep within 30 minutes of taking the supplements.

If melatonin does have a downside, it is on two counts: First, researchers have not discovered the optimal dose of melatonin supplementation. Thus, people taking this hormone generally need to experiment with different dosages before finding the right one for their needs. Second, the long-term effects of melatonin supplementation are unknown. As with any hormone replacement therapy, there is a chance the endocrine system (in this case the pineal gland) could stop producing its own melatonin if you supply it from an external source; this could cause the gland to atrophy. Additionally, most of the melatonin in supplements is synthetically derived and is slightly different than natural melatonin; this may have detrimental long-term effects. If you're considering supplementing with melatonin, seek out a source of bioidentical melatonin, which is exactly like the melatonin the body produces; you may need to work with a health-care practitioner on this.

Cautions: While melatonin has been shown to be very safe in short-term use, people with severe allergies, severe mental illness or depression, autoimmune diseases, and immune-system cancers such as lymphoma and leukemia are advised to avoid melatonin supplements since the hormone may exacerbate these conditions.[58] Pregnant or nursing women should not take melatonin, as its impact on fetal and newborn development is not known. Women who are trying to conceive should avoid high doses of melatonin (10 mg or more), which can prevent ovulation.[59] Melatonin is also not recommended for healthy children (who have naturally high levels of melatonin) and people taking steroid drugs such as cortisone (as melatonin may counteract their effectiveness).[60] Men taking high doses of melatonin should consider supplementing with vitamin E, as this will reverse melatonin's suppressive effects on testosterone production.[61]

Hence, we advise against self-dosing melatonin supplements on a long-term basis or in certain conditions without first consulting a health-care practitioner who can monitor your levels of melatonin. Never take melatonin supplements during the day unless advised by your doctor, as this will further disrupt your circadian rhythms. Do not operate machinery or drive after taking melatonin supplements. One additional warning: Expect vivid, even bizarre dreams for up to two months upon starting melatonin supplements, as this hormone stimulates REM sleep.

Using Melatonin for Insomnia

Numerous studies have found melatonin supplements very effective for insomnia, especially in the elderly.[62] For sleep onset and other types of insomnia, the standard dosage of melatonin is between 0.2 and 10 mg, taken approximately 30 minutes before bedtime. As discussed above, optimal dosages vary, so begin by taking 1 to 2 mg and increasing or decreasing as necessary to reach the lowest dose that induces sleep. It's best to take melatonin at the same time each night to properly reset your body clock. The duration of supplementation depends on your sleep problem. If you suffer from chronic insomnia and other lifestyle modifications don't help, you may need to take melatonin supplements every night. On the other hand, if you experience occasional insomnia due to stress, illness, or other factors, use melatonin supplements only as needed.

Using Melatonin for Jet Lag

In studies on people traveling by plane across time zones, those treated with melatonin supplements reported less severe symptoms of jet lag than those given a placebo. They also returned more rapidly to their normal sleep patterns, experienced less daytime fatigue, and reported reaching normal energy levels more rapidly.[63]

While most doctors agree that melatonin is effective for jet lag, the best time to take melatonin is debatable. Sleep researcher Alfred Lewy, MD, advises that you start taking melatonin the day before travel, and early in the day to start shifting your clock forward or backward. For example, if you're traveling from the West Coast to the East Coast of the United States, you will need to advance your body clock by 3 hours. So you can take a small dose of melatonin (0.5 mg, just enough to shift your body clock without causing excessive daytime drowsiness) at 2 P.M. the day before you travel (5 P.M. at your destination). Then take the same dose at 2 P.M. the day of travel, and at 5 P.M. the first full day on the East Coast. This will help you feel tired on Eastern time. The day before you return home, and for the next two days, take melatonin first thing in the morning. This will delay your body clock so you will be able to stay up on Pacific time.

Ray Sahelian, MD, author of *Melatonin: Nature's Sleeping Pill*, advises taking melatonin when you get to your destination in the evening of the new time zone, especially when traveling west to east. He advocates increasing the dosage by about 1 mg for every hour earlier you want to sleep. For example, if you take a day flight from Los Angeles to New York, by midnight in New

York it will be only 9 P.M. in Los Angeles, so it may be hard for you to go to sleep. Because of the 3-hour difference, you would take 3 mg of melatonin sometime between 10 P.M. and 11 P.M. Eastern time.[64]

A third strategy is to take 0.5 mg of melatonin on the plane when it's 8:30 P.M. or 9 P.M. at your destination. Then, when you arrive, take between 0.5 and 5 mg (as much as needed to fall asleep quickly) the first night or two at the local bedtime. You can also use sunlight to help your body make the shift. When traveling west to east, avoid daylight until after 10 A.M., and then get out in the sun for about 30 minutes at midday. In traveling east to west, avoid daylight after 6 P.M.

Using Melatonin for Shift Work

Endocrinologist and melatonin expert Russel Reiter, Ph.D., recommends that shift workers take 1 to 5 mg of melatonin at the beginning of their desired sleep time, or as needed. Wearing dark wraparound sunglasses or sleeping in a dark room is important too, to avoid exposure to light, which suppresses melatonin production. Dr. Lewy, however, discourages shift workers from self-treatment because the circadian rhythms can be difficult to reset, especially in the case of rotating-shift work. He advises that shift workers find a doctor with expertise in chronobiology (resetting body clocks) to help them—with light therapy and melatonin—shift their body clocks to a stable rhythm.

Using Melatonin for Sleep Phase Syndromes

Two other sleep-wake disturbances are caused by disruptions in the melatonin production cycle: advanced sleep phase syndrome (ASPS), in which people fall asleep in early evening and then wake up well before dawn, and delayed sleep phase syndrome (DSPS), in which people habitually stay up until 2 A.M. or later and sleep until 11 A.M. or noon. ASPS sufferers tend to be elderly, while people with DSPS are often in their teens or early twenties.

Dr. Lewy has successfully treated both advanced and delayed sleep phase syndromes with a combination of light therapy and low-dose melatonin supplements.[65] People with ASPS can undergo light therapy in the early evening, when the body is just about to start its melatonin production. The light will delay melatonin buildup and keep the person awake. Then, upon awakening in the early morning, the person would take 0.5 mg of melatonin to promote melatonin secretion in the predawn darkness.

DSPS patients need to reverse the process: doing light therapy first thing in the morning and taking 0.5 mg of melatonin in early evening or 7 hours after they get up. One study showed that taking 1 to 2 mg of melatonin 2 hours before the desired bedtime helped people with extreme DSPS (who were falling asleep at 5 A.M.) reset their body clocks in eight weeks.[66] With all cases of sleep phase syndrome, patients can discontinue melatonin supplementation once they've achieved their ideal sleep-wake pattern.

Using Melatonin for REM Behavior Disorder

Melatonin has shown great promise in eliminating REM behavior disorder (RBD), a sleep problem characterized by head banging and other repetitive body movements during the REM stage of sleep. Because melatonin is involved in immobilizing the body during REM sleep, RBD indicates a melatonin deficiency and specifically a desynchronization of melatonin secretion and sleep stages. In one study, six people with RBD were administered 3 mg of melatonin 30 minutes before bedtime. Within one week, five patients experienced a dramatic reduction of RBD episodes; after six weeks, these patients slept normally.[67] In another study, a man fully recovered from RBD after five months of melatonin treatment (3 mg daily). When melatonin supplementation was discontinued, his RBD symptoms reappeared, only to vanish when the melatonin treatment was restored.[68]

success story

Melatonin Lets a Chronic Insomniac Sleep Again

INTEGRATIVE HEALTH PIONEER William Lee Cowden, MD, has had excellent success using melatonin supplements in treating insomnia. He reports that one of his former patients had suffered from insomnia for 10 years, sleeping only 3 hours a night. The patient had visited numerous sleep disorder centers as well as dozens of sleep specialists, and had tried virtually every prescription drug for insomnia—all to no avail. Over the years, the chronic insomnia had made the man extremely irritable and difficult to live with.

Dr. Cowden, believing the insomnia was due to an imbalance in melatonin, instructed his patient to take certain steps to boost his melatonin production: avoid sugar and caffeine, sleep in a totally darkened room, and remove all electrical devices such as clocks, radios, and televisions from his bedroom. He recommended that the patient take melatonin supplements between 10 P.M. and midnight every night for two weeks, then every other night for two months.

Dr. Cowden also gave the patient supplements of vitamin C and omega-3 essential fatty acids, which are instrumental in producing prostaglandins, hormonelike substances that aid in melatonin synthesis. After a few nights on this regimen, the patient was sleeping 7 to 8 hours a night, and after two months, he reported that he was sleeping as well as he had during childhood.

Beating the Winter Blues

In recent decades, the "winter blues" have gained scientific credibility. Physicians now diagnose seasonal affective disorder (SAD)—the measurable negative effects that sunlight deprivation produces in some people. The symptoms of SAD's winter doldrums are no doubt familiar to many. It is estimated that more than 10 million Americans experience SAD every year, and another 25 million get milder depressive symptoms on a seasonal basis. Additionally, the more northern the latitude at which you live, the shorter your days and the more susceptible you are to SAD. In the United States, cases of SAD increase the further north you go, with estimates ranging from 1.4% of the population in Florida to 9.7% in New Hampshire.[69]

What does SAD feel like? Typically, it entails chronic depression and fatigue, which may leave you bedridden; hypersomnia (increased sleep by as much as 4 hours or even more per night) and reduced quality of sleep, leaving you feeling less refreshed; and cravings for carbohydrates and candy, which sometimes can lead to significant weight gain. Some women with SAD report that their premenstrual symptoms are aggravated. Similar seasonal behavioral changes, particularly increased sleep and variations in appetite, are seen in other mammals.

How does a shortage of sunlight cause these changes? According to naturopathic physician and educator Michael T. Murray, ND, author of *Natural Alternatives to Prozac*, the cause may be in your hormones. "The key hormonal change may be reduced secretion of melatonin from the pineal gland and an increased secretion of cortisol by the adrenal glands." Both of these hormones affect mood; studies have found decreased melatonin and increased cortisol in depressed patients. Reduced duration and intensity of sunlight in winter throws off the body's internal clock and its levels of melatonin, the sleep-inducing hormone. It's like a season-long case of jet lag.

Sleep Rituals

Once you have reset your circadian rhythms and find that your body is responding to natural cues for sleep, such as waning light in the evening, you may want to consider establishing a sleep ritual. A sleep ritual is a conscious effort to set aside adequate time to allow yourself to relax and release the day's activities. A sleep ritual can help reduce nighttime stress, minimizing the adverse effects of cortisol on melatonin production. It can also take on the status of zeitgeber with your body clock, providing temporal cues that it's almost time to go to sleep. Sleep researcher Sonia Ancoli-Israel, Ph.D., recommends integrating these steps into your own sleep ritual:

■ **Set aside a specific time for worrying.** Many of us tend to worry about the day's events or next day while in bed. Dr. Ancoli-Israel recommends spending time in the daytime to process your concerns. "We suggest that people find 30 minutes earlier in the day when they can sit down quietly, put out the Do Not Disturb sign, and worry. That's your chance to sit and think about all the things that you're concerned about. We also recommend getting it out of your head and onto paper or your computer. Make a list of all that is on your mind. Get it out of your system so that once you get into bed at night, or if

you wake up in the middle of the night, you don't have to start thinking about all of it."

■ **Clear your head of thoughts.** To dispel the internal chatter of anxiety and other sleep-inhibiting thoughts at night, Dr. Ancoli-Israel recommends employing some sort of meditative process. She says that this can range from counting sheep to more elaborate forms of meditation. Concentrating on your breathing will help clear your mind. Simply breathe deeply and count each breath.

■ **Relax before bedtime.** Don't engage in stimulating activities before going to bed. Avoid working, spending time on the computer, perhaps even watching TV. Do things that are relaxing and allow your mind and body to unwind and slow down. Read, knit, or listen to soothing music.

■ **Don't rush the sleep ritual.** Set aside a specific time window for the sleep ritual and give yourself adequate time to do all of these activities. It will be counterproductive to rush through your meditation or anything else and still expect to drop off to sleep easily. Any activity, whether physical or mental, that is stimulating or creates arousal is likely to interfere with your sleep.

Numerous studies show that light therapy with natural or full-spectrum lights drastically reduces the symptoms of SAD. Spending 1 hour outside in the morning light can eliminate SAD in 50% of patients.[70] Of course, this isn't always an option, so light box therapy may be useful (see "Light Therapy," page 114). Studies have shown that the efficacy of light box therapy on SAD may vary according to time of day. In one study, for instance, 10,000-lux light therapy for 30 minutes in the morning was 69% effective in reversing SAD, while evening exposure was up to 80% effective.[71] However, other studies have shown converse results. Regardless timing, symptoms usually begin to improve after two to four days of treatment, with full improvement evident in two weeks.[72]

Light therapy also seems to help people who are concerned about gaining weight in the winter. The carbohydrate cravings that frequently accompany SAD are associated with serotonin deficiency, a possible outgrowth of cortisol increase. Serotonin, a neurotransmitter believed to play a role in regulating appetite, is produced during light exposure.

SAD No More with Light Therapy

DECADES AGO, Sherrie Baxter left sunny Oklahoma, her native state, for Vancouver, Washington, in the Pacific Northwest. As the years went by, Sherrie would become tired and depressed and find herself craving carbohydrates as soon as autumn arrived, with its characteristic overcast skies and dark mornings. Around that same time of year, she'd also start staying up late and having trouble getting up in the morning. But her depression and fatigue always mysteriously lifted by April or May. "One of things I always vividly remember happened during Christmas: I was walking through a store and they were playing holiday music, and I just started crying for no reason. I didn't have problems like that in spring or summer," she recalls.

In 1985, both Sherrie, then 28, and her mother, who had the same symptoms, signed up as research subjects for a study on seasonal affective disorder at Oregon Health Sciences University in Portland. For three weeks, the two women lived in special quarters where the amount of light was strictly controlled. Technicians took regular blood samples day and night to monitor their levels of melatonin. The researchers were testing whether the lack of light in the morning allowed melatonin to be produced later in the day, causing the women's SAD symptoms.

The first week of the study, Sherrie and her mother were kept mostly in near-darkness except for one dim lightbulb. The only break was at 2 P.M., when they were told to stay in front of 4 by 6-foot, 2,500-lux light boxes for about 2 hours. In the second week, they used the light boxes at progressively earlier times. The third week, they woke at 6 A.M. and used the light boxes immediately upon awakening. By the fourth day of that regimen, Sherrie and her mother were no longer depressed and were full of energy. Blood test results revealed that the positive changes were occurring because the morning light had normalized their melatonin production cycle.

"I tend to be skeptical of things until I see proof," says Sherrie, now 43. "But we were able to see this was a physical thing happening, and that was useful to me." After the study, Sherrie made a light box for herself, and, several years later, started her own business, Enviro-Med (see Resources), to sell them.

six

Step 4: Resolve Emotional Issues

Stress is a common part of everyday life, but it can become harmful to the body when it is prolonged or chronic. It affects the body in very real physical ways by influencing the immune and endocrine systems. One result can be poor sleep quality, restless nights, and development of sleep disorders. A basic premise of mind-body medicine is that chronic stress and other emotional issues contribute to illness and that relaxation techniques and learning positive ways of coping with these issues will improve your health. In this chapter, we examine how stress, suppressed emotions, and related lifestyle choices can contribute to sleep problems. We also explore a number of therapies that can help you change negative thought patterns into more healthful ones, deal with stress in a positive way, and incorporate habits for relaxation into your life.

success story

A Return-to-Sleep Strategy

BY THE TIME JEAN FOUND HER WAY to a sleep disorders center, she had been having trouble sleeping for six years. The problems started when she went into training for a new job. The training required that Jean work the swing shift, 3 P.M. to 11 P.M., for several months, a

Mind-Body Therapies for Better Sleep

- Meditation
- Biofeedback
- Hypnotherapy
- Visualization and guided imagery
- Counseling

- Cranial electrical stimulation
- Herbal therapy
- Homeopathic remedies
- Aromatherapy
- Flower therapies

change from her normal 8:30 A.M. to 4:30 P.M. work schedule. Unable to get to sleep when she came home from the swing shift, Jean often ended up staying up quite late then sleeping until midmorning. When she resumed her normal work schedule, her sleep schedule remained disrupted, so she began to fall asleep at about 11 P.M. but would wake up at 2:30 A.M., unable to fall back to sleep.

After two years of only getting about 3 hours sleep on many nights, Jean developed what psychologist Robert E. Becker, Ph.D., calls "anticipatory anxiety." The person starts to worry early in the day about how they will sleep that night. "They start thinking, 'How am I going to do tonight? What time shall I got to bed?'" he says.

In Jean's case, her anticipatory anxiety grew for the next four years until, at age 31, she was so distraught that she enrolled in Dr. Becker's sleep disorders program. By this time, Jean was losing mental concentration and was emotionally on edge, and her marriage was shaky, all due to the sleeping problems. She told Dr. Becker she didn't want to take sleep medication or other drugs.

According to Dr. Becker, by the time they enroll in a sleep disorders program, most people have tried the full range of home remedies, from warm milk to herbal tea to a glass of wine to hot baths. The ones who try sleeping pills or other drugs find they only work for a short period of time and then the insomnia returns. They've also tried listening to music, talking to their spouse, and talking to themselves—strategies that work for the general population, but don't work once people have developed anticipatory anxiety.

"What we need to do is to stop the anticipatory anxiety as much as we can," Dr. Becker says. "For Jean, we needed to get a return-to-sleep strategy in place, because as soon as she wakes up in the night, her body chemistry starts to become alert again." People make themselves even more alert, he says, by reading, watching television, or working at their computer when they wake up in the middle of the night. Those activities can increase mental stimulation, instead of inducing relaxation. Dr. Becker established Jean's return-to-sleep strategy as follows:

1. Have a guided imagery tape in a tape recorder and ready to play. The tape includes descriptions of floating in a balloon, walking in the woods, lying on the beach, or floating in a boat. This type of visualization is right-brain activity, which shuts off the left brain's worry and anxiety about not getting enough sleep.

2. Start diaphragmatic (belly) breathing. The normal resting breathing rate is 15 breaths a minute, but when people wake up and start worrying, their breathing rate goes up to about 20 breaths a minute. Diaphragmatic breathing uses your diaphragm and belly muscles instead of your intercostal, or chest, muscles. The purpose is to slow the breathing rate down. Dr. Becker taught Jean how to do diaphragmatic breathing and also gave her a video to help her practice the technique. He instructed her to use the visualization tape and start diaphragmatic breathing immediately upon awakening and continue for 30 minutes or until she fell asleep.

> **"Those who try sleeping pills or other drugs find they only work for a short period of time and then the insomnia returns."**

3. Change sleep location. If Jean did not fall back asleep in 30 minutes, she was instructed to get up and move to another bed that was already set up and waiting in another part of the house. The reason for the change was to get Jean away from any cues in her primary bedroom that signal her to be awake. Getting into a different bed, with different textures, temperature, and smells, can help break down any conditioned responses she had in the other bedroom.

4. If the new location didn't induce sleep, then Jean was to get up and do some kind of mindless activity, such as sitting and sipping a cup of warm milk, and not thinking about anything. She could also replay the visualization tape or have a small snack, such as a banana or some turkey or other protein. Then she was to go back to the new location and try to sleep.

After one week on the program, Jean had slept 7 hours on four nights and 6 hours on three nights. The first two strategies—visualization tape plus diaphragmatic breathing—were successful in getting Jean back to sleep. She kept on using the four strategies, and her sleep continued to improve. Her next goal was to have 10 consecutive nights of solid sleep. After she achieved that, Dr. Becker allowed her to relax a bit on the strategies, but he helped her remain alert to whether she was slipping back into worry about whether her insomnia would come back, particularly during stressful times. He monitored her closely over the next three months, and when Jean did relapse, which most people do, she went back on the return-to-sleep program.

Stress and Your Sleep Problems

Although the concept of stress—being "stressed-out" or "under constant stress"—may be commonly discussed today, its role as a contributing factor in many diseases is underappreciated. Some estimates suggest that as many as 60% to 90% of all visits to physicians' offices are for stress-related problems.[1] Chronic stress directly affects the immune system, and if not effectively dealt with, it can seriously compromise health.

Stress is a pervasive problem among Americans. According to a 2001 poll, more than one-third of workers said their job was detrimental to their physical or emotional health, and 42% said that their job was having a negative effect on personal relationships. Half of those surveyed said their workload demands had increased over the past year.[2] The number of days employees called in sick due to stress tripled between 1996 and 2000, and by some accounts, "problems at work are more strongly associated with complaints than are any other stressor—more so even than financial problems or family problems."[3]

Stress can be defined as a reaction (to any stimulus or interference) that upsets normal functioning and disturbs mental or physical health. It can be brought on by internal conditions such as illness, pain, emotional conflict, or psychological problems, or by external circumstances, such as bereavement, financial problems, loss of a job, divorce or death close family member, relocation, food allergies, and electromagnetic fields. Even positive events, such as marriage, a promotion, or the birth of a child, can cause stress. When stress becomes chronic, it often goes unrecognized by the person experiencing it; one begins to accept it as a fact of life, without being aware of how it is actually compromising all bodily function and laying the foundation for illness.

More specifically, research confirms that high levels of emotional stress increase one's susceptibility to illness. Unrelieved chronic stress taxes and eventually weakens or even suppresses the immune system. Stress can also lead to hormonal imbalances, which in turn interfere with immune function. Of all the body's systems, immune function is the most damaged by stress. It does so by overly activating the sympathetic nervous system, the part of the autonomic nervous system that controls the fight-or-flight response and initiates release of adrenaline and cortisol.

Research in psychoneuroimmunology, a field of medicine that is specifically concerned with the influence of emotional states and the nervous system on immune function, has shown that the immune and nervous systems are linked by extensive networks of nerve endings in the spleen, bone marrow, lymph nodes, and thymus gland (a primary source of the immune system's T cells). At the same time, receptors for a variety of chemical messengers—catecholamines, prostaglandins, thyroid hormones, growth

How to Do Diaphragmatic Breathing

1. Lie on your back and place your hands on your abdomen immediately below your navel, with your middle fingertips touching.

2. Breathing through your nose, inhale slowly and push your abdomen out as if it were a balloon expanding: your fingers should separate.

3. As your abdomen expands, your diaphragm muscle, at the base of your rib cage, will move downward, allowing fresh air to enter the bottom of your lungs.

4. As the inhalation continues, expand your chest. More air should now enter, filling the middle part of your lungs.

5. Slightly contract your abdomen, raise your shoulders and collarbones; this will fill your upper lungs.

6. Hold your breath for a few seconds (a slow count to seven) without straining.

7. Slowly exhale through your nose, drawing in your abdomen. Exhaling completely will expel all of the stale air. At the end of the exhalation, hold for a count of seven.

Diaphragmatic breathing may take some practice or cause slight dizziness at the beginning; this is normal. The most important thing is not to strain or force yourself to breathe slower than is comfortable.

Common Causes of Stress

- Illness
- Pain
- Emotional conflict
- Financial problems
- Death in the family
- Job or career pressures
- Allergies
- Poor diet
- Substance abuse
- Fatigue
- Environmental pollution

hormone, sex hormones, serotonin, and endorphins—have been found on the surfaces of white blood cells. Such connections serve to integrate the activities of the immune, hormonal, and nervous systems, enabling the mind and emotional states to influence the body's resistance to disease.[4]

Stress and the Adrenal Glands

The adrenal glands, part of the body's endocrine system, are located atop the kidneys. The adrenals are composed of two types of tissue: the adrenal medulla and the adrenal cortex. The adrenal medulla, comprising 10% to 20% of the gland, is located in the interior portion and is responsible for the production of the hormones epinephrine (adrenaline) and norepinephrine (noradrenaline). These hormones are released in direct response to the sympathetic nervous system, which is responsible for the fight-or-flight response to stress or physical threats. The adrenal cortex, the outer layer, surrounds the medulla and accounts for 80% to 90% of the gland. It is responsible for the production of corticosteroids (also called adrenal steroids). Over 30 different steroids have been isolated from the adrenal cortex, including cortisol and cortisone.

As mentioned in chapter 5, secretion of cortisol (as well other adrenal hormones) occurs in daily cycles, peaking in the morning and having the lowest values at night. In response to stress, high amounts of cortisol are released. The body is designed to deal with this, but when stress is frequent or ongoing, imbalances usually result. Chronic high levels of cortisol are linked with low energy, inflammation, muscle dysfunction, impaired bone repair, thyroid dysfunction, immune system depression, sleep disorders, and poor skin regeneration.

A number of studies have found a connection between stress and disturbed sleeping patterns. In one study, comparisons between good and poor sleepers showed that stress and insufficient coping skills contributed to ongoing sleep disorders.[5] Another study indicated that, on average, 41% of insomnia cases were related to stress or other emotional factors.[6] And, though it makes sense that overstimulation due to stress hormones would interfere with sleep, there's also scientific proof of this: A study of 15 chronic insomniacs found that elevated levels of the stress hormones cortisol and adrenaline were inversely related to the amount and quality of sleep.[7]

This dynamic can create a vicious cycle wherein stress leads to sleeplessness, and sleeplessness, in turn, creates a wide variety of problems that can further exacerbate stress. Fortunately, mind-body medicine offers many methods for reducing stress or enhancing your ability to cope with it, ranging from meditation to biofeedback to counseling to aromatherapy. Among the many options you're sure to find something that's a good fit for your lifestyle and personality. And take heart, just as stress and sleep problems can create a terrible negative feedback loop, the opposite is also true: Many mind-body techniques for stress reduction have also been proven to improve sleep. In 1995, a panel of the National Institutes of Health announced that their review of the clinical data showed that meditation and other relaxation techniques (such as biofeedback and hypnosis) can be effective treatments for insomnia and chronic pain. The panel was made up of experts in behavior, pain and sleep medicine, nursing, psychology, and neurology.[9]

The Fight-or-Flight Response

Pioneering stress researcher Hans Selye, MD, a Canadian physiologist, noted a consistent pattern of response to stress and termed these the general adaptation syndrome, commonly referred to as the fight-or-flight response. This response occurs in three stages: the alarm reaction, the stage of resistance, and the stage of exhaustion.

Initially, the body's biochemistry tends to react to stress in an orderly fashion. Stimulation of the sympathetic nervous system activates the secretion of hormones from the endocrine glands and constricts both the blood vessels and the involuntary muscles of the body. When the endocrine glands, particularly the adrenals, are stimulated, heart rate, glucose metabolism, and oxygen consumption increase. The parasympathetic nervous system is also stimulated, which begins a process of relaxation. The pituitary gland responds by releasing a variety of hormones throughout the body to influence the defensive and adaptive mechanisms. Endorphins, the body's own natural painkillers, are also released.

Dr. Selye points out, however, that chronic stress eventually depletes the body's resources and its ability to adapt. If stress continues for a long period, the body's coping functions will be compromised and illness will result.[8]

Are You Stressed-Out?

If you answer yes to more than five of the questions below, it indicates that you have too much stress in your life. In parenthesis after each question are some potential underlying causes for the problem.

- Do you often grind your teeth? (digestive dysfunction, parasites)

- Is your breath shallow and irregular? (low metabolic energy, food allergies)

- Are you hands and feet cold? (hormonal imbalance, adrenal or thyroid weakness)

- Do you have trouble sleeping or tend to wake up tired? (liver dysfunction, food allergies)

Symptoms Associated with Stress

Countless symptoms are associated with stress. Here are some of the most pervasive among them:

- Insomnia
- Headaches
- High blood pressure
- Chest pain
- Indigestion and other digestive problems
- Muscle aches and spasms
- Anxiety
- Depression
- Mood swings
- Forgetfulness
- Weight loss or gain
- Premenstrual syndrome (PMS)
- Bad breath or body odors
- Substance abuse

- Do you often have an upset stomach? (food allergies)

- Do you get mad or irritated easily? (liver dysfunction)

- Do you feel worthless? (low metabolic energy, chronic fatigue)

- Do you constantly worry? (hormonal imbalance)

- Do you have problems concen trating and articulating your thoughts? (low metabolic energy, digestive dysfunction, or hor monal imbalance)

- Do you frequently fidget, chew your fingers, or bite your nails? (food allergies, digestive dysfunc tion)

- Do you have high blood pressure? (food allergies, digestive dysfunc tion)

- Do you eat, drink, or smoke excessively? (low metabolic energy, poor diet)

- Do you sometimes turn to recreational drugs just to get away? (low metabolic energy, poor diet)

Are Your Adrenal Glands Stressed?

The Adrenal Stress Index (ASI; see Resources) evaluates how well one's adrenal glands are functioning by tracking hormone levels over a 24-hour cycle. Four saliva samples taken at intervals throughout the day are used to reconstruct the adrenal rhythm in the laboratory. Saliva has been shown to closely mirror blood levels of hormones, and a saliva test is also less invasive. These samples are used to determine whether two main stress hormones (cortisol and DHEA) are being secreted in proper proportion to each other, and at the right times. Based on the results, a health-care practitioner can prescribe the appropriate treatment to restore the balance of hormones and correct the circadian rhythm.

Mind-Body Therapies for Better Sleep

According to Hans Selye, MD, whether a person experiences stress as a positive motivational force or as a negative detrimental one depends on their perception of the stress.[10] People who perceive that they are in control of their lives (referred to as an inner locus of control) and generally feel good about themselves will use life's stressors in a positive fashion. However, those who feel that their life circumstances are controlled by outside forces and other people (outer locus of control) tend to react negatively to stress. The locus of control can be consciously shifted by deliberately reprogramming the mind with positive instead of negative thoughts, using techniques such as meditation and cognitive therapy. Relaxation therapies, such as biofeedback, hypnotherapy, guided imagery, cranial electrical stimulation, flower remedies, and aromatherapy, among others, can help reduce your stress levels and relieve your sleep problems.

Meditation

Meditation is a safe and simple way to balance physical, emotional, and mental states. It is easy to learn and can have many benefits beyond treating stress and sleep disorders. In the broadest sense, meditation is any activity that keeps the attention focused in the present. When the mind is calm and focused in the present, it is not reacting to past events or preoccupied with future plans, two major sources of chronic stress. The concept of "being here now" can be very important for reversing insomnia, because insomnia, by its nature, creates the opposite state—a person who is lost in the "mental movies" of the mind, out of touch with the body, and stressed. There are many forms of meditation, but they can be categorized into two main approaches, concentrative meditation and mindfulness meditation.

Concentrative meditation focuses the "lens of the mind" on the breath or on one object, sound (mantra), image, or thought to still the mind and allow greater awareness or clarity to emerge. The breath is one of the most popular objects of focus in this type of meditation. As the person focuses on the ebb and flow of their breath, the mind is absorbed in the rhythm and becomes more placid, tranquil, and still. Mindfulness-based meditation entails turning off the mind's internal dialogue and simply receiving whatever exists in the environment without judgment. The meditator attempts to experience each unfolding moment fully, whether this involves visual observations, sounds, tastes, aromas, or sensations. When distracting thoughts

A Simple Meditation Exercise

The first step to practicing meditation is learning to breathe in a manner that facilitates a state of calmness and awareness. Dr. Kabat-Zinn recommends the following exercise for achieving a sense of calmness:

1. Find a quiet place where you will not be disturbed.
2. Assume a comfortable position lying on your back or sitting. If you are sitting, keep your spine straight and let your shoulders drop.
3. Close your eyes if it feels comfortable to do so.
4. Bring your attention to your belly, feeling it rise or expand gently as you inhale and fall or recede as you exhale. Keep the focus on your breathing.
5. When your mind wanders off your breath, notice what it was that took you away and then gently bring your attention back to your belly and the feeling of your breath moving in and out. If your mind wanders away from your breath, your job is simply to bring it back to the breath every time, no matter what it has become preoccupied with.

Practice this exercise for 15 minutes every day, whether you feel like it or not, for one week and see how it feels to incorporate a disciplined meditation practice into your life.

and judgments arise (as they inevitably will), the person simply witnesses these as well, not reacting or becoming involved with thoughts, memories, worries, or internal images. This helps the person gain a more calm, clear, and nonreactive state of mind.

Transcendental Meditation (TM), a popular form of concentration meditation, is the most well-documented regarding the physiological effects of meditation, with over 500 clinical studies conducted to date.[11] Research shows that during TM practice, the body gains a deeper state of relaxation than during ordinary rest or sleep.[12] Brain wave changes during TM also indicate a state of enhanced awareness and coherence. TM has been found to increase intelligence, creativity, and perceptual ability, and to reduce blood pressure and rates of illness by 50%.[13] TM also causes decreased blood levels of the stress hormone cortisol,[14] and increased alpha waves, a brain wave associated with wakeful relaxation.[15]

Meditation has been finding its way into the mainstream for quite some time now. In 1979, Jon Kabat-Zinn, Ph.D., a leading proponent of mindfulness meditation and an expert in behavioral medicine, established the Stress Reduction Clinic and Center for Mindfulness Programs at the University of Massachusetts Medical Center. The clinic's programs teach people how to meditate, reduce stress, and use other mind-body techniques to heal themselves. In one experiment at the clinic, 22 patients suffering from panic attacks and anxiety went through an eight-week course in mindfulness meditation. When the course ended, 20 of them felt significantly less depressed and anxious. In other studies at the clinic, patients with chronic pain reported a 50% reduction in their suffering after learning how to meditate.[16]

"Through meditation, we can learn to access the relaxation response and to be aware of the mind and the way our attitudes produce stress," according to Joan Borysenko, Ph.D., a pioneer in the field of mind-body medicine and cofounder of the Mind-Body clinical programs at two Harvard Medical School teaching hospitals. "By quieting the mind, meditation can also put one in touch with the inner physician, allowing the body's own wisdom to be heard." Instead of running to the doctor for sleeping pills, for example, Dr. Borysenko advises us to pay attention to the body and ask ourselves, "What is going on in my mind or what's happening in my life that I need to attend to?"[17]

Biofeedback

Biofeedback training is a method for learning how to consciously regulate normally unconscious bodily functions (such as breathing, heart rate, and blood pressure) through the use of simple electronic devices. It's particularly useful for learning to reduce stress, eliminate headaches, reduce muscle spasms, and relieve pain. Biofeedback can intercept a chronic fight-or-flight response and aid in revitalizing adrenal gland function. By teaching patients relaxation techniques, biofeedback helps them reduce or eliminate sleep problems.

Biofeedback devices give immediate feedback in the form of information about the biological system of the person being monitored, so that they can learn to consciously influence that system. For example, a person seeking to regulate their heart rate would train with a biofeedback device set up to transmit one blinking light or one audible beep per heartbeat. Electrodes are placed on the person's skin (a simple, painless process), and the person is instructed to use various techniques such as meditation, relaxation, and visualization to effect the desired response (muscle relaxation, lowered heart rate, or lowered temperature). The biofeedback device reports the person's progress by a change in the speed of the beeps or flashes. By learning to alter the rate of the flashes or beeps, the person would be subtly programmed to control their heart rate.

The idea of biofeedback training is that the person will learn how to relax during the sessions with the machine, then use those relaxation techniques by themselves, in daily life, whenever stressful situations arise. For insomnia, biofeedback can be successful if the practitioner uses the biofeedback machine that corresponds to the patient's type of insomnia, according to Melvyn Werbach, MD, an expert in both biofeedback and nutritional medicine. "Biofeedback is appropriate when insomnia is due to overactivation of the autonomic nervous system," Dr. Werbach says. "I use it particularly with people who have a problem with obsessive thinking when they try to go to sleep. This is when EEG biofeedback is most effective."

Similarly, sleep expert Peter Hauri, Ph.D., says that biofeedback about muscle tension can be helpful for those people who are kept awake by extreme muscle tension. In two experiments, Dr. Hauri found that biofeedback had a lasting effect on insomnia. In the first study, at Dartmouth Medical School, 45 insomniacs kept written logs of their sleep habits and then spent three nights in the sleep laboratory. They were given biofeedback training and then continued with biofeedback at home. They returned to the lab for checkups after several weeks and again after nine months. The study showed that insomniacs who were tense and anxious were helped by biofeedback, but it didn't help those whose muscles were relaxed but still couldn't sleep. The second study involved 16 people who had suffered from chronic, severe insomnia for at least two years. The subjects were evaluated during three nights at the Dartmouth Sleep Disorders Center and given a series of questionnaires and interviews. Then they participated in biofeedback training. All 16 experienced improved sleep after the biofeedback training, and this continued through the nine-month checkup. But, again, Dr. Hauri emphasizes that this type of biofeedback works best for people who have insomnia due to tense muscles.[18]

Hypnotherapy

Hypnotherapy has therapeutic applications for both psychological and physical disorders. A skilled hypnotherapist can facilitate profound changes in respiration and relaxation to create positive shifts in behavior and an enhanced sense of well-being. A physiological shift can be observed in a hypnotic state, as can greater control of autonomic nervous system functions normally considered beyond one's ability to control. Stress reduction is a common occurrence, as is a lowering of blood pressure. Hypnotherapy can be a key to switching off insomnia because it provides a way to contact the deeper, unconscious self, let go of old anxiety patterns, and create healthy lifestyle changes in their place.

Hypnosis works by accessing the unconscious mind and training it to react in a positive way, such as inducing an immediate sense of relaxation. It can be a nurturing and highly relaxing experience. Certified hypnotherapists do not attempt to control your mind or take you into a state so deep that you don't have control over yourself. Most people are aware of everything that transpires during a hypnotherapy session, yet they are able to mobilize deeper levels of their mind to facilitate healing.

Hypnotherapy is currently taught in several allopathic medical programs and has been approved by the American Medical Association as a clinical adjunct in the management of chronic pain.[19] Some states certify the profession of hypnotherapy by requiring a certain level of training. Other types of practitioners, such as psychotherapists and bodyworkers, may also use hypnosis as a tool to help their patients relax.

Self-Hypnosis for Relaxation and Sleep

Here's a basic procedure you can use to induce a state of self-hypnosis:

1. Think of an affirmation and place it in the back of your mind. An affirmation is a simple statement of a goal about the future, stated in the present tense as if that goal had already been achieved; for example, "As I sleep soundly, I feel refreshed" or "Each breath enhances my relaxation" or "Every day, I feel calmer and calmer, stronger and stronger, healthier and healthier." The purpose of putting the goal in the present tense is so the subconscious knows it must make what is stated into a reality. The subconscious finds the best and fastest way to that goal.

2. Take three slow, comfortable breaths. Close your eyes.

3. Signal to your body to relax from head to toe. You can suggest that each part feel relaxed, heavy, or warm, or that it is letting go. Say to yourself, "My forehead is relaxed . . . The muscles around my eyes and mouth are relaxed . . . My jaw releases and drops open slightly, releasing all the tension in my face . . . My neck and shoulders are relaxed . . . My arms and hands are heavy and warm . . . My chest and belly are relaxed, as my breathing becomes smooth and calm . . . My hips and buttocks feel heavy and relaxed . . . My knees, calves, ankles, and feet feel heavy and warm . . . My toes are relaxed."

4. Count backward from 100 to 55. Visualize the numbers as you count, either on a large screen coming into focus and fading or seeing the numbers appear in changing colors.

5. Imagine a special place where everything is exactly as you would like it to be. Is it a mountain forest with sunlight filtering through the trees? Is there a rippling stream or a sparkling lake or wildflowers in a field? Is it a tropical beach with crystal clear blue water? Fill in all the details (colors, sounds, textures, and smells) of this place. You may want to build a shelter of some kind there, as simple or as elaborate as you like. Imagine the details of your shelter.

6. Repeat your affirmation three times.

7. Offer thanks to the universe for your creation or a positive occurrence.

8. When you feel ready, say good-bye mentally to your special place and slowly open your eyes. The new thought, feeling, or goal is now part of your subconscious.

Visualization and Guided Imagery

By using the power of the mind to evoke a positive physical response, guided imagery and visualization can modulate the immune system and help with insomnia. These techniques are similar to meditation, except that instead of focusing on the breath or a mantra, you allow your mind to dwell on a positive vision of what you would like to bring into your life; this can, in turn, elicit positive physiological responses. By directly accessing emotions, imagery can help a person understand the needs that may be represented by an illness and can help develop ways to meet those needs. Imagery is also one of the quickest and most direct ways to become aware of emotions and their effects on health, both positive and negative.

Imagery is simply a flow of thoughts that one can mentally see, hear, feel, smell, taste, or experience. According to Martin L. Rossman, MD, cofounder of the Academy for Guided Imagery, while the sensory phenomenon that is being experienced in the mind may or may not represent external reality, it always depicts internal reality.

What Dr. Rossman means is that the sensations in the body that imagery creates are very real phenomena that can be measured via laboratory devices. Research using brain scans indicates that imagery activates part of the cerebral cortex and centers of the primitive brain. During visualization, the visual cortex is active, and when sounds are imagined, the auditory cortex is active. It appears that the cortex can create imaginary realities and that the lower centers (and perhaps every cell in the body) respond to this information. "If you are a good worrier," states Dr. Rossman, "and especially if you ever 'worry yourself sick,' you may be an especially good candidate for learning how to positively affect your health with imagery, as the internal process involved in worrying yourself sick and 'imagining yourself well' are quite similar." This is the same technique that some elite athletes successfully use to visualize winning tennis matches, being strong and poised at the finish line, or breaking world records.

Here's an example of a visualization for someone with sleep problems: You are filling a tub with warm, aromatic, sudsy water. You get in and soak for 20 minutes. Then you get out, dry off with a fluffy towel, yawn, and put on flannel pajamas. You pick up a cup of warm herbal tea and sip it for a few minutes at your bedside. Then you climb into your warm, comfortable bed and easily fall asleep. You sleep soundly and deeply through the night, and your body is nourished by all the deep rest. Then, in the morning, the sun streams through your window and you wake up feeling completely rested and refreshed, full of energy and vitality.

The whole visualization process could take up to 20 minutes. Try to repeat the visualization once or twice a day for a few days; as you're visualizing, feel free to elaborate and add more details. Then, see if you can reproduce the same script in real life.

Counseling

Each person with sleep problems has individual reasons—physical, emotional, or chemical—for disturbed sleep. In many cases, people can resolve sleep problems with nothing more than counseling in what types of behavioral, dietary, or physical changes they need to make and some support in making those changes. Cognitive therapy and cognitive-behavioral therapy can be very helpful for those with sleep problems. First, let's take a look at the purely cognitive aspect of this approach: It has been estimated the average human being has around 50,000 thoughts per day, according to Dr. Richard

Carlson, author of *Don't Sweat the Small Stuff . . . And It's All Small Stuff*. Unfortunately, he reminds us, many of those thoughts are also going to be negative: angry, fearful, pessimistic, or worrisome. Up to 85% of the thinking we regularly engage in is negative and self-defeating.[20]

The basis of cognitive therapy is to identify—through maintaining a journal and by introspection—the negative, self-defeating inner dialogue of thoughts (what cognitive therapists refer to as "automatic thoughts"). Positive, coping thoughts can then be used to counter the negative thoughts. The goal is to pull yourself out of reflexive self-destructive mental behavior that may be exacerbating your sleep problems and to bolster the positive, self-reliant aspects of your personality. Cognitive therapy does not focus on the root causes of psychological problems; rather, it seeks to support health by interrupting the flow of negative thoughts. Countering each negative thought with a list of positive responses to the same situation enables the mind to reframe the situation.

Now let's take a look at the behavioral component of cognitive-behavioral therapy. Many people have disruptive habits that disturb their sleep or contribute to sleep disorders. Identifying the problematic behaviors and changing them can often make a huge difference. People who tend to have conditioned responses to certain stimuli, such as anxiety, when they go into the bedroom might try the following strategies:

● Go to bed only when sleepy.

● Use the bed only for sleeping; do not read, watch TV, or eat in bed.

● If you're unable to sleep, get up and move to another room. Stay up and do something relaxing until you're really sleepy, then return to bed. If sleep does not come easily, get out of bed again. The goal is to associate the bed not with frustration and sleeplessness, but with falling asleep easily and quickly. You may need to repeat this step as many as 10 times a night at first, but that will lessen as your condition improves.

● Don't look at the clock. Awareness of how long you've been trying to fall asleep can contribute to anxiety, making it harder to sleep.

● Set an alarm and get up at the same time every morning, regardless of how much or how little you sleep during the night. This helps the body to establish a constant sleep-wake rhythm.

● Do not nap during the day.

Sleep Checklist

Each morning, check off the recommendations you followed the night before to prepare your mind and body for sleep:

____ Ate an early dinner

____ Filled out worry cards at least 3 hours before bedtime

____ Took a short walk after dinner

____ Avoided focused work after dinner

____ Avoided TV before bed

____ Did light, relaxing activities before bed

____ Drank herbal tea

____ Took a warm bath

____ Set an alarm for 6 A.M. to 7 A.M. or earlier

____ Got in bed before 10 P.M. If later, record time: _____

____ Did breathing exercises to relax in bed

____ Did self-hypnosis to relax in bed

____ Woke up by 6 A.M. to 7 A.M. If later, record time: _____

Those who feel stressed in general or feel they have no control over their lives, which is not uncommon among people who suffer from insomnia, may need to try different strategies. The following technique may be useful: Schedule 30 minutes or more of worry time at least 3 hours before bedtime. Write down what you are worrying about on index cards, then write solutions at the bottom of the card. The purpose is to get these thoughts out of your head and onto paper. Next, put the cards into categories: financial, business, personal, children, spouse, parents, and so on. After you have written the cards, organized them, and given them some attention, deposit all of them in a worry box before you go to bed. At the next scheduled worry time, take them out again, review them, add to them, or change them as need be. If you find the worries creeping back into your mind as you're trying to sleep, say to yourself, "I've already worked that out."

Cranial Electrical Stimulation

Experimentation with low-level electrical stimulation of the brain was started in France in the early 1900s. It was originally called "electrosleep," as it was thought to be able to induce sleep. Newer names developed, such as transcranial electrotherapy and neuroelectric therapy. Research on the use of what is now called cranial electrical stimulation (CES) for treatment of anxiety began in the Soviet Union during the 1950s.[21]

According to Eric Braverman, MD, a specialist in biochemical brain disorders, CES devices work by stimulating brain tissue to produce essential neurochemicals that may have been depleted due to stress or anxiety. These neurochemicals act to increase levels of beta-endorphins in the brain—the substances that produce a feel-good relaxed state or a runner's high.[22] The U.S. Food and Drug Administration has approved CES devices for treatment of insomnia, depression, and anxiety.

In 1996, Daniel Kirsch, Ph.D., a neurobiologist, reviewed 103 studies of CES involving 4,848 subjects. He found there were significant changes in relaxation levels in the subjects who received CES treatments, including slower electroencephalograms and reductions in blood pressure, respiration, and heart rate. In a survey of health-care practitioners who used CES on their patients, 71 of 74 patients who had insomnia reported 95% improvement after using the device.[23]

Some minor side effects reported with CES use are burning at the electrode site or dizziness for a short time afterward. For insomnia, Dr. Braverman recommends using the CES device before bed, but other physicians caution it can be too stimulating and should be used at least 3 hours before bedtime to induce sleep.

Herbal Therapy

Specific herbs with sedative effects can ease stress and anxiety and help with insomnia. Clinical herbalist Terry Willard, founder of the Wild Rose College of Natural Healing, recommends the following seven herbs for people with insomnia: valerian, hops, passionflower, kava, lemon balm, reishi mushrooms, and skullcap.[25] Chamomile or St. John's wort may also be helpful. Most of these herbs are available at health food stores or through your health-care practitioner. Although herbs are natural substances, they do contain powerful compounds (one reason they can help you sleep!). Some of the herbs discussed below can cause drowsiness or interfere with medications. If you're taking prescription medications, make sure you discuss herbal supplements with your doctor.

Acupuncture for Stress Reduction

To help patients cope with stress, as well as correct other imbalances that may be contributing to sleep disorders, practitioners of mind-body medicine often adjust a patient's energy fields. These fields, generally ignored by mainstream practitioners, link the emotions, consciousness, and physical body. "Other cultures recognize that there is a kind of energy that animates us," says Kristy Fassler, ND, a practitioner of both homeopathy and naturopathy. "It's called qi in China, prana in India."

In the Chinese model, qi is considered to be the life force that flows along specific pathways, called meridians, throughout the body. Points of heightened energy along the meridians are called acupoints. Sometimes the flow of qi in the body can become blocked, causing illnesses to develop. An acupuncturist uses the acupoints to stimulate the flow of qi and thus restore health to the body. In addition to its physical effects, acupuncture has a positive psychological effect as well. Acupuncture has effects equivalent to those of drug-based therapies in cases of depression, insomnia, and other nervous disorders, and its action is swift and lasting without the side effects of drugs.[24]

Valerian

The odorous root of valerian (*Valeriana officianalis*) has been used in European traditional medicine as a natural tranquilizer for centuries. In Germany, valerian root and its teas and extracts are approved as over-the-counter medicines for states of excitation and difficulty in falling asleep owing to nervousness.[26] A scientific team representing the European community has reviewed the research on valerian and concluded that it is a safe nighttime sleep aid. These scientists also found that there are no major adverse reactions associated with the use of valerian and, unlike barbiturates and other conventional drugs for insomnia, valerian does not have a synergy with alcohol, meaning it is not dangerous to mix the two.[27] Possessing warming qualities, valerian is also effective in easing muscle pain when applied topically.[28] A randomized, double-blind study of 121 insomnia patients showed that those given 600 mg of valerian extract daily for four weeks slept better and were more rested than those in the control group. About 3% of the subjects in both groups reported side effects.

Willard recommends a dose of 300 to 400 mg of valerian extract (standardized to 0.5% of essential oil) taken about 1 hour before bedtime. It can be mildly habit-forming, with stronger doses required over time to get the same effect, so Willard recommends taking valerian for no more than a month at a time, or for occasional sleepless nights.[29] Rob McCaleb, founder of the Herb Research Foundation, says valerian root extract is his top choice for treating insomnia, and he does not believe valerian is addictive. He says studies have shown that the extract reduces the time it takes to fall asleep and improves sleep quality. He recommends taking valerian 30 to 45 minutes before bed at one of the following doses: 1 to 2 grams of the root in tea; 150 to 300 mg of standardized herb extract; or 1 teaspoon of tincture. He cautions that 10% of people are stimulated, not sedated, by valerian.[30]

Hops

Hops (*Humulus lupulus*) has been used as a bittering and preservative agent in brewing for centuries. In Germany, hops is licensed for use in states of unrest and anxiety as well as sleep disorders due to its calming and sleep-inducing properties. European medicinal plant researchers have approved the use of hops for such conditions as nervous tension, excitability, restlessness, and sleep disturbances, and as an aid to stimulate appetite. Unlike many other sedatives, hops is not associated with either dependence or withdrawal symptoms, nor are there any reports of adverse side effects. Hops tea is effective just before bedtime; use 1 heaping teaspoon of whole hops per cup of water for tea.[31] Christopher Hobbs, cofounder of the American School of Herbalism, recommends a valerian-hops preparation as a daytime sedative because it will not interfere with or slow reflexive responses[32]—again, unlike conventional pharmaceuticals.

Passionflower

Passionflower (*Passiflora incarnata*) has enjoyed a long tradition of use for its mildly sedative properties. In Germany, passionflower is approved as an over-the-counter drug for states of nervous unrest.[33] It is often used in combination with other calming herbs, usually valerian and hawthorn. Pharmacological studies indicate that passionflower extract has antispasmodic, sedative, and antianxiety qualities and that it can also help lower blood pressure.[34] Passionflower is said to help in quieting worry and giving a feeling of well-being. For the anxiety and stress associated with sleep disorders, this can be an effective herb. For a tea, steep ½ teaspoon of the dried herb in 1 cup of steaming hot water; or use a tincture or extract.

Kava

Extracts of the kava plant (*Piper methysticum*; a slow-growing bushy perennial) act as a natural tranquilizer. In one study, 29 patients diagnosed with anxiety (including panic disorder and general tension) took 100 mg of kava three times daily for four weeks. At the beginning and end of the trial, they were evaluated using three standard psychological profiles of anxiety, and all measures were significantly lower at the end. No side effects or adverse reactions occurred, and benefits were noted as early as the first and second weeks.[35] In another study, a subgroup of 101 people taking 100 mg of kava extract three times daily experienced significant improvement in anxiety and tension; the effects were noted from the eighth week of supplementation. Specifically, 20% of those taking kava were rated "very much improved" according to a standard anxiety scale, while only 10.5% of the placebo group received a similar rating. After 24 weeks, the percentages were 53.1% for the kava group and 30.2% for those taking a placebo.[36]

Kava is useful when anxiety is a contributing factor in insomnia or other sleep problems. A typical recommended dose is 100 mg of kava extract (standardized to 70% kavalactones, the active ingredient) daily, divided into three equal doses.

Caution: It's best to consult with a medical professional before taking kava. It can be toxic to the liver, so it is not advised for those with compromised liver function; it also may interact with some pharmaceutical drugs.

Lemon Balm

Lemon balm (*Melissa officinalis*), an herb in the mint family, has long been used as a folk remedy for insomnia. This calming herb is used to relieve tension, anxiety, and other nervous disorders, and to reduce fevers and headaches. To make a tea, Willard recommends steeping 1 to 2 teaspoons of the herb in a cup of hot, but not boiling, water; lemon balm can also be mixed with other sedative herbs.

Reishi Mushroom

For thousands of years, the reishi mushroom (*Ganoderma lucidum*) has been used as a sedative and immune system tonic. It contains a complex of phytochemicals proven to have antiallergenic, anti-inflammatory, and antioxidant

Herbs Can Be Used in Many Forms

Whole herbs: Dried plants or plant parts that are cut or powdered. Depending on their source, whole herbs can have varying degrees of potency and contamination. Buy whole herbs from reputable manufacturers.

Teas: In loose or tea bag form. Steeping herbs in steaming hot water for a few minutes releases their fragrance, aromatic flavor, and medicinal properties.

Capsules and tablets: A convenient and popular form of herbs. Some herbs, such as goldenseal, have repulsive flavors, which can be hidden in a capsule or tablet.

Extracts and tinctures: Highly concentrated herbal preparations that are more quickly assimilated by the body than tablets. Alcohol or glycerin is used as a solvent to extract non-water-soluble compounds from the herb and as a preservative. Tinctures usually contain more alcohol than extracts (sometimes 70% to 80% alcohol). Herbal tinctures and extracts should have the color and taste of the herbs or plants they were derived from.

Essential oils: Oils distilled from various parts of medicinal and aromatic plants. Essential oils are highly concentrated, and many aren't safe for internal use, so make sure you're well informed before using them internally, and even then, use them sparingly. For topical use, dilute essential oils in water or in oil, except eucalyptus and tea tree oils, which can be applied directly to the skin without causing irritation.

Salves, balms, and ointments: Used for muscle aches, insect bites, or wounds. These are usually available in a vegetable oil base.

properties. It is used in traditional Chinese medicine for the treatment of high blood pressure, arthritis, and insomnia and other nervous disorders, and to increase longevity. Reishi is Willard's herb of choice for insomnia because it is calming during the day, reduces anxiety, and is helpful in regulating sugar metabolism. He typically recommends three 1-gram tablets of reishi three times a day.[37]

Skullcap

Skullcap (*Scutellaria lateriflora*), also a member of the mint family, has traditionally been used as a nerve tonic and sedative. Skullcap's calming action comes mostly from the component scutellarin, which is antispasmodic.[38] Willard recommends using this herb in combination with reishi, hops, and valerian, or alone in tincture form (15 to 40 drops two to three times daily). To make a tea, steep 1 to 3 teaspoons of the root in a cup of steaming hot water.

Chamomile

Two different species of chamomile are used in herbal medicine: German or wild chamomile (*Matricaria recutita*) and Roman chamomile (*Anthemis*

Chinese Herbal Formulas for Insomnia

Chinese medicine offers at least six premade herbal formulas (also known as "patent remedies") for restlessness and insomnia, according to acupuncturist and herbalist Lesley Tierra, L.Ac., Dip.Ac. These remedies are available at Chinese pharmacies or by mail order from Chinese herbal suppliers. Dr. Tierra offers the following list of insomnia symptoms matched with the appropriate formula:

Mental agitation. This type of insomnia is accompanied by exhaustion, anxiety, mental agitation, excessive dreaming and thinking, red or irritated eyes, and poor memory. Remedy: Anmien Pien 4 pills three times daily); do not eat hot, greasy foods while using this remedy.

Night sweats. Symptoms include restlessness, anxiety, palpitations, night sweats, vivid dreaming, and nocturnal emissions. Remedy: Emperor's Tea (Tian Wang Bu Xin Wan: 8 pills three times daily). This formula can also help students during times of prolonged study. Dr. Tierra cautions that this formula should not be used for more than two weeks at a time; discontinue for one week, then resume for two weeks if needed. Do not eat hot, greasy foods while using this remedy.

Nightmares. This type of insomnia is characterized by nightmares, restless sleep, night sweats, dizziness, ringing in the ears, palpitations, and fatigue. Remedy: Shen Ching Shuai Jao Wan (20 pills twice daily). Dr. Tierra advises that this formula should not be used for more than two weeks, as overuse can impair digestion; if necessary, resume again after a two-week hiatus. Do not consume cold foods while using this formula.

Uneasiness. The accompanying symptoms include palpitations, poor memory, a sense of unease, excessive dreaming, restlessness, and dizziness. Remedy: An Shen Bu Xin Wan (15 pills three times daily).[39]

nobilis). The flowers of both species produce a calming effect, easing anxiety and reducing tension.[40] It can thus be helpful with overall anxiety, sleep disorders, and muscle tension. Its calming property has a beneficial effect on the gastrointestinal system as well. In Europe, chamomile is recognized as a digestive aid, a mild sedative, and an anti-inflammatory, notably in antibacterial oral hygiene and skin preparations.[41]

St. John's Wort

Long used as an anti-inflammatory, wound-healer, mild sedative, and pain-reliever, St. John's wort (*Hypericum perforatum*) has attracted medical attention in recent decades. Traditionally used to treat neuralgia, anxiety, tension, and similar problems, more recently it has been recommended in the treatment of depression.[42] In Germany, St. John's wort is widely prescribed for depression—by some estimates accounting for as much as 50% of the antidepressant market. In 23 separate clinical trials involving 1,757 patients who reported mild to moderately severe depression, taking 500 to 900 mg daily of St. John's wort extract (containing up to 2.7% hypericin, the active component of the herb) was three times more effective than a placebo and as effective as standard antidepressants such as Prozac and Zoloft. The researchers noted that it generally takes two to four weeks of steady use before the mood-elevating benefits of St. John's wort takes place.[43]

Christopher Hobbs has found St. John's wort useful in sleep disorders as well. He credits this to the same action behind the herb's antidepressant properties—maintaining serotonin levels in the brain. Serotonin is a neurotransmitter that influences mood and helps produce sleep.

Caution: St. John's wort can have negative interactions with some pharmaceutical drugs, and it may increase the side effects of antidepressant medications. If you're taking pharmaceutical drugs, it's best to consult with your doctor before taking St. John's wort.

success story

Homeopathy Cures Insomnia

DOLORES, A 38-YEAR-OLD HOSPITAL DESK CLERK, had tried almost all the traditional and alternative cures for her insomnia, which had been plaguing her for the past five years. She would either fall asleep easily and then wake up at 3 A.M. or 4 A.M., unable to fall back asleep, or if she had trouble falling asleep, she would be up until 3 A.M. Sometimes, she would fall asleep easily but wake up every hour starting around 1 A.M., and then by early morning be awake for good. By the time she came to Thomas Kruzel, ND, Dolores had tried many things, including enrolling in a hospital sleep clinic, sampling several sleep drugs, taking the herb valerian, and supplementing with melatonin, but none of these had helped. Her lifestyle didn't appear to be the issue: She liked her work and had a good relationship with her husband, and she exercised moderately, ate a balanced diet, and had cut down on coffee, which she avoided completely after 10 A.M.

Dr. Kruzel tested Dolores's adrenal function using a salivary cortisol test. He found that she had high cortisol levels late at night. Normally, cortisol levels are highest at about 8 A.M., but Dolores's levels were highest at midnight. She also had higher-than-normal levels of cortisol throughout the day. After taking Dolores's case history, Dr. Kruzel prescribed a single homeopathic remedy: Carcinosin 30C, once per day (two pellets). Although insomnia is one of the indications for Carcinosin, the prescription was based not so much on Dolores's symptom profile as on her family history of cancer, diabetes, and tuberculosis. (The name Carcinosin is derived from carcinoma, a type of cancer. According to the principles of homeopathy, Carcinosin is indicated when there are symptoms of various cancers in the family.[44])

Dr. Kruzel also prescribed phosphatidylserine, a phospholipid that is often successful in inducing sleep (500 mg twice a day), and pituitary glandular supplements (two tablets twice a day with meals, for the first month only). Based on Dolores's blood type, Dr. Kruzel also recommended a vegetarian diet. Although Dolores's diet wasn't particularly an issue, he recommends that all of his patients eat according to their blood type system.

His greatest concern was Dolores's high cortisol levels, which indicated a maladaptive stress syndrome. Even though she appeared happy and calm, her body was signaling that she was under a great deal of stress. After following her new regimen for one month, Dolores was sleeping through the night about half the time, and getting about 6 to 8 hours of sleep per night. Her insomnia patterns persisted on the other nights, but she began to feel much better because she was getting some rest, if not perfect sleep.

> **"Even though she appeared happy and calm, her body was signaling that she was under a great deal of stress."**

Over the next year, Dolores saw Dr. Kruzel at six weeks, at eight weeks, at three months, and then at six months. After 10 weeks, Dr. Kruzel increased the potency of the Carcinosin to 200C to speed up her progress. Dolores stayed on the phosphatidylserine for three months and continued with the diet. After about eight months, Dolores no longer needed either the homeopathic remedy or the supplement and was sleeping through the night almost every night.

Homeopathic Remedies

Homeopathy was founded in the early 1800s by German physician Samuel Hahnemann. Today, an estimated 500 million people worldwide receive homeopathic treatment. Homeopathy is now practiced according to two differing concepts: classical and complex. In classical homeopathy, only one single-component remedy is prescribed at a time, in a potency specifically adjusted to the patient; the physician waits to see the results before prescribing anything further. In complex homeopathy, a prescription involves multiple substances given at the same time, usually in low potencies.

Since there are more than 3,000 homeopathic remedies, derived from everything from plants to minerals to animals, choosing the right remedy can be a challenge. The key is uncovering the pattern of behavior or feelings that accompany the insomnia. In the short-term, some basic remedies can be helpful for occasional insomnia. For chronic insomnia, however, you need what is called a constitutional formula—one that addresses not only the symptoms, but also your underlying life pattern. For a constitutional formula, see a classical homeopath, who will normally thoroughly examine your lifestyle, habits, and medical history before prescribing a remedy.

Homeopathy is based on the principle of "like cures like." This means that the same substance that in large doses produces the symptoms of an illness can cure it in very minute doses. Homeopathic remedies are "potentized" from tinctures, meaning they are diluted and shaken, sometimes 200 times or more. The result is that the final remedy is diluted such a degree that it contains no molecules of the original substance, only its energetic vibration. According to homeopathic theory, the more times the remedy is potentized, the more powerful it is and the deeper effect it will have.

In classical homeopathy, symptoms or disturbances clear up in the reverse order that they occurred, usually beginning with the symptom that caused the patient to seek treatment, such as insomnia. As the more recent symptoms are resolved, new layers of underlying symptoms often present themselves for healing and the practitioner will adjust the remedy accordingly. The underlying layers are often residues of fevers, trauma, or chronic disease that were unsuccessfully treated or suppressed by conventional medicine.

Homeopathic remedies for sleep vary depending on symptoms. For chronic insomnia, you will need to see a classical homeopathic practitioner (or one that is able to use that approach) to get a constitutional remedy. Some basic remedies for occasional, acute, or short-term insomnia are listed below, along with the symptoms each is appropriate for. Take them in 30C potency, in the dosage recommended on the label (usually 3 tablets or 10 drops) 1 hour before going to bed for 10 nights. Repeat the dose if you wake and cannot get to sleep again.[45]

- *Aconite:* Restlessness, nightmares, fear of dying, sleep problems that are worse after shock or panic

- *Arsenicum Album:* Waking between midnight and 2 A.M., restlessness, worry, apprehension, foreboding dreams of fire or danger

- *Belladonna:* Restlessness, irritability, excitement, anger, difficulty falling asleep, overly sensitive to stimuli including light, noise, and touch

- *Chamomilla:* Feeling wide awake and irritable during the first part of night; especially useful for children

- *Cocculus:* Too tired to sleep, giddy

- *Coffea Cruda:* Overactive mind as the result of good or bad news, inability to switch off

- *Ignatia Amara:* Yawning but can't sleep, dread about not being able to sleep (especially after emotional upset), frequent nightmares, grief

- *Lycopodium:* Mind very active at bedtime (repeatedly going over work done during the day), frequent dreaming, talking and laughing while asleep, waking around 1 A.M.

- *Natrum Muriaticum:* Anxiety, anxious dreams, becoming ill after emotional trauma, sensitivity to sudden noise and heat

- *Nux Vomica:* Sleeplessness due to great mental strain, overindulgence in food or alcohol, or withdrawal from alcohol or sleeping tablets; waking around 3 A.M. or 4 A.M., then falling asleep just as it is time to get up; nightmares; irritability during the day

- *Opium:* Sharp senses, bed too hot

- *Pulsatilla:* Restlessness in early sleep; feeling too hot, throwing the covers off, then feeling too cold and lying with the arms above the head; not thirsty; insomnia worse after rich food

- *Rhus Toxicodendron:* Irritability, restlessness, walking about, inability to sleep, especially if there is pain or discomfort

In addition, homeopath and integrative medicine specialist Robert Milne, MD, traces many cases of insomnia to grief. For grieving individuals whose symptoms include irritability, sobbing, and muscle spasms, Ignatia Amara, is often used. Another remedy, Muriaticum Acidum, is recommended for grief-stricken insomnia patients who are marked by extreme emotional sensitivity (another symptom may be an intolerance of sunlight).

Although there is some disagreement on this point, many practitioners believe homeopathic remedies can be rendered ineffective if people consume or expose themselves to strong substances such as coffee, marijuana, mint, camphor, other strong tastes or scents, electric blankets, and dental procedures.

Aromatherapy

Essential oils from plants contain healing agents that are quite powerful. The word *aromatherapy* doesn't do them justice because it makes it sound as though the smell is the full treatment. "In actuality, the oils exert much of their therapeutic effect through their pharmacological properties and their small molecular size, making them one of the few therapeutic agents to easily penetrate bodily tissues," says Dr. Kurt Schnaubelt, director of the Pacific Institute of Aromatherapy. Dr. Schnaubelt says the chemical makeup of essential oils gives them a host of desirable pharmacological properties, including the following:

- Antiviral
- Antibacterial
- Antispasmodic
- Diuretic
- Vasodilation (widening blood vessels)
- Vasoconstriction (narrowing blood vessels)
- Endocrine effects through action on the adrenals, ovaries, and thyroid gland
- Gastrointestinal effects by energizing, pacifying, detoxifying, or facilitating the digestive system
- Treating infections and affecting the immune response
- Interacting with the nervous system
- Harmonizing moods and emotions

Essential oils are usually extracted from the plants by a special distillation method. Pure oils, without any extenders, are the most desirable and have the highest therapeutic value, but they are usually quite expensive. According to certified aromatherapist Marta Schreiner, many of the oils sold at health food stores have some type of synthetic or natural extenders added. People may get minor results from those oils, but if they want a true healing treatment, they need to buy the pure oils. "It takes a large amount of plant materials to make pure oils," says Schreiner. "But the pure essential oils are 75% more potent." She cautions that some manufacturers who advertise "pure oils" actually do use natural extenders. Since it is impossible to verify the purity without chemical analysis, she advises people to buy from reputable sources and expect to pay more for a small bottle of oil.

For insomnia, lavender is the most frequently prescribed oil, either in a diffuser near the bed before sleep or in a bath before bed. Schreiner says her three favorite oils for insomnia are lavender, German chamomile, and marjoram. According to aromatherapist Peter Holmes, MH, L.Ac., lavender is well-known for its actions on the nervous system and particularly the brain. "It will act as a sedative or as a stimulant, depending on actual needs," Dr. Holmes says. "It will act as a sedative in conditions of emotional agitation and unrest, calming the mind, comforting and alleviating fears. With emotional depletion and depression, lavender has a distinctly stimulating effect, transforming depression and reviving the spirits as well as consciousness."[46] Along with lavender, oils of neroli (orange blossom), spikenard, Roman chamomile, and ylang-ylang may be useful for insomnia.

How to Use Aromatherapy

Drops of essential oil can be placed on a heat diffuser to disperse the essence and aroma into the air. Another option is to use an aromatherapy ring, which is placed over a lightbulb to heat the oils. Both are available at health food stores and through mail order. Here are some other ways to use essential oils:

- Add a few drops to massage oil for an aromatherapy massage.

- Add a few drops to the bathtub for a therapeutic soak.

- Add a few drops to hot and cold compresses to soothe minor aches and pains.

- Spray floral waters into the air or on skin that is too sensitive to be touched.

- Apply diluted oils topically. As a general rule, don't apply undiluted oils to the skin because they might elicit an allergic reaction or rash.

- Place a few drops on a pillow or eye shades to waft the fragrance in while you sleep.

Flower Remedies

By balancing negative feelings and stress, flower remedies can effectively remove the emotional barriers to health and recovery. Flower remedies are subtle liquid preparations made from the fresh flowers of various plants, bushes, and trees to address emotional, psychological, and spiritual issues underlying physical and medical problems. The approach was pioneered by British physician Edward Bach in the 1930s, when he introduced the 38 Bach Flower Remedies, based on English plants.

Today, an estimated 20 different brands of flower remedies based on plants native to many landscapes, from Australia to India to Alaska, offer about 1,500 different blends for a diverse range of psychological conditions. Each flower remedy addresses a particular emotional issue. For example, Vine helps to increase feelings of self-worth, Impatiens is recommended for feelings of impatience with others and yourself, and Aspen is for feelings of fear. An individualized formula can be made by combining four to six of the remedies. Flower remedies are taken orally or rubbed into the skin. They can be taken for a short time to cope with a crisis or for a period of months.

Flower essences are made by floating fresh blossoms in spring water and letting them sit in the morning sun for 3 hours (or heating them by fire, as with some English essences). The blossoms are removed and what is left is the mother essence, which carries the vibratory energy—although no actual physical trace—of the flower. The essence is then diluted to the stock level, which is the form generally available commercially; the stock level can be diluted again to the dosage level. To use the essence directly from stock, place 4 drops under your tongue or in a little water; this dosage usually is taken four times a day. Another way to take the essences, especially if you are taking more than one, is to mix 4 drops of each into a large glass of water, stir, and sip it throughout the day. For baths, use about 20 drops of stock essence per tub. Stir the water to help potentiate the remedies, then soak for about 20 minutes. For topical use, add 8 to 10 drops of stock essence per 1 ounce of cream, oil, or lotion.

Flower remedies are often selected according to their ability to work with a specific imbalanced emotional pattern rather than a physical complaint such as insomnia, as the imbalanced pattern is usually what is causing the physical symptoms. However, there are specific remedies that can be helpful for insomnia, often because they address anxiety: Aspen, Black-Eyed Susan, Chamomile, Chaparral, Dill, Lavender, Mugwort, Red Chestnut, St. John's Wort, and White Chestnut.[47] Flower essences can be useful for insomnia in the following ways:

- They can help to ground and embody, bringing mental and spiritual components in alignment with a physical relaxation response.

- They can open and clarify, to awaken consciousness. Sometimes when we awaken the consciousness, that allows the physical part of the body to go to sleep.

- They can help resolve repressed emotions and fears. They can also help deal with deep-seated fears that hinder the body's ability to relax (fears due to trauma, such as physical injury or the death of a loved one).

- They can help hypersensitive people or highly allergic people, who overreact to their environment.

- They can help people who are reacting to geopathic stress by fostering the development of a healthier immune system.

seven

Step 5: Protect Yourself from Environmental Factors

Chapter 4, on detoxification, discussed "the usual suspects" in regard to toxicity: synthetic chemicals, heavy metals, and other pollutants in the air, water, and soil, as well as inner toxins. However, some less familiar environmental factors can also have negative effects on the body and play a role in disrupting sleep, particularly electromagnetic fields (EMFs), geopathic stress, and qi. EMFs, a type of low-level radiation generated by computer monitors, televisions, fluorescent lights, electronic devices, and sometimes wiring, are generated when electric currents flow through wire coils, so every time you turn on an electric current, EMFs are produced. Although you can't see, hear, or feel them, they're very real, and they do have impacts on the body. They can pass through almost anything except lead barriers, but their strength does diminish with distance. Most common household and office devices emit very low frequency (VLF) or extremely low frequency (ELF) electromagnetic fields.

The earth itself produces some energy fields that can be detrimental to human health as well; this is commonly referred to as geopathic stress. While the intensity of these fields is small, studies continue to show that they may be a factor in a number of chronic illnesses, including cancer, heart disease, and sleep disorders. And while qi, the life force energy central to the philosophy of traditional Chinese medicine, is innately benign and positive, blockages in qi, both in environments and in the body, can have negative effects. In this chapter, we'll look at how these various types of energy affect the body, how to detect them, and therapeutic options for protecting yourself from their harmful effects.

Alternative Medicine Plan for Reducing Toxic Exposure

- Prudent avoidance of EMFs
- Feng shui for fostering sleep
- Relieving geopathic stress
- Creating a comfortable bedroom environment
- Sleeping on a body-friendly mattress

success story

Combating the Side Effects of Technology

EVERY NIGHT, Janice, a 34-year-old executive secretary, had trouble staying asleep. She would wake up several times during the night, tense and stressed, unable to fall back to sleep for 30 minutes or more. Tired all the time from such restless nights, Janice also suffered from headaches, red and irritated eyes, and frequent colds and flu. After months of trying different approaches on her own without success, Janice sought help for her sleeping problems.

Janice spent her workdays surrounded by electronic equipment such as computers, cell phones, and fax machines, all of them generating electromagnetic fields (EMFs). Her symptoms and a complete medical evaluation pointed to chronic overexposure to electromagnetic fields. Janice was given two protective devices to use at work. The first was a screen that Janice placed over her computer monitor, designed to shield her from some of the electromagnetic fields generated by the monitor. (A flat-panel monitor is another good option for reducing EMF exposure—if you or your employer are willing to invest in upgrading). Janice also installed a QLink ClearWave device (see Resources) in her office, designed to neutralize random EMFs emitted by electronic devices. The night after she installed the ClearWave device, she began to sleep better. In three months, all her symptoms were gone, including the insomnia and restless sleep. QLink also offers a pendant with a crystal chip that is said to boost the body's bioelectric field and help offset the negative effects of EMFs. It also increases energy, focus, and concentration, and is believed to boost melatonin as well.

Electromagnetic Fields—The Dark Side of Technology

An electromagnetic field can be likened to an invisible energy web (shaped somewhat like the contour lines on a topographical map) produced by electricity that, in turn, creates a magnetic field. While EMFs are part of nature and in fact are radiated by the human body and its individual organs, the quality and intensity (called respectively frequency and gauss field strength) of the energy forming this contoured web can either support or undermine health. As a general rule, EMFs generated by technological devices tend to be more harmful than naturally occurring EMFs.

Researchers once thought EMFs, especially very low frequency and extremely low frequency EMFs, were safe because they were of such low strength compared to other forms of radiation, such as those from a nuclear reactor or X-rays. But now, as technology proliferates and people are using more electronic devices, some researchers suspect EMFs are contributing to a subtle assault on people's immune systems and overall health.

Electromagnetic changes in the environment can adversely affect the energy balance of the human organism and contribute to disease. We are surrounded by stress-producing electromagnetic fields generated by televisions, computers and video terminals, microwave ovens, overhead lights, power lines, electrical wiring, and motors that can generate higher-than-normal magnetic energy. EMFs interact with living systems, affecting cell division and multiplication, enzymes related to growth regulation, and the functioning of the pineal gland, which regulates the sleep hormone, melatonin.

In 1979, Nancy Wertheimer, Ph.D., and Ed Leeper, Ph.D., epidemiologists at the University of Colorado, found that children who had been exposed to high-voltage lines in their early childhood had a two to three times higher than normal risk of developing cancer, especially leukemia.[1] That was the first study to establish the direct link between EMFs and cancer. In 1987, a large-scale study conducted by the New York State Department of Health confirmed Dr. Wertheimer's findings and added that EMFs from high-voltage power lines also affect the neurohormones of the brain.[2] Since then, various studies have indicated that electromagnetic fields may be linked to increased incidence of heart disease, Alzheimer's disease, high blood pressure, headaches, sexual dysfunction, and blood disorders—the latter including a 50% increase in white blood count.[3]

However, it's important to note that this topic is extremely difficult to research, and newer research seems to contradict some of these findings. While childhood leukemia and sleep disturbances do appear to be linked with EMFs,[4] recent studies indicate that there may be less cause for concern in regard to other health conditions.[5] Part of the uncertainty stems from the difficulty in isolating single environmental factors as causes of health problems.

This does not mean that a stressor such as EMF does not contribute to health issues, but rather that it is difficult to quantify its effects. We are beings of frequencies, and given the amounts of EMF radiation that we have to deal with on a daily basis, it is possible that there's a danger to our human physiology. But as to the potential for harm from EMFs emitted by your toaster or hair dryer, the rules and guidelines are still being established.

And there's actually yet another side to this complex issue. Some researchers and medical professionals see promise in using very low currents of electromagnetic radiation to heal the body instead of harm it. Dr. Robert Becker discovered that a small electrode implanted inside the body next to an unhealed bone fracture could speed healing.[6] Becker has also explored the possibilities for using electrical current to heal other conditions, including cancer, but he cautions that more work needs to be done to establish solid scientific evidence.[7] Other medical professionals, such as physical therapists, acupuncturists, physicians, and chiropractors, use various therapies, such as TENS (transcutaneous electrical nerve stimulation) or electroacupuncture, that involve sending a very small electromagnetic current into an injured part of the body, usually to reduce pain.

Electromagnetic Fields Are Part of Nature

Electromagnetic energy is not solely a phenomenon of technology. The life force itself, the earth that we live on, and all living things are intricately connected to and by electromagnetic energy fields. Dr. Becker, twice nominated for the Nobel Prize in Medicine, proved in a series of animal experiments that human and animal bodies carry their own electromagnetic currents, complete with positive and negative charges. In addition, he showed that trauma to the body creates an electromagnetic "current of injury" that stimulates the healing process and, in some animals such as salamanders, initiates regeneration. It was those experiments that led to his findings about how electric currents could be used to heal bone fractures.[8]

Millennia ago, the Chinese recognized our intimate link with energy fields by identifying energy pathways, known as meridians, in the body. They use the word *qi* to describe the electromagnetic life force that flows through these meridians. Much of traditional Chinese medicine consists of finding ways to keep the natural electromagnetic energies of the human body in alignment and in balance with each other. The Chinese also honor the earth's life force and electromagnetic energies through their science of feng shui (pronounced FUNG-shway), which studies ways of creating natural energy flows in a given environment that are beneficial to people and in harmony with nature. Its purpose is to create the most beneficial flow of qi, or life force energy, in an environment (home, office, or other setting) by arranging furniture, plants, decorations, buildings, or rooms in ways that are most in line with the natural energy field.

But although electromagnetic energy is part of nature, there is concern about the health effects of the artificial, technology-generated electromagnetic fields. Some researchers think the artificial EMFs are upsetting the natural balance of our bodies as the number of EMF-generating devices increases.

Sources of EMFs

The greatest concern about EMFs is not from a one-time use of a hair dryer or an hour in front of a computer, but from cumulative exposures: continuous high levels of EMFs hour after hour, day after day. For example, people who travel extensively in airplanes can have high exposure rates, up to 85 milligauss in the airplane cabin. EMF exposure from hair dryers, heaters, electric shavers, and other appliances can be injurious to health over time. Food mixers, hair dryers, and vacuum cleaners emit EMFs that are 30 to 100 times greater than the suggested safety limit.[9] Ordinary household appliances tend to generate larger cumulative EMF exposures than power lines. The reason is proximity: Most people do not live close enough to power lines to be greatly affected by their EMFs, but the situation is different with kitchen appliances, computers, cell phones, televisions, even electrical outlets if they're located behind the head of a bed. Although the EMFs from appliances drop off rapidly with distance and are usually at minimal levels at a distance of 4 to 8 feet. However, people often stand or sit closer than this to the source of EMFs—typically 18 inches from computers, a few feet from televisions, and almost no distance at all from cellular phones.[10]

A unique type of EMF exposure is from electric blankets, which give you close-up exposure at high levels (50 to 100 milligauss) all night long. According to noted brain researcher Russel J. Reiter, Ph.D., electric blankets are dangerous because they are close to the body and they expose the entire body to EMFs, which are thought to lower levels of melatonin, the hormone secreted by the pineal gland to control the sleeping and waking cycle and regulate the body's internal clock, or circadian rhythm. Because electric blankets are used at night, when the pineal gland is producing its highest amount of melatonin, they have the greatest chance of disrupting melatonin production and sleep.[11]

Another concentrated source of EMFs is the breaker box, where the electric power line enters your home. That fuse box—which connects the utility company's line with the inside wiring—generates large amounts of EMFs on a continual basis. Another potential EMF source is the wiring in your home. Older wiring sometimes generates high amounts of EMFs at the electrical outlets, whether or not anything is plugged in. Check your outlets with a gauss meter, and if levels are high, consider installing new wiring or having a professional reconfigure the existing wiring pattern.

Outside the home, electric power lines can also be a major EMF source. As mentioned above, some scientists believe that exposure to EMFs from electric power lines is responsible for a wide variety of health conditions. And some activist groups are so concerned that that they're advocating the closure of public facilities such as schools that are located near power lines, and even suggesting overhauling the electric power delivery infrastructure.[12] Dr. Becker says we are constantly exposed to a background level of EMFs generated by the electric power delivery system. In urban areas, this so-called ambient field level, which exists both inside and outside the home, could exceed 3 milligauss. In the suburbs, the ambient field ranges from 1 to 3 milligauss. Dr. Wertheimer and others said in their studies on power lines that constant surrounding levels of 3 milligauss or more were significantly related to increases in the risk of childhood cancer. Dr. Becker advocates 1 milligauss as a safe limit for continuous exposure to 60-hertz fields (the usual kind generated by electric power systems).[13]

Electromagnetic Fields and Sleep Disorders

Researchers suspect artificial EMFs cause sleep problems in a number of ways. First, the fields have a higher strength and rate of oscillation (meaning they vibrate at a higher number of cycles) than the natural electromagnetic energy fields of the body at rest. In addition, EMFs can disrupt the body's production of the sleep hormone melatonin.

High Oscillation Rate and Strength Disrupts Sleep

The frequency at which an EMF pulses determines whether or not it is harmful. For example, the voltage of the electric current used in homes in the United States is 60 hertz (Hz). In contrast, the ideal frequency of the human brain during waking hours ranges from 8 Hz to 20 Hz, while in sleep the frequency may drop to as low as 2 Hz. The higher frequencies of EMFs generated by artificial electrical currents may disturb the brain's natural resonant frequencies and, in time, lead to cellular fatigue, according to John Zimmerman, Ph.D., president of the Bio-Electro Magnetics Institute.[14]

While common household electric currents oscillate at a rate of 50 to 60 Hz, this is slow compared to an FM radio station broadcast that comes to you on waves that oscillate at 100 million times per second, or 100 megahertz. Generally, the higher the frequency of the wave, the more energy it has and also the more potential it carries for damage.

But even 60-hertz EMFs are vibrating much faster than the human body's brain wave patterns at rest. For example, if you have an electric clock radio on your bedside nightstand, it is generating 60 Hz EMFs at a distance probably not more than 1 or 2 feet from your head. This is a problem because your brain waves in deep sleep oscillate at 2 to 4 cycles per second (2 to 4 Hz). The EMFs from the clock radio could interfere with your brain's rest pattern and prevent you from falling asleep or from staying in deep sleep. Some alternative practitioners recommend removing all electric appliances from your bedroom, or at least from close proximity to the bed.

Equally as important as the oscillation frequency of the EMFs is their strength (measured in gauss). Most common appliances generate very low frequency or extremely low frequency EMFs measured in units of milligauss (thousandths of a gauss). The strength of the field decreases with increasing distance from the appliance or device. For instance, an electric fan may have an EMF of up to 900 milligauss at 4 inches, but at 3 feet it is only 5 to 20 milligauss. A computer monitor may have an EMF measuring up to 600 milligauss at a 4-inch distance, but at 1 foot it is only 3 to 30 milligauss. A microwave oven may have an EMF up to 90 milligauss at 1 foot, but at 3 feet it drops to 3 to 5 milligauss.[15]

EMFs Can Disrupt Melatonin Production

One of the main reasons why medical professionals and others are concerned about EMF exposure levels is a growing body of research showing that EMFs have a negative impact on melatonin production in the body. EMFs from household sources are so weak that the electrical currents they induce in the human body are actually weaker than those induced by the electrical activity in nerve and muscle cells. Yet even these low-frequency EMFs can alter gene expression, the activity of enzymes involved in growth regulation, calcium balance in the cell, and the brain's metabolism of the hormone melatonin.[16]

Melatonin, a hormone produced by the pineal gland in the brain, was once thought to be unimportant. However, in recent years, researchers have found that it is present in every cell of the body and is essential in regulating the body's clock, or circadian rhythm, the mechanism that controls our sleep-wake cycles. Your pineal gland registers the amount of light in your surroundings, and if it finds no light, it increases the melatonin level, signaling your body that it's time to go to sleep. If light is present, melatonin production decreases and you feel more awake. Thus, restoring and maintaining adequate amounts of melatonin is crucial for people with sleep disorders. Other factors besides light decrease the body's production of melatonin, including aging, certain prescription drugs, stress, poor nutrition, and EMFs.

Researchers have discovered that an adequate level of melatonin does much more than regulate sleep; it also improves immunity, has anticancer and antiaging effects, can relieve depression, and may boost sexual function. Those types of health conditions are the same ones that researchers say may be caused or exacerbated by EMF overexposure. The connection between melatonin and EMFs appears to be getting more solid evidence. For example, in 1996 a team of researchers found that blood melatonin levels in female rats decreased after exposure to 50 Hz magnetic fields, about the same frequency as most household appliances. Many similar studies on melatonin are now underway.[17]

At the same time, not being exposed to naturally occurring EMFs can have a negative impact on health, for they function as a kind of energy nutrient. Kyoichi Nakagawa, MD, one of the world's foremost researchers in the field of magnetic treatment of disease, observes that the amount of time people now spend in buildings and cars (tightly enclosed spaces) reduces their exposure to the geomagnetic field of the earth and may interfere with their health. Dr. Nakagawa calls this condition "magnetic field deficiency syndrome" and notes that it can cause headaches, dizziness, muscle stiffness, chest pain, insomnia, constipation, and general fatigue.

Geopathic Stress and Sleep Disturbances

The concept of geopathic stress has been well researched and substantiated in Germany since the 1920s. The theory is that in some locations, the earth (*geo*) generates energies that are detrimental (*pathic* as in *pathological*) to humans living or working in structures immediately above their source. These energies—electromagnetic or more subtle in nature—can put chronic stress on the body, eventually producing sickness.

Geopathic stress is an abnormal energy field, usually of an electromagnetic nature, generated deep underground by large mineral deposits, water streams, or geological faults. As British researcher Jane Thurnell-Read explains in *Geopathic Stress*, this abnormal energy occurs "when the earth's magnetic field is disturbed, either naturally or artificially, and the background field we normally experience is changed."[18] Artificial disturbances can be produced by mining, foundations for tall buildings, subways, and public utility pipes, such as for sewers and water, says Thurnell-Read.

European research indicates that if you work or, especially, sleep over an area of geopathic stress, you may get sick from continuous exposure to this abnormal energy. Sleep disorders are common in this situation, as are symptoms such as unaccountable irritation or depression, susceptibility to colds, waking up tired, and a slow deterioration in vitality, health, and mood.

While most of the emphasis on EMF exposure has to do with artificial EMFs (generated by utilities, appliances, and electronic devices), natural patterns of electromagnetic energy can also affect people—for both good and ill. The earth itself has an electromagnetic field of about 0.5 gauss. Compared to the magnetic strip that holds your refrigerator door closed, which has about a 200-gauss strength, the earth's field is weak. However, living things are able to sense even minute fluctuations in the earth's field. Experiments with homing pigeons and even bacteria have shown this to be true, and scientists have identified magnetlike mechanisms in people and other creatures that act to align our energies with those of the earth.[19]

Researchers around the world have documented cases where currents of energy coming from the ground caused sleep disorders, headaches, depression, and other symptoms. The concept of geopathic influences from the earth took root in Germany in 1929, when Baron Gustav Freiherr von Pohl made a systematic tour of the community of Vilsbiburg. It had 565 houses, 3,300 residents, and an unusually high rate of cancer. Von Pohl was acting on a hunch inspired by a survey of Stuttgart in the 1920s that showed a clear correlation between major geological faults in the city and those districts that had the highest cancer mortality rates. His tentative conclusion was that an unknown but noxious radiation emanating from the faults might be an important and overlooked factor in the cancers.

Baron von Pohl located all the major subterranean water veins (lying at a depth of 144 to 164 feet with a width of 10 to 13 feet) under Vilsbiburg, then mapped their courses onto a map of the city streets. Next, he cross-checked this with the residences of the 54 people who had recently died of cancer and arrived at a startling conclusion: "The completed check of my map confirmed all the beds of the 54 cancer deaths were where I had drawn the radiation currents," von Pohl wrote in 1932 in *Earth Currents: Causative Factor of Cancer and Other Diseases.*[20] Von Pohl also presented dozens of cases in which rapid, perhaps miraculous, cures of numerous complaints, from insomnia to heart spasms, were achieved by simply moving the sleeper's bed out of the geopathic zone.

"The effects of geopathic stress undermine and weaken a person's life force," says Thurnell-Read. "This does not mean that geopathic stress causes illness; rather, by weakening the body, it provides a fertile ground in which ill health can flourish." She says strong earth energies can specifically influence brain rhythms, cellular renewal, functioning of specific body parts, the blood, and electrical activity in the body.[21] These effects can have a detrimental influence on sleep.

In 1971, the theory of geopathic stress was supported by research showing that water flowing underground, especially subterranean streams that cross, produces measurable increases in magnetic anomalies; these conditions also increase electrical conductivity in the air and soil and cause other physical changes. While the changes may be small (in the vicinity of 10 inches square), they are still capable of contributing to the development of serious illness.

"The magnetic field of the earth is an important physiologic factor for living organisms," says Dr. Becker. "It appears that behavioral changes of an undesirable nature, either quite evident or subtle, may result from environments having lower or higher field strengths than normal."[22]

It is possible to measure earth energies using a machine called a magnetometer. Dr. Scott-Morley, an alternative medicine practitioner extremely knowledgeable about geopathic stress, says that if people are particularly sensitive to geopathic stress, it can make it difficult for them to maintain their normal balance of health. Geopathic stress zones may be tiny, but according to Dr. Scott-Morley, shifting a bed a few feet in a geopathically troubled bedroom can make the difference between sleep and insomnia for the susceptible individual. The growing popularity of feng shui, the Chinese science of landscape interpretation and household exterior and interior design, is bringing the concept of geopathic stress to a larger audience in the West.

success story

Bedroom Feng Shui Helps a Child Sleep

DAVID, AN 8-YEAR-OLD BOY with brain damage from birth, was a restless and fitful sleeper. He had trouble falling asleep, and when he did sleep, he would wake up every 2 hours and be unable to fall back asleep for at least 30 minutes. David's parents, afraid he would hurt himself through tossing and turning or banging his head against the wall, were afraid to let him sleep alone and had to take turns sleeping with him.

David attended special physical therapy sessions during the day and took muscle relaxants, but his parents did not want to put him on sleeping pills. Hoping that changes in his physical environment might help, they consulted with a feng shui practitioner. The practitioner determined that David was closely aligned with the earth element, meaning he would be most comfortable around items related to nature, such as natural fabrics, earth-toned colors, plants, crystals, terra cotta pottery, trees, and stones. He would also be most comfortable sleeping close to the ground. Unfortunately, David's bedroom, was unsuited to his personality profile. It was entirely white because David's parents believed he was unable to perceive colors. His bed was high off the floor, and there were very few decorations. The overall effect was one of being in a sterile hospital room.

The first thing the feng shui consultant did was move David's bed onto the floor, to give him a feeling of being grounded. Then, she and David's parents painted the walls of the room a rich earthy yellow. They added items from nature on the walls and ceiling, such as feathers, crystals, and Native American animal totems and symbols of peace. They placed a handmade Native American tapestry on the bed and plants in terra cotta pots around the room. They covered the pillows with colorful handmade fabric and replaced the carpet with a tile floor to give a feeling of being outdoors. Finally, they added a window that opened out onto the family's garden, to give a feeling of freedom and connection with nature.

Within a week after the bedroom was redesigned, David was sleeping comfortably by himself. His periods of sleep began increasing in length until, by the end of the month, David was sleeping 8 hours straight, without waking up in the middle of the night.

Alternative Medicine Plan for Reducing Toxic Exposure

A number of therapeutic options are available for dealing with EMFs and geopathic stress and returning to restful sleep. Reducing your daily exposure to electrical devices and EMFs is the simplest way to help yourself. Feng shui, the Chinese art of placement, can help you realign your bedroom for better sleep. Finally, make sure that your bedroom environment and bedding materials are conducive to sound sleep.

Prudent Avoidance of EMFs

For many people, it is not that easy to control the surrounding EMF field, unless they move to a home away from any power lines or transformer boxes.

The safest and most effective strategy is "prudent avoidance"—taking steps to reduce your personal exposure to EMFs from appliances, tools, electronic devices, and office equipment. There are some simple steps you can take immediately to reduce your EMF exposure. As you consider these suggestions, be aware that the degree of exposure depends on both distance from the source and duration of exposure:

- In the bedroom, place all electric devices at least 3 feet from the bed, including lamps, alarm clocks, televisions, and heaters. (You may even want to try turning off all circuit breakers before going to bed for three nights to see if there is any improvement in your sleep.) If you sleep on a water bed, turn off the heater before you go to bed and, in cold weather, preserve the heat in the water with an insulating pad. Don't use an electric blanket except to heat the bed. Be sure to unplug it before you get in; don't leave it on through the night.

- In the bathroom, avoid or reduce use of a hair dryer. Use a safety razor instead of an electric one.

- In the kitchen, don't stand in close proximity to the microwave, dishwasher, or other appliances while they are in operation. Consider converting to a gas range if your stove is electric.

- Vacuum cleaners and portable electric heaters generate fairly strong EMFs, as do power tools.

- Turn off computer monitors, TVs, and other electronic devices when not in use.

- When possible, avoid or minimize proximity to transmission lines, especially high-voltage lines.

It's a good idea to find out what levels of EMFs you are actually exposed to in your home or office. This can help you decide where to place furniture you use often, which devices to turn off when not in use, and so on. You can check EMF levels with a gauss meter, an inexpensive handheld device that can measure the EMFs emitted by any electrical equipment. If you live in an apartment or condominium, be sure to check any shared walls around your bed for the presence of hidden junction boxes. (Your electric utility may also do this for you.) This will help you determine which sources pose the greatest danger and guide you on avoidance strategies.

Researchers disagree as to whether monitor screens are needed. Some say they are more important for older monitors, since newer models have been engineered to reduce the user's exposure to EMFs. The need for a screen may also depend on the person using the computer: some people are highly sensitive to the EMFs computer monitors generate, while others report no adverse effects.

In her book *Radiation Protection Manual*, enzyme specialist and researcher Lita Lee, Ph.D., says that most screens block only the monitor's electric energy fields and not its magnetic energy fields. The dominant type of emission from computer monitors is extremely low frequency (ELF) magnetic fields. Thus, many protective screens may not be offering complete protection from EMFs. If you purchase such a screen, check as to whether the screen blocks glare, electric fields, magnetic fields, or some combination of these three.[23] Robert O. Becker, MD, who has done decades of research in the area of electromagnetic energy, says the best advice is to put some distance between you and the monitor. He recommends using a detachable keyboard that can be placed further from the computer and the monitor.[24]

A number of devices are available that may provide protection from harmful EMFs. Products include fabrics, pendants, bedding, headsets, and paint. See the Resources section for more information.

Feng Shui for Fostering Sleep

The term *feng shui*, which literally means "wind and water," is drawn from the ancient Chinese philosophy of Taoism, which linked energies of the solar system and earth with human habitation and activities. Feng shui embodies ideals for placement of objects and structures in inhabited environments. It can also be used to document the flow or impedance of basic life force energy, or qi, through environments, homes and other structures, and rooms and their benefits or disadvantages for inhabitants.

Qi is a Chinese word variously translated to mean "vital energy," "essence of life," and "living force." In Chinese medicine, the proper flow of qi along energy channels (meridians) within the body is crucial to a person's health and vitality. There are many types of qi, classified according to source, location, and function, such as activation, warming, defense, transformation, and containment. However, qi has two essential qualities: yang (active, fiery, moving, bright, energizing) and yin (passive, watery, stationary, dark, calming). According to this view, everything in the universe is subject to a constant interaction of yin and yang. Location, shape, size, color, weather, and other subtle influences all produce various levels of yin and yang energies. Feng shui seeks ways to harmonize and balance these energetic patterns.

These energies are categorized into five basic energy movements linked to the five elements of traditional Chinese philosophy: south (fire), center (earth), west (metal), north (water), and east (wood). As you can see on the accompanying table (see "The Five Elements of Feng Shui," page 169), these energy movements correspond with certain colors, shapes, and seasons of the year. Thus, in feng shui, objects, furniture, rooms, and buildings are not static but have particular energetic qualities that can affect our responses to them.

For example, most people have a favorite color. Perhaps you naturally favor a particular shade of blue. One way of looking at your preference is that the cool energy of blue corresponds to your attitude or personality type in some way. These subtle influences of color, shape, and space are the purview of feng shui. "Ordinarily our senses perceive the most obvious forms of motion—traffic passing by in the street or the cool rush of the wind against the skin," says Master Lam Kam Chuen, author of the *Feng Shui Handbook*. "We are less conscious of the subtle movements of energy as it passes invisibly through the space of an open room or the vibration of the patterns of energy in the walls and furnishings."[25]

The Nine Basic Cures

In feng shui, the cure or remedy for spaces that don't feel comfortable is to add items that help to stimulate, moderate, or move the qi. These cures can be very simple, such as adding a mirror, but on a subtle energy level they will create a difference that people will feel. In a bedroom, for example, it is advisable to add yin elements, such water sounds, and to avoid overly stimulating yang items, such as a television. Here are the nine basic cures:

1. Bright or light-refracting objects: A mirror, a crystal ball, or lights. Mirrors are considered the "aspirin" of feng shui because they cure many ills.

2. Sounds: Wind chimes or bells.

3. Living objects: Plants such as bonsai and flowers or an aquarium or fishbowl.

4. Moving objects: A mobile, miniature windmill, or fountain.

5. Heavy objects: Stones or statues.

6. Electrically powered objects: An air conditioner, stereo, TV. These are not recommended for the bedroom because they are too stimulating.

7. Bamboo flutes.

8. Colors: Most auspicious are red, green, blue, yellow.

9. Other items: For example, chalk under the bed to cure a backache.[26]

The Energy Friendly Bedroom

Here are some ways to make your bedroom a health-enhancing, not health-draining, environment:

The Five Elements of Feng Shui[27]

	Fire	Earth	Metal	Water	Wood
Direction	South	Center	West	North	East
Season	Summer	Indian summer	Fall	Winter	Spring
Color	Red	Yellow	White	Blue/black	Green
Shape	Triangular	Square	Round	Horizontal and curving	Rectangular
Representations	Candles, red objects	Terra cotta, ceramics, yellow objects	Wind chimes, metallic objects	Aquarium, fountain, black or blue objects	Plants, flowers, green objects

- One factor to consider is where the bedroom is located within the house. Since sleep is considered a yin activity, bedrooms should be on the yin, or nonsolar, shady side, which is usually north (in the northern hemisphere) or east. The solar side, usually west or south, gets more sun exposure and is better for rooms for yang activities, such as an office, living room, or kitchen. If it is not possible to have your bedroom on the nonsolar side of the house, you could add some trees or water sounds, such as a fountain outside the window, to provide cooling, yin energy.

- Where you put the bed is very important in feng shui. Ideally, it should be diagonally across from the room entrance so that people in the bed have a full view of anyone coming in the door.[28] If you move your bed to straddle the corner, be sure to put a headboard or shelf behind it with plants, candles, stones, or other nurturing items. Corners are considered a place where qi can stagnate unless you add items that keep the qi flowing. If you can't place the bed kitty-corner to the entrance for some reason, add a mirror to reflect the entryway or place a wind chime between the entrance and the bed and keep a mirror opposite the entrance. Also, try to have the bed face the morning sunlight, if possible.

- Avoid placing your bed next to a window because you will lose too much vital energy (qi) out the window during the night. Also, the

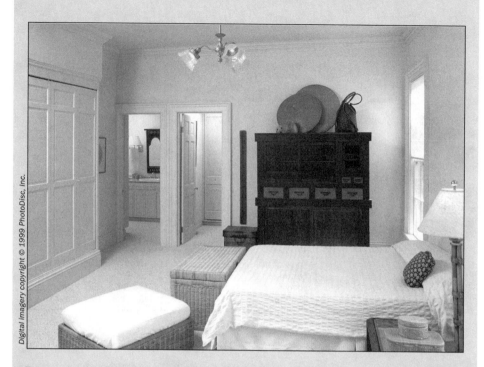

Feng shui aims to maximize the flow of basic life force energy, or qi, through environments, homes and other structures, and rooms for the benefit of inhabitants. For sleep problems, it is important to create a soft, calm, and nurturing atmosphere in the bedroom. For example, the bed should be diagonally across the room from the entrance so that people in the bed have a full view of anyone entering. Other doorways (to the bathroom, for instance) should not be in direct line with the bed. Also, the bed should not be placed directly beneath a window, as too much vital energy will be lost during the night. In general, avoid sharp angles and clutter, which can agitate the flow of energy in the room.

energy coming in the windows at night could disrupt your body's yin energies and prevent sleep. But allow as much air and sunlight as possible into the bedroom during the day to accumulate qi; this will help replenish your body during sleep.

● Besides the position of the bed, also pay attention to other details of flow of qi. If you have a bathroom off the bedroom, for example, be sure to buffer the qi of the bathroom from the qi of the bedroom with a curtain, mirror, or other divider. If you have a desk in the bedroom, have it screened off or away from the main flow of qi.

● Don't place your bed under an exposed beam. If it runs lengthwise down the bed, it may alienate the couple sleeping in the bed; if it crosses the bed at chest level, it may create health problems.

- Don't place a mirror at the foot of the bed. When you wake up in the middle of the night, you may mistake your own visage for a ghost's.

- Don't use your bedroom as a storage area, especially under the bed. Negative or detrimental qi can accumulate.

- Place something pleasant and attractive or a beautiful scene (either a painting or a window view) beside your bed or in the line of vision from your bed so that, upon waking, you are greeted by this and start the day on a bright note.

- Avoid harsh angles. Never place your bed under a low slanting ceiling or any other angular protrusion in your bedroom. These features can contribute to headaches, confused thinking, illness, and possibly financial or career problems.

- Do not face sharp edges. The sharp edges from bookcases, dressers, and other furniture in the bedroom should not face where you lie in bed. The energy coming off the edges is sharp and can harm your health and create irritability.

- Avoid "poison arrows." A bedroom with an irregular shape (in which edges such as a closet jut out) generates, geometrically speaking, "poison arrows." A sleeper regularly exposed to these influences is subject to minor health problems, mood swings, and loss of concentration. If you're stuck with a poison-arrowed corner or sharp-edged furniture, hang a crystal from the ceiling in front of the sharp edge or position a plant or folding screen to block any edges.

- Remove electronic devices, such as a television, from the bedroom; they are too stimulating. This applies especially to office equipment, such as a computer.

- Try to use cooling colors, such as blues and greens, in darker shades for your curtains and bedspreads. Bright colors such as red or bright pink are too stimulating. In general, try to create a soft, nurturing atmosphere.

- Keep the qi fresh. Ultimately, feng shui is about managing the flow of qi for the best advantage of people within a given environment. In *Feng Shui: Secrets That Change Your Life*, Li Pak Tin and Helen Yeap say that qi is "the animating life force that is everywhere; it permeates your home, physical surroundings, the rivers, roads, trees, and all people." The goal of feng shui is to constructively employ this qi and to "disperse, disrupt, or remove obstructions" in its free flow.[29]

Relieving Geopathic Stress

How can you know if you suffer from geopathic stress? You could engage a skilled dowser, kinesiologist, or feng shui expert to assess your home; or, if you suspect the influence of geopathic stress, implement some of the following recommendations and see if you feel better. (Some of these recommendations will require the expert advice of a qualified dowser, who can confirm and pinpoint the existence of problem areas underneath the house.)

- Move your bed: The average person spends 6 to 8 hours a day in the bedroom sleeping, making this part of the house the one most likely to transmit geopathic stress if it exists underground. As geopathic stress often occurs in thin bands, relocating the bed elsewhere in the room may take you out of the zone of influence.

- Hang where the dog lies: Cats tend to sleep in places of geopathic stress, while dogs assiduously avoid them. If your dog has a favorite spot in the bedroom, relocate your bed there. If you suspect you have geopathic stress in your bedroom and your cat likes perching on your bed, move the bed. Feng shui experts also observe that ants, termites, bees, and wasps (as well as bacteria, viruses, and parasites) thrive in areas of geopathic stress, while chickens, ducks, and most birds do not.

- Use cork tiles and plastic sheets: Lay untreated cork tiles under the bed or between the box spring and mattress for a few weeks. The cork is said to neutralize the detrimental energies, at least temporarily. Plastic sheeting will also screen out geopathic energies for about a week, but then must be replaced, according to Karen Kingston in *Creating Sacred Space with Feng Shui.*[30]

- Get a new bed: Kingston notes that if you have a metal bed frame or a mattress with metal springs and your bed sits over an area of geopathic stress, "the metal will conduct the harmful radiation throughout the bed."[31] She recommends trading in your heavy metal box springs for a wood-framed bed with a natural cotton mattress.

- Pile crushed marble or quartz in specific locations: Placing small piles (4 to 7 pounds each) of either crushed marble (such as garden centers sell) or quartz crystals at specific locations within your bedroom and house may offset geopathic stress, according to Jane Thurnell-Read, an expert in geopathic stress. (The precise locations must be identified by an expert dowser, kinesiologist, or feng shui consultant.) It is believed that these stones somehow absorb the detrimental or negative energies. It is necessary to wash the crystals or marble regularly to remove any accumulations of such energy, she advises; soak the stones in a bucket into which cold water flows for 30 minutes.

- Install copper coils: Thurnell-Read suggests placing several pairs of copper coils as high as possible in the house, even hung from the ceiling or placed in a loft; these will accumulate the detrimental energies. Each coil should consist of 10 revolutions of copper wire; in a pair, one is coiled clockwise; the other, counterclockwise. Like the marble and crystals, the coils need to be refreshed regularly, in the same manner. (The coils can be quite small, just several inches long.)

- Mirror it back down: Placing small mirrors in strategic locations in the bedroom can directly offset, neutralize, or reflect back to their source the "rays" of unfavorable energies. In some cases, strips of aluminum foil (multiple layers work best) can also deflect detrimental energies, says Thurnell-Read. Often, both mirrors and foil work even when blocked by furniture or wallpaper, provided their size and positioning are correct.

- Put magnets on the water pipes: It can be helpful to affix two to four magnets (800- to 1,200-gauss strength) on an incoming water pipe with the magnets' south-seeking poles pointing inward to the pipe, advises Thurnell-Read. Magnets may also be attached to walls, ceilings, or floors to work against geopathic stress.

- Neutralize underground water streams: Australian engineer and architect George Birdsall cites the case of a bedroom in which three underground streams crossed under the bed of a child who was chronically sick. The presence of three "black streams," as feng shui experts call such streams, amplified the unhealthy energy. To correct this, Birdsall recommends inserting a ½-inch thick copper pipe into the ground at the upstream end of the water flow, as determined by a skilled dowser. "After correction, the negative effects dissipate for some distance up and down stream," he says in *The Feng Shui Companion*.[32]

- Copper pipes yield sleep: Birdsall also advises using ½-inch copper pipe for removing the energy influences of a geological fault. He corrected a bedroom in which a seven-year-old boy had insomnia due to two geological faults beneath the room. Birdsall notes that the copper pipes pounded into the ground at the upstream end of the fault (in terms of its energy flow) should have a few twists at their tops.

Creating a Comfortable Bedroom Environment

Once you have your bedroom arranged in a manner conducive to sleep, you can take care of sensory elements such as light, sound, and temperature. First, the right room temperature during sleep can be crucial. For most people, the best sleeping temperature is between 60°F and 70°F. If the temperature is above 75°F, you may have nighttime awakening, increased movement in bed, and shallower sleep. Cold feet can also keep you awake. If your feet get cold, warm them in a foot bath or tub before going to sleep, then wear socks in bed to keep your feet warm.[33] Although it may be tempting to use a heating pad, there are contraindications for this—including the EMFs it will generate. A hot water bottle or something similar is a better bet.

Be sure your bedroom is quiet and completely dark at night. Ear plugs and eye masks, available at most pharmacies and department stores, are options for blocking noise and light. An eye mask can be useful if your window curtains or shades don't block enough light. For noise, another option is a white noise machine, which produces ocean sounds or other calming background sounds to mask any disruptive noise.

Snoring is a nighttime noise problem that ruins not only sleep, but relationships as well. If you have a partner whose snoring is disturbing your sleep, your partner needs to get treatment, or at least be evaluated by a medical professional. Snoring, especially heavy snoring, may be a symptom of sleep apnea, in which a person temporarily stops breathing and has frequent awakenings during the night. Derek S. Lipman, MD, author of *Snoring From A to ZZZZ*, says snoring used to be thought of as little more than a social handicap or nuisance, but it's now considered a legitimate medical problem. As a first line of treatment, snorers who are overweight can try losing weight to see if that allows air to move through the throat and sinuses more easily. If not, the snorer can try some of the antisnoring gadgets available, including a wrist bracelet that gives sleepers a mild electric shock if they snore.

Sleeping on a Body Friendly Mattress

Part of making your bedroom a restful sleep haven is to have a bed that is firm enough to support your body weight but cushioned enough to let you sleep through the night. Mattresses generally start to deteriorate after about eight years. If yours is relatively new, you may only need to add a top layer of extra cushioning. Try spreading a sleeping bag on top of your mattress to see if you sleep better and feel more comfortable. If so, you can buy an inexpensive foam pad or mattress pad that will cover your mattress and give you the extra cushioning you need. Besides cushioning, you also want to test your mattress for sag. Try putting a sheet of plywood under the mattress. If you feel better after sleeping on it for a few nights, you need a firmer mattress—or you can just leave the plywood in place.

If you decide you need a new mattress, you have many options: You can buy a ready-made mattress and box spring off the shelf, or you can have one custom made. Although a water bed can feel soft and warm, they generally don't breathe and they tend to sag under your body's heaviest parts. Air beds are more adjustable, but they can be expensive; plus, sometimes the vinyl core is hot. A high-density foam mattress is firm, but some people may find it too hot, as well. Because of these reservations, most people choose an innerspring mattress because they're widely available, offer many choices in firmness, and are cooler and drier because air can circulate around the coils.

An innerspring mattress consists of rows of tempered steel coils sandwiched between insulation and cushioning. Firmness and durability are based on the thickness of the wire and number of turns per coil. The thicker the wire and the more turns per coil, the stronger and firmer the mattress. In general, the higher the coil count, the firmer the mattress. A standard 500-coil mattress is considered somewhat soft. Look for thicker wire and more coils if you want a firmer mattress.

Memory foam is another option you might consider. This technology was first invented by NASA to help astronauts more comfortably withstand the enormous pressures they experience on liftoff. Mattress companies have taken this technology and put a great deal of money and research into developing it into some of the most comfortable mattresses available. However, people have different responses to memory foam; some love it, while others can't stand it. If you're unsure, briefly lying on a memory foam mattress in a showroom is unlikely to be enough to help you make your decision. Fortunately, you can begin by purchasing a memory foam topper that can be placed on top of your current mattress. If it has a positive impact on your sleeping experience, this may be all you need to do. If you feel there's still room for improvement, you might consider purchasing a memory foam mattress. In either case, consider going with memory foam the next time you purchase a mattress.

Beyond helping with sleep, memory foam has allowed some people to resolve long-standing issues such as chronic back pain. In truth, the two issues are interrelated; if you have less discomfort, you'll sleep better. Because memory foam supports the curves of the body and provides the support the body, it can help eliminate restless, pain-filled nights and provide relief from back pain the following day.

The top layers of cushioning in a mattress are important not only for their firmness, but also for their ability to breathe and prevent overheating. Even though metabolism slows during sleep, our bodies still produce up to 80 watts of heat per hour. Often the top layers of mattresses are polyester and cotton on top of polyurethane foam—materials that don't have very good absorption and breathability. The optimum material for these layers is wool, which wicks moisture away from the body.[34]

When you're in the store buying a mattress, lie down in the position you usually sleep in and have a companion check your alignment for sags or a scrunched posture. Most people do well with a medium-firm mattress with a medium-soft top layer of padding to cushion their hips and shoulders. However, if you sleep on your side or stomach, you might prefer a medium-firm top. And if you sleep on your back and have a lot of curve in your low back, you might need a softer mattress to support and cushion your spine.

Avoid Bedding Materials That Make You Sick

People who are sensitive to chemicals and synthetic fabrics can get severe allergic reactions to toxic materials in certain types mattresses, pillows, and even sheets. For some people, the reaction can develop into a syndrome called multiple chemical sensitivity (MCS). Symptoms could include headaches, nausea, breathing problems, and joint pain, according to Lynn Marie Bower, author of *The Healthy Household: A Complete Guide for Creating a Healthy Indoor Environment.*

And now, thanks to overzealous regulation, all of us are being shoehorned into buying mattresses that contain toxic chemicals that can make anyone sick, not just those with MCS. All new mattresses have to conform to guidelines in a federal law passed in 2006 designed to ensure your mattress won't accidentally catch fire from a dropped cigarette.[35] In a test that vastly exceeds the power of the average cigarette, mattresses must now pass a rigorous high-intensity flame test in which they're subjected to a two-foot-wide flame from a blowtorch for 70 seconds. To make mattresses that can withstand this test, manufacturers must use excessive amounts of toxic, carcinogenic fire-retardant chemicals. Mattress companies are under no obligation to tell the pubic about these chemicals; all they have to do is label the mattresses "flame-retardant."

These toxic materials can and will leach out of the mattress and into your body,[36] and as a result, the time you spend in bed may be contributing to a future cancer or some other degenerative illness rather than being a restorative time that contributes to your well-being. This is especially true for those with chemical and other environmental sensitivities or weak immune systems. Even cribs mattresses must contain these chemicals.

But in reality, a federal law passed in 1973 served the same purpose, but with lower standards that didn't require saturating mattresses with such high amounts of toxic chemical. It's a shame that people who don't smoke (and even those who do) are being exposed to this health risk; if health were really the uppermost concern, they should have passed a law against smoking in bed! But as of February 2006, if you wish to purchase a mattress that doesn't contain these harmful chemicals, you must obtain a doctor's prescription and then actively search for a company that manufactures mattresses free of such chemicals.

Look for other ways to reduce toxicity in your bedroom, too. Whenever possible, buy your bedding and carpets from companies that use natural fabrics, such as wool and cotton. Make sure the companies don't coat their fabrics with fire-retardant chemicals or other chemicals to keep them from wrinkling. For example, avoid polyester and polyester-blend percale sheets, which are coated with formaldehyde to resist wrinkling. The formaldehyde gives off gases for the life of the sheets. In people with formaldehyde sensitivity, the gases can cause coughing, throat and eye irritation, headaches, nausea, nosebleeds, and, insidiously, insomnia. Look instead for high-density, combed-cotton percale sheets, without a "no-iron" or "easy-care" designation. Similar problems exist with mattresses and pillows stuffed with polyurethane foam; consider a natural cotton mattress or futons and pillows stuffed with cotton or buckwheat.[37]

eight

Step 6: Balance Your Hormones

Hormone levels can have a profound influence on sleep. Indeed, one of the primary symptoms of midlife hormonal changes for both men and women is disturbed sleep. In addition to aging, other factors that can contribute to hormonal imbalances are stress and our increasingly toxic environment. Rebalancing hormone levels through nutrition, hormone therapy, and herbs may help you return to getting a good night's sleep.

Hormonal Imbalance and Sleep Disorders

The word *hormone* comes from the Greek *hormon*, meaning "to stir up." Hormones are released by the various endocrine glands in the body in order to regulate energy production, growth, sexual development, stress responses, and many other functions. Because minute quantities of hormones can "stir up" so many activities in the body, when they are thrown out of balance the results can affect the entire body. A common symptom of hormonal imbalance is insomnia and other sleep problems.

Hypothyroidism, or low thyroid hormone levels, a condition that's surprisingly common, is a prime example of the interactions between hormones and sleep. The thyroid gland is located in the throat, just below the larynx. The thyroid is the body's metabolic thermostat, controlling body temperature, energy use, the rate at which organs function, and the speed with which the body uses food; it affects the operation of all body processes and organs. Of the hormones the thyroid synthesizes and releases, T3 (triiodothyronine) represents 7% and T4 (thyroxine) accounts for almost 93%. The secretion of both these hormones is regulated by thyroid-stimulating hormone (TSH), which is secreted by the pituitary gland, located in the brain.

The thyroid plays a key role in the interaction between REM and non-REM sleep cycles and patterns of hormone secretion from the endocrine system during the night. Both

Alternative Medicine Plan for Balancing Hormones

- Dietary recommendations
- Natural hormone therapy
- Herbal therapy
- Traditional Chinese medicine
- Homeopathic remedies

TSH and T4 show a definite circadian pattern, and levels of TSH directly affect the onset of REM sleep periods.[1] Researcher and enzyme specialist Lita Lee, Ph.D., says that people with low thyroid function generally also have low blood sugar. When blood sugar is low, the body produces adrenaline to compensate, which induces the fight-or-flight stress response. Low blood sugar often occurs at night (because we eat less frequently then), and the resulting adrenaline surge can wake a person up and make them tense. The end result can be sleep maintenance insomnia.

Common symptoms of hypothyroidism are chronic fatigue, aches and pains, depression, weight gain, cold limbs, poor hair and skin quality, and insomnia. For this condition, Dr. Lee often prescribes a thyroid glandular extract, such as Armour Thyroid (a glandular extract is a purified nutritional and therapeutic product derived from animal glands). According to Dr. Lee, when people with both hypothyroidism and insomnia improve their thyroid function, they usually start sleeping better in a short time.

Women's Hormones and Sleep Disorders

For women at midlife, the natural interplay between the two primary female hormones, estrogen and progesterone (see "A Hormone Glossary," page 184), takes on a new significance. As a woman approaches menopause, her hormone levels begin to shift, and this can start to occur as much as 10 to 15 years before menopause. Many women don't realize that they may start having some symptoms of menopause long before what is still referred to as "The Change" is due; this phase of changing hormone levels and its symptoms is called perimenopause. These symptoms, which include insomnia, night sweats, fluctuating moods, little interest in sex, and memory loss, are indications that levels of the basic female hormones are shifting or out of balance.

Perimenopause affects every woman differently, but some liken it to "PMS from hell"—an apt comparison because both are brought on disproportionately high estrogen levels in relation to lowered progesterone. Perimenopause

Peaks and Troughs of Estrogen Secretion throughout a Woman's Life

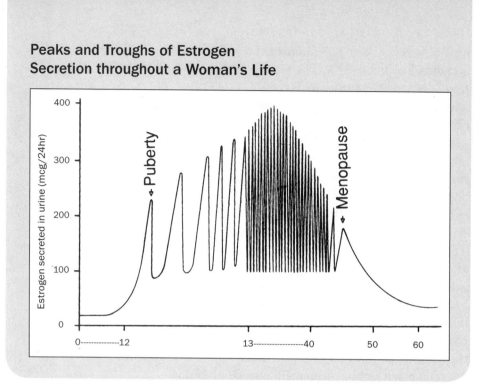

has been associated with a significant increase in sleep disturbances.[2] In fact, disturbed sleep is one of the primary complaints that causes women to seek treatment for menopause and perimenopause. It's estimated that about two-thirds of women who visit the Yale Mid-Life Center are afflicted with insomnia.[3]

Although levels of both estrogen and progesterone diminish as a woman approaches menopause, progesterone usually falls off more rapidly. The resulting imbalance is known as estrogen dominance, a condition that women's health expert John R. Lee, MD, describes as "toxic to the body.[4] If the liver is overburdened by other toxins, this will exacerbate the situation; one of the many jobs of this hardworking organ is to break down excess estrogen and neutralize its metabolites. Estrogen-dominant women also tend to retain fluids and salt and to crave carbohydrates, which can lead to blood sugar problems and insulin imbalances, both factors in disturbed sleeping patterns. This imbalance can also cause cascading effects throughout the endocrine system, and as a result, throughout the body. For example, it can interfere with the function of the thyroid and the action of thyroid hormones, causing hypothyroidism, yet another factor that can contribute to sleep problems.[5]

Adrenal function, stress, and the balance of estrogen and progesterone are also intimately intertwined. As described in chapter 6, stress causes the adrenals to release cortisol and other stress hormones. Chronic stress can lead to adrenal exhaustion, which leads, in turn, to reduced progesterone, and any of these factors can have a negative effect on sleep.

Estrogen is necessary for the smooth functioning of the sleep cycle, so when women enter menopause and their estrogen levels start to fluctuate and diminish, they are likely to experience disturbances in their sleep. Levels of estrogen can directly alter the circadian pattern of neurotransmitters affecting sleep, particularly serotonin and norepinephrine (adrenaline). In one study, 25 menopausal women classified as "bad sleepers" (based on questionnaires about their sleep patterns) were placed on a program of hormone replacement therapy with an estradiol transdermal gel. After three months, 18 of those women were rated as "good sleepers," a 72% response rate.[6] A randomized, double-blind study involving 63 postmenopausal women over a seven-month period found that hormone therapy "improved sleep quality, facilitated falling asleep, and decreased nocturnal awakenings and restlessness."[7]

Hormone fluctuations influence body temperature and as a result can cause insomnia indirectly because of the increased frequency of hot flashes and night sweats during perimenopause and menopause.[8] In a recent study, over 81 percent of women with severe, frequent hot flashes showed signs of insomnia, including unsatisfying sleep patterns and problems falling asleep. Therefore, treating hot flashes could be an important way to ease the symptoms of insomnia for menopausal women.[9] For night sweats and hot flashes, wearing clothing that wicks absorbs sweat and wicks moisture away may help the sleeper feel more dry and comfortable (see Resources section).

Signs of Imbalanced Female Hormones

The symptoms of hormonal imbalance are almost without number, especially during menopause and perimenopause. These symptoms are also highly individualized. Here are a few of the most common and troublesome symptoms:

- Insomnia
- Fluid retention
- Hot flashes
- Loss of libido
- Night sweats
- Moodiness
- Memory loss

Men's Hormones and Sleep Disorder

A man's testosterone levels start to slowly decrease beginning around age 30, then decline more rapidly around age 60. Signs of andropause (sometimes referred to as "male menopause") are usually noticeable by the time men reach their midfifties, though some men may experience symptoms sooner. The andropause complex of symptoms includes lack of energy, loss of muscle mass, weight gain, a loss of interest in sex and possibly some sexual dysfunction, depression or emotional malaise, irritability, panic attacks, decrease

Signs of Decreased Male Hormones

- Insomnia
- Weight gain (particularly around the abdomen)
- Loss of lean muscle mass
- Fatigue
- Depression
- Heart disease
- Hair loss
- Loss of sexual interest
- Infertility or impotence

in short-term memory, and insomnia, among others.

These are signs that a man's hormones—their levels and ratios to one another—are in flux, shifting into a new configuration at midlife. "Men experience a 'lite' version of menopause, physically," says Theresa L. Crenshaw, MD, author of *The Alchemy of Love and Lust*. "Their hormones and neuropeptides diminish, albeit less abruptly. Their bodies sag and change shape. Sexual functioning is often compromised by hormonal imbalance, disease, medications, mind, or mood. Their stamina and temperament alter as well. Yet often they are less well-equipped to deal with these extremes than women."[10]

This hormonal shift can lead to sleep problems in a number of ways. Testosterone is involved in blood sugar control. Decreased levels of the hormone are associated with increased insulin output, a factor for the development of sugar imbalances and insomnia. Decreased testosterone levels can also lead to an increase in blood levels of the stress hormones adrenaline and cortisol. If this state persists for an extended period of time, sleep disturbances can result. "Testosterone has been shown to be an antagonist of the stress hormones," says Eugene Shippen, MD, author of *The Testosterone Syndrome*. "More testosterone, less stress hormone production."[11]

There also appears to be a direct relationship between testosterone levels and REM sleep, according to a clinical study. Testosterone levels in four male subjects were measured at 10- to 20-minute intervals throughout the night. Researchers found a pattern of increases in testosterone concentrations just prior to the onset of periods of REM sleep.[12] Researchers on another study confirmed this finding, stating that there were "positive associations . . . between sleep efficiency, decreased latency to onset of REM, and a number of REM episodes, and circulating testosterone."[13] Thus, fluctuations in testosterone during andropause could have a profound effect on sleep.

Causes of Hormone Problems

A number of factors can cause hormone imbalances in women and men. Hormone levels generally decline as a result of aging, but they can also be affected by dietary choices, mineral deficiencies, environmental toxins and synthetic chemicals, medications, smoking, and stress.

Causes of Hormone Imbalances in Women

Estrogen dominance (excessive estrogen in relation to progesterone) can be created by numerous factors. Eating a diet high in estrogenic foods can be a major cause, because many foods are high in estrogen or compounds similar to estrogen. When you consider that eggs are a reproductive structure, and that a fair amount of the milk in the United States is produced by pregnant cows, you can understand that these foods are full of hormones—including estrogen—that can affect human physiology. Even eggs and dairy products from animals raised organically will contain these hormones. Plant foods also contain estrogen-like compounds, referred to as phytoestrogens (*phyto* means "plant"). However, we can control these dietary sources of estrogen if we avoid these foods or minimize our intake of them. More insidious is flood of synthetic estrogen-mimicking chemicals, known as environmental estrogens or xenoestrogens, which are increasingly pervasive in our food, air, and water. Herbicides, pesticides, by-products of plastics manufacturing, and many other synthetic chemicals mimic estrogen once they enter the body. The body responds as if it is real estrogen, resulting in estrogen dominance and all the problems that imbalance carries with it.

Environmental estrogens aren't just a problem in highly polluted areas. These chemicals have penetrated even into seemingly remote and pristine environments, like the Arctic, where they are affecting reproduction and other physiological functions of polar bears. Once in the body, they accumulate and persist for decades. There is no doubt that something is seriously interfering with normal human hormonal and endocrine functioning, states Theo Colborn, Ph.D., a senior scientist with the World Wildlife Fund and an environmental scientist. Since 1945, synthetic chemicals (such as DDT, DES, PCBs, dioxins, among many others) have been released into the air, water, soil and have found their way into our food and ultimately our bodies. At least 51 of these have been conclusively shown to disrupt the human endocrine system. Each year, an estimated 2,000 new synthetic chemicals enter the world market, swelling the planetary total to well over 100,000. All of these are completely foreign and potentially harmful to endocrine function, but almost none have been thoroughly tested for long-term, transgenerational health effects. Evidence is accumulating that these chemicals, even at very low concentrations and exposures, can, by disrupting the endocrine system, cause hormonal havoc.[14]

Progesterone normally exerts a balancing effect on estrogen that neutralizes it, but stressful situations can disrupt the estrogen-progesterone

A Hormone Glossary

Estrogen: a female sex hormone produced mainly in the ovaries, regulates the menstrual cycle. Estrogen is important for adolescent sexual development, prepares the uterus for receiving a fertilized egg, and affects all the body's cells; its levels decline after menopause. Estrogen slows down bone loss, helps reverse the incidence of heart attacks, and acts as an antiaging factor.

Progesterone: A female sex hormone produced in the ovaries that prepares the uterus for a fertilized egg and then stops cell proliferation in the uterus if pregnancy does not occur. When estrogen is high (days 7 to 14 of a woman's cycle), the level of progesterone is at its lowest. Its levels climb to a peak around days 14 to 24 and then drop off again just before the start of menstruation. Around age 35, a woman usually starts producing less progesterone.

Pregnenolone: The parent hormone for DHEA and other key hormones. It has powerful effects on the brain, enhancing memory, improving concentration, reducing mental fatigue, and generally helping to keep the brain functioning at peak capacity.

DHEA (dehydroepiandrosterone): Naturally produced by the human adrenal glands and gonads, with optimal levels occurring around age 20 for women and age 25 for men. As an antioxidant, hormone regulator, and the building block from which estrogen and testosterone are produced, DHEA is vital to health. Low DHEA levels have been associated with diabetes, hypertension, obesity, heart disease, Alzheimer's, and immune dysfunction illnesses. Test subjects using supplemental DHEA reported improved sleeping patterns, better memory, an improved ability to cope with stress, and decreases in body fat.

Testosterone: The primary male sex hormone, important for the development of male sexual characteristics. Testosterone can help reverse male impotency, heighten virility, and increase muscle mass. After andropause at midlife, testosterone levels decline.

Cortisol: Secreted by the adrenal glands, which are located atop the kidneys. Secretion of cortisol (as well as other adrenal hormones such as DHEA, adrenaline, and aldosterone) occurs in daily cycles, peaking in the morning and having the lowest values at night. Cortisol promotes protein building, regulates insulin and blood sugar metabolism, and helps produce prostaglandins, fatty acids with hormonelike functions. Under conditions of stress, high amounts of cortisol are released; chronic excess secretion is associated with obesity and suppressed thyroid function.

balance. Betty Kamen, Ph.D., psychologist, nutritionist, and author of *Hormone Replacement Therapy: Yes or No?*, says that under prolonged stress, the body uses progesterone to make cortisol, one of the adrenal hormones.[15] As progesterone is used up in cortisol production, there is nothing left to balance or offset the effects of estrogen.

Both women and men can be affected by all of these various environmental and dietary factors involved in estrogen imbalance, but for a woman, an additional factor may be involved—her own body. If a woman has chronic constipation or toxic buildup in her intestines, any excess estrogen is reabsorbed by her body instead of being eliminated, further adding to the imbalance.

Another contributing factor to estrogen dominance is perimenopause (the 10 to 15 years before the actual cessation of menses), which depletes progesterone supplies and skews the estrogen-to-progesterone ratio.

Chronic stress can also be a factor. The adrenal glands respond to stress by producing the hormones adrenaline and noradrenaline. Progesterone is the primary raw material the glands use for producing the adrenal hormones; the more adrenaline, the more progesterone needed. This is how chronic stress can lead to a state of progesterone deficiency (or estrogen dominance). Emotional disturbances, along with many other symptoms that may arise as a result, can potentially lead to sleep disturbances.

Causes of Hormone Imbalances in Men

The concept that men go through major midlife physiological changes, potentially with an impact equal to that of menopause, is beginning to gain acceptance. But most men still remain unaware that they will experience a predictable decline in hormone production at midlife, notes Julian Whitaker, MD, a nationally recognized alternative medicine educator and cofounder of the California Orthomolecular Medical Society. As noted above, a man's testosterone levels naturally start to decrease around age 30, with a more rapid decline around age 60.

Dietary factors can influence a man's hormone levels as well. The typical Western diet, with its high levels of dietary fat and low levels of fiber may have a direct influence on testosterone production, according to clinical studies.[16] Other foods that have been found detrimental to hormone balance include saturated fats (commonly found in fast foods, processed foods, and red meats), hydrogenated oils, preservatives, and products containing refined sugar.

10 Reasons Why Women's Hormones May Be Imbalanced

Estrogen dominance (too much estrogen in relation to progesterone) can be created by either an excess of estrogen or a deficiency of progesterone, or both. Here are some of the key causes too much estrogen may caused by:

1. Foods that are high in hormones, particularly animal products, but also soy products

2. Herbs that have estrogenic effects in the body, such as licorice, black cohosh, and damiana

3. Birth control pills that have high levels of estrogen

4. Environmental toxins that mimic the actions of estrogen (xenoestrogens), most notably pesticides

5. Exposure to radiation, which increases estrogen levels in the blood

6. Chronic constipation, which interferes with the body's ability to eliminate estrogen properly

7. Supplemental estrogen as part of hormone replacement therapy for menopausal symptoms

Too little progesterone may be caused by:

8. An underactive thyroid gland (hypothyroidism)

9. Chronic stress

10. Frequent anovulatory cycles (menstruation without ovulation)

The minerals zinc, copper, and selenium are necessary for normal hormone production in men. In one study, a group of patients was given 1.4 mg of zinc daily while a second group received 10.4 mg per day. While blood levels of zinc did not vary between the groups, the low-zinc group had significantly lower levels of testosterone.[17] Selenium, in addition to being required for testosterone production, helps protect the male sex glands against free radicals and heavy metals.[18] If these minerals are lacking in the diet, hormone imbalances may occur. Copper is a little tricky, because excessive levels are much more likely and can be toxic. If you're eating a well-balanced whole foods diet, copper deficiency shouldn't be a problem.

As with women, men's hormones may be thrown out of balance by environmental estrogens, synthetic chemicals that mimic the effects of estrogen. Also called xenoestrogens, these chemicals are widespread and ever more present in our environment; some of the most common are pesticides (such as DDT, PCBs, and dioxins) and industrial by-products. According to some researchers, environmental estrogens may contribute to testicular cancer, urinary tract disorders, and low sperm count. In men, a high level of estrogen slows down the production of testosterone.[19] Exposure to lead, mercury, cadmium, and other heavy metals also inhibits testosterone production.[20]

Men's hormone levels can be adversely affected by certain lifestyle choices. Smoking, in particular, may be a factor in reduced production of testosterone. Animal studies have shown that nicotine and related substances in cigarettes increase the activity of enzymes that deactivate male hormones, including testosterone.[21] Excessive consumption of alcohol decreases levels of testosterone and increases estrogen levels in men. However, modest alcohol intake has not been shown to affect hormone levels.[22] In addition, physical, mental, or emotional stress can inhibit production of hormones, particularly the adrenal hormone DHEA. Under conditions of chronic stress, the adrenal glands switch from producing DHEA to producing cortisol. Since DHEA is a precursor of the male hormones, less DHEA can severely limit testosterone production. A high level of cortisol also leads to blood sugar imbalances, depressed immune function, and sleep disturbances.[23]

Are Your Hormones Imbalanced?

The first step in treating a hormonal imbalance is to get an accurate measurement of your hormone levels. Blood tests or 24-hour urine tests, which can be ordered by your physician, are the standard conventional method of determining hormone levels. However, saliva tests provide a noninvasive and simple alternative to a blood test and are more easily used during the therapeutic process to determine your progress.

Sleep, Hormones, and Body Weight

There's no doubt that obesity is reaching epidemic proportions. While poor diet and lack of exercise undoubtedly play a role, the sheer number of people who are overweight suggest there may be other factors at work. All of us have heard overweight people say things like "I just can't stop eating the wrong foods," "I'm out of control. I can't resist my cravings for fat and sugar," or "I diet and exercise, but I still can't lose weight." Many of these people have repeatedly sought help without success, but all too often they're condemned for lack of discipline or not trying.

Groundbreaking studies by three major medical universities have revealed a previously unsuspected culprit: insufficient sleep. These studies determined that sleep-deprived people (those who sleep less than the 7.9 recommended hours) may be ravenously hungry, and worse, that they may crave the richest, most fat-producing foods. People who routinely sleep 5 hours a night or less are at the greatest risk for elevated weight gain. The mechanism involves two hormones—ghrelin and leptin—that play an important role in regulating appetite. Ghrelin stimulates the appetite and may make a person more hungry for calorie-dense, high-carbohydrate foods. Leptin diminishes appetite by signaling the brain that the body is full. Studies at the University of Chicago found that sleep deprivation led to elevated levels of ghrelin and decreased levels of leptin.[24]

The National Sleep Foundation estimates that as many as 63% of Americans get at least 1 hour less than the recommended amount of sleep. Though no definitive link exists, it's interesting to compare this with statistics indicating that about 65% of the U.S. population is overweight or obese.

"We know that the obesity epidemic is due to overeating—too big portions, too much rich food, and too little activity—but why do we crave too much of these rich foods?" says Eve Van Cauter, lead investigator on one of the new studies. Based on the results of her study, she postulates that it may be because "we are sleep deprived and unable to curb our appetites."[25]

These recent studies offer new hope for the overweight and may motivate people to establish more healthful sleep patterns. As discussed throughout this chapter, the endocrine system and the body's other systems are complexly intertwined. Many feedback mechanisms play a role in this finely tuned orchestra of physiological functioning. Though we may never fully understand all of these interactions, we've learned that not only can hormones have a profound influence on sleep, but sleep or lack of sleep can have a strong effect on hormones.

Home test kits are widely available; these involve sending samples to a laboratory, which will send you a detailed report of the results. However, some states require that a doctor order the test kit. If you are able to order a home test kit, it's important to go over the results with your health-care practitioner. Healthy hormone levels can vary immensely from person to person, so the baseline values laboratories provide for comparison can only reflect averages, not what's best for you. Also, hormone levels can fluctuate greatly over the course of time, and throughout the day. Should you discover that you have an imbalance, you'd be well-advised to work with a medical professional who specializes in the complex field of endocrinology.

Whether you do a saliva test independently or through your doctor, it has several advantages over traditional blood testing for hormones. It is painless

Aging: Sleep Problems Are Not Inevitable

It is commonly believed that people should expect to sleep poorly as they get older, but we disagree with that conclusion. How well you will sleep as you age depends to a large extent on your lifestyle. If you have spent most of your life drinking alcohol and caffeinated beverages, not exercising, and eating poorly, your body will pay you back with sleep problems later in life. But many people in their seventies and eighties sleep wonderfully well because they have had a healthy lifestyle. Here are some lifestyle changes that you can make to improve your sleep in the long run:

- Get plenty of exercise each day.

- Go to bed at a regular time each night and get up at the same time every morning.

- Eliminate distractions at bedtime. Turn off lights and the television.

- Avoid caffeine prior to bedtime, and preferably after 10 A.M.

- Don't smoke. Nicotine is a stimulant.

- Avoid sleeping pills. If you must use them, never do so for more than three nights in a row.

- Avoid alcohol.

- Don't use your bed for eating or watching television.[26]

"The most consistent change with aging is in sleep quality, not in sleep duration," says Charles M. Morin, Ph.D., author of *Relief from Insomnia: Getting the Sleep of Your Dreams*. The proportion of time spent in deep sleep (stages 3 to 4) decreases from about 20% to 25% of the night during young adulthood to 5% to 10% during your sixties. "This deep slumber virtually disappears," Dr. Morin says.[27] He adds that, as the deep sleep disappears, the lightest sleep (stage 1) increases, meaning people are more easily awakened by noise, movements of a bed partner, or a full bladder. He says it is not unusual for a 65-year-old to be awakened two to five times a night, for only a few minutes or as much as 30 minutes.

Not only is sleep not as deep, it is not as efficient with aging. Older people spend more time in bed, but a lesser percentage of that time is spent in sleep. "For example, a 20-year-old without insomnia sleeps on average about 95% of the time spent in bed; in contrast, a 70-year-old without insomnia sleeps just over 80% of that time," Dr. Morin says.[28] He says those are normal changes with aging, but true insomnia does not have to happen as we age.

Another common problem with aging is advanced sleep phase syndrome, or falling asleep too early and then awakening before dawn. About one-third of adults over 65 tend to fall into that pattern, says James Perl, Ph.D., author of *Sleep Right in Five Nights*. This problem can be corrected with light therapy, melatonin supplements, or napping. Dr. Perl says that if you're gong to nap, don't nap after 3 P.M. and don't nap for more than 1 hour. Also, try to stay up until 10 P.M. to 11 P.M.; if you get sleepy earlier, take a walk or do indoor exercise.[29]

Older adults also tend to have less dramatic ups and downs in their body clock, or circadian rhythms. "The polarity between nighttime sleep and daytime wakefulness decreases as night and day blend together," says Dr. Perl. The core body temperature of a young adult is about 2°F lower during the night, while a 75-year-old may have a temperature difference of only 0.5°F or less. This lessening of circadian temperature variation is a factor in sleep disturbances.

As we age, melatonin levels decline; since melatonin is the hormone that puts the body to sleep, it makes sense that older adults would have more sleep problems.[30] In a study of elderly insomniacs, researchers found a connection between deficient levels of melatonin and an increased prevalence of sleep disorders with advancing age. The study involved 95 elderly patients with insomnia, 25 elderly patients without sleep disorders, and 12 young men without sleep disorders. The melatonin levels in the elderly insomniacs were only half those of either the young men or the elderly people without insomnia. "Melatonin deficiency seems to be a key component in the incidence of sleep disorders in elderly subjects and melatonin replacement therapy may be of benefit," the researchers concluded.[31]

and noninvasive, and tests can easily be performed at any time or place. Because levels of many hormones, including DHEA, cortisol, estrogen, progesterone, and testosterone, are highest in the morning, it is far more convenient to be able to test them at home. And, because saliva tests are less expensive than blood testing, you can monitor your levels more frequently to adjust your levels of any supplemental hormone therapy, or to see what effects various interventions (such as diet, exercise, herbs, stress reduction, or acupuncture) are having. (For more information on the Adrenal Stress Index saliva test, see chapter 6, page 134.)

Alternative Medicine Plan for Balancing Hormones

If your hormones are imbalanced, one of your priorities should be to detoxify your body systems of accumulated toxins. Both the liver and the gastrointestinal system are involved in processing and eliminating excess levels of hormones. When these organs are not functioning properly, your hormones may become imbalanced, contributing to a number of health problems, including sleep disorders. Holistic practitioners generally recommend tending to these systems first in order to normalize the body's functions. (For full details on detoxification, see chapter 4, Detoxify Your Body.) Beyond detoxification, alternative medicine offers a number of therapies that can help balance hormones, including dietary and nutritional support, natural hormone therapy, herbal medicine, and homeopathic remedies.

success story

Hormone Therapy for Better Sleep

PHYLLIS BRONSON, PH.D., and Harold Whitcomb, MD, report that almost all of the perimenopausal women they see are suffering from either depression, anxiety, or other emotional disturbances caused by hormonal imbalance. Bronson and Dr. Whitcomb relate the following case which illustrates the powerful influence hormones have on mood and how insomnia can be reversed with the proper balance of supplements and natural hormone therapy:

Margaret, age 50, was nearing menopause and had irregular periods. She had sleeping difficulties and a lack of clarity in her thinking, a condition referred to as brain fog. She also suffered from chronic depression, for which she had been prescribed numerous antidepressants over the last 10 years. She experienced persistent sadness, cried frequently, and continually gained weight and retained water. Other symptoms included hot flashes, loss of sex drive, and mood swings.

Finally, Margaret visited a clinic specializing in preventive care and environmental medicine. They measured her estrogen status and found that she had low levels of estradiol; this was the likely cause of her insomnia and emotional disturbances. Her estrogen level was 54.3, whereas a woman her age should have a level between 90 and 130. Margaret's progesterone level was 0.2; a normal reading for her would have been 25. Her testosterone was around 14, at the low end of the acceptable reference range for women (14 to 76). However, her new doctor preferred to see levels closer to 40 to 60 for menopausal women. With a low level of 14, Margaret had no sex drive.

> **"Margaret had sleeping difficulties and a lack of clarity in her thinking, a condition referred to as brain fog.**

Her doctor also checked her DHEA level, which was 90. For a woman of Margaret's age to be optimally healthy and have a low risk of degenerative disease, that number should be above 400 and preferably 500 to 600. Low DHEA levels are often correlated with extreme exhaustion and flulike symptoms that have no apparent medical basis. Estrogen-deficient women are also often low in pregnenolone, an hormone that's a precursor to progesterone. Pregnenolone appears to have a significant calming effect because it activates receptor sites in brain cells for GABA (itself a calming agent), enabling more GABA to be absorbed by the cells.

Using a procedure called electrodermal screening, in which a blunt, noninvasive electric probe measures minute electrical discharges from acupuncture points on the body, her doctor discovered that Margaret had many food sensitivities, specifically to grains such as wheat, rice, rye, Kamut, and spelt. In addition, a blood test showed that she was deficient in histidine, an amino acid associated with allergies; histidine deficiencies are often correlated with hormonal imbalances.

To address her food allergies and depression, the doctor prescribed histidine (200 mg once daily) and another amino acid, tyrosine (500 mg before meals), along with vitamin B_5 (500 mg with meals), and a supplement with a blend of amino acids needed for the body to produce serotonin, a key brain chemical involved in sleep. Margaret's doctor also prescribed a bioidentical estrogen supplement, progesterone in cream form, and a transdermal DHEA gel.

To resolve her sleeping problems, Margaret's doctor recommended melatonin, but she felt agitated after each dose, as sometimes occurs in women with preexisting hormonal imbalances. So in its place, her doctor recommended inositol, a nutrient considered part of the vitamin B complex (650 mg at bedtime).

After the first six weeks on her new regimen, Margaret's energy picked up and she started sleeping deeply and woke feeling refreshed. She also reported a marked improvement in the clarity of her thinking as one of her most significant symptoms, brain fog, lifted. Her libido returned and, with it, interest in a romantic relationship. Four months into the program, Margaret's progesterone level had climbed to 5.6. Her estrogen level came up more slowly, which is often the case when supplementing with natural estrogens. After a year, Margaret's estrogen was at 95, progesterone at 8, DHEA at 350, and testosterone at 42. Margaret says she feels great and has plenty of energy. Her insomnia, emotional disturbances, and other symptoms were all resolved by rebalancing her hormones naturally.

Therapies for Women

Rather than artificially manipulating your estrogen levels with synthetic hormones and ignoring the reasons behind any imbalances, it is more valuable to determine why you have hormonal imbalances in the first place. Depending on the reason, restoring hormonal balance may be more effectively achieved with dietary changes, nutritional supplements, natural progesterone cream, herbal therapy, or traditional Chinese medicine.

Dietary Recommendations
Eating soybeans and soybean-derived products, particularly fermented soy foods such as tempeh and miso, can help counteract the negative effects of

excess estrogen. These foods contain high levels of genistein, a substance that has a chemical structure similar to estrogen. Genistein and other similar compounds known as phytoestrogens are plant compounds that can block the body's more potent estrogens (and xenoestrogens) from attaching to cell receptor sites—the places where estrogens exert their effects on the body. Phytoestrogens tend to balance estrogen in the body.[32]

Soy foods have received a lot of attention, and accolades, because they're thought to play a role in the healthy aging of many Asian populations—and the low incidence of breast cancer among Asian women. But be aware that these cultures use soy foods in moderation, and mostly in fermented forms. Because soy foods are so rich in phytoestrogens, it's best introduce them slowly, and to monitor your response. Those with a severe deficiency of progesterone may not benefit, or could even experience health problems as a result. In conventional agriculture, genetically modified strains of soy are often cultivated, and the crop may be heavily treated with herbicides. It's best to consume organic soy products whenever possible. It's also a good idea to avoid processed forms of soy, such as soy protein isolates, meat substitutes, and soy milk; these contain high levels of compounds that can interfere with thyroid function. Other than soy, foods high in phytoestrogens include flaxseeds, whole grains, and nuts and seeds.[33]

If you're not fond of soy or are concerned about eating it, other dietary approaches exist. Ellen Brown and Lynn Walker, Pharm.D., M.Ac., DHM, authors of *Menopause and Estrogen*, suggest the following foods to help balance estrogens: raw fruits, fresh fruit and vegetable juices (especially green juices), leafy green vegetables, garlic, figs, dates, cabbage, avocados, grapes, apples, beets, spirulina, chlorella, seaweed, wheat germ, and wheat germ oil.[34]

Supplementing with essential fatty acids (EFAs) can be important for balancing your hormones. "Many women actually eat themselves into hormonal dysfunction," says clinical nutritionist Ann Louise Gittleman, who specializes in natural hormone therapy. "They overindulge in carbohydrates and they don't get enough protein, which is needed to support the adrenal glands. They deprive themselves of needed fats and end up lacking the building blocks of the essential sex-related hormones, which derive from fats." In the effort to cut down on fats, many women don't get enough of the fats their bodies need.[35] There are two principal types of EFAs required in the diet: omega-3 and omega-6. Only 1 or 2 tablespoons per day of EFAs is often all it takes to restore hormonal balance. Flaxseed oil (1 tablespoon) and evening primrose oil (500 mg twice daily) are excellent sources of EFAs. If you use flaxseed oil in or on foods, be aware that this oil is extremely vulnerable to oxidative damage from both heat and light. Never cook with flaxseed oil or other oils high in EFAs. They can, however, be added to salads, salad dressings, smoothies, and other uncooked foods; you may also stir them into a warm foods, such as a bowl of soup.

John Lee, MD, author of *What Your Doctor May Not Tell You about Menopause*, recommends taking the following antioxidant vitamins to help cleanse the body of harmful toxins that can lead to excessive estrogen: 1 to 2 grams of vitamin C daily; 400 IU of vitamin E daily; 500 mg of quercetin (a bioflavonoid) twice daily; a B complex supplement daily with about 50 mg of the major B vitamins, and 500 to 1,000 mg of magnesium (in the gluconate or citrate form).[36]

Natural Progesterone Therapy

To restore progesterone levels in the body, Dr. Lee recommends supplementing with progesterone, which can help turn fat into energy and reduce water retention.[38] While progesterone is available in sublingual (under-the-tongue) drops and capsules, using a progesterone skin cream or oil is best. Applying progesterone to the skin allows it to be absorbed into fat beneath the skin, where it can be taken up by the blood as needed. If taken in a capsule form, it is more difficult for the body to regulate the amount of progesterone entering the blood.

Natural progesterone can be manufactured in the laboratory from a substance called diosgenin, which is found in wild yam or soybeans. However, the body cannot manufacture progesterone from the raw diosgenin found in these foods. Dr. Lee therefore recommends using products that have been preconverted in the laboratory into progesterone, rather than trying to obtain it from dietary sources. He advises consumers to check labels to make sure that a product lists the actual concentration of progesterone.

The recommended application of progesterone cream is between ⅛ and ½ teaspoon per day, or 3 to 10 drops of the oil. Premenopausal women with average menstrual cycles (28 days) should apply the cream during days 12 to 26 of their cycle. Those with longer cycles should apply it from days 10 to 28. For menopausal women, Dr. Lee indicates that there can be

Dietary Guidelines for Balancing Your Hormones

Women's health expert John R. Lee, MD, who coined the term estrogen dominance, offers the following general dietary recommendations for maintaining balanced hormone levels:

- Avoid refined sugars and processed foods; instead, eat organic whole foods, emphasizing fresh vegetables and fruit, whole grains, legumes, and nuts.

- Consume modest amounts of meat (chicken, beef, or pork) two or three times per week at most; preferable sources of protein are eggs, yogurt, and cold-water ocean fish (four to five servings per week).

- Avoid hydrogenated oils (in margarine and processed foods); use primarily olive oil instead. Limit total dietary intake of fat to 20% to 25%.

- Eliminate colas and other sodas and reduce alcohol consumption; drink plenty of purified water daily.[37]

more flexibility in applying the cream. He recommends using it for 14 to 21 days of each month. The cream can be applied to the palms, face, neck, upper chest, breasts, insides of the arms, and behind the knees. Alternating applications among these sites will increase absorption.[39]

Various creams are available in health food stores and by mail order. When you purchase a product, there are two points to keep in mind: First, make sure it contains natural progesterone, not just wild yam (*Dioscorea villosa*). Don't be misled by claims that wild yam creams are the same as progesterone creams. As an herbal supplement, wild yam can have a mild hormone-balancing effect, but it does not provide natural progesterone. Second, make sure you use a brand of cream that has enough natural progesterone in it to make a difference. Dr. Lee advises using only creams that have at least 400 mg of progesterone per ounce.

Herbal Therapy

Herbs that are helpful for balancing women's hormones include unicorn root, an herb used in folk remedies for premenopausal women, and black cohosh. These herbs promote the normal production of estrogen and contribute to the proper balance of estrogen and progesterone. Other herbs that may be helpful include dong quai, licorice (to avoid any potentially toxic effects, use deglycyrrhizinated licorice supplements), and Siberian ginseng, all of which help balance hormone levels.[40]

Linda Ojeda, CNC, Ph.D., author of *Menopause Without Medicine*, generally suggests using certain herbs for their hormone-stimulating properties. Unlike synthetic hormone replacement therapy, the action of herbs is safe and gentle. Dr. Ojeda cites the following herbs as estrogen-stimulating: black cohosh, alfalfa, hops, sweetbriar, horsetail, buckwheat, sage, rose, and shepherd's purse. Among the herbs she recommends to support progesterone are wild yam, chasteberry, sarsaparilla, and yarrow. The herbs can be taken as supplements or teas.[41]

Traditional Chinese Medicine

In traditional Chinese medicine, insomnia is seen as an imbalance between the yin and yang energies of the body. Yin is the calming, slow, quiet, wet, dense, feminine life energy, while yang is the fast, bright, strong, loud, expansive, masculine life energy. In menopause, a decrease in a woman's kidney essence, or reproductive force, can trigger a yin-yang imbalance in the associated organ systems, such as kidney, liver, or heart. If a woman does not maintain a lifestyle that keeps her kidney energy strong—good nutrition, exercise, plenty of rest, low stress, positive outlook—she could develop menopausal symptoms, including insomnia.

In addition to a healthy lifestyle, Chinese herbal supplements can be very helpful in strengthening the kidney essence, says Harriet Beinfeld, L.Ac. She recommends the herbs ginseng, lotus seed, and longan fruit for a woman with a kidney essence weakness that results in a heart yin deficiency. Symptoms of this condition are insomnia, hot flashes, anxiety, palpitations, emotional instability, unusual thirst or perspiration, and premenstrual buildup with scanty, bright flow. For women with a kidney essence deficiency that results in a liver weakness, Dr. Beinfeld recommends white peony root and lycii berries. Symptoms of this imbalance are irritability or hypersensitivity, headaches, muscle tension or cramping, dizziness or vertigo, uneven or intermittent menstrual flow, and dry eyes, skin, hair, nails, or vaginal mucosa.[42]

success story

Acupuncture and Herbs Outperform Drugs

LYNN, A 28-YEAR-OLD WOMAN, was three months pregnant when she developed insomnia that kept her awake all night. Initially, she used conventional sedatives to try to get some sleep, but she was concerned about potential side effects, ranging from memory loss to headaches to poor muscle coordination. She was also worried about potential harm to the baby; plus, the medications weren't even working for her! After two more months of insomnia, Lynn decided to see an acupuncturist Edythe Vickers.

As soon as Dr. Vickers inserted the hair-thin acupuncture needles into Lynn's body, Lynn fell asleep on the table, which Dr. Vickers felt was a favorable sign because it showed Lynn's body responded well to acupuncture. Dr. Vickers used 21 needles: 10 on Lynn's back and 11 on the front side of her body at her feet, hands, knees, neck, and forehead. The needles were placed at specific points along energy pathways called meridians. At any acupuncture point, the needle helps unblock the qi, or life force energy, that circulates in the body's meridians. Qi can become blocked by various traumas or stress, such as poor diet, overwork, emotional tension, viruses, or, as in Lynn's case, changes due to pregnancy.

After the treatment, Dr. Vickers gave Lynn a Chinese herbal formula featuring the herbs ginseng and longan to strengthen Lynn's kidney and heart energies so that the two systems could work together. In Lynn's case, the kidney energy, a water element in traditional Chinese medicine (TCM), was being diverted to care for the baby, which left the heart energy, a fire element, blazing out of control, causing anxiety, restlessness, and insomnia. In addition, Dr. Vickers gave Lynn zizyphus, a Chinese herb used for insomnia because it strengthens the yin, the cooling, feminine energy of the body. Yin is the energy that governs sleep and rest, while yang refers to the active, masculine, bright qualities of energy. In general, TCM practitioners say that most types of insomnia are due to either too much yang energy or not enough yin. Lynn took 1 teaspoon of the herbs before bed and 1 teaspoon every time she woke up.

Dr. Vickers often recommends that pregnant women with insomnia take the naturally calming minerals calcium and magnesium in liquid form before bed. (The liquid form is more readily absorbed.) Supplementing with minerals is a good choice for treating insomnia during pregnancy, when women need to avoid taking drugs and must also be careful with herbal supplements.

That night, Lynn fell asleep within 20 minutes without any medications, which was an unusually short time for her, and she slept for 4 hours straight. Thereafter, Lynn slept through the night, aided by the herbs and supplements and, initially, acupuncture treatments three times a week. After the first few weeks, Lynn continued once-a-week acupuncture treatments until her baby was born. Her insomnia did not return until she became pregnant again two years later, when she again sought treatment from Dr. Vickers.

Therapies for Men

Once you've determined that your hormones are imbalanced, a number of alternative therapies are available to normalize them. Dietary adjustments can have a significant impact on hormone levels, especially when combined with nutritional supplements, hormone therapy, herbs, or homeopathic remedies.

Dietary Recommendations

To help rebalance the hormones, reduce consumption of refined sugar products, saturated fats, and food preservatives. Eat more fresh fruit and vegetables with a high nutrient content. Increase your intake of legumes (especially soy), dark leafy greens (for their protective antioxidant content), essential fatty acids (flaxseed, evening primrose, and borage oils), and nuts and seeds (a good source of zinc).

During andropause, declining levels of testosterone may lead to a relative excess in estrogen; this female hormone can, in turn, reduce the effects of testosterone in the body. Dr. Eugene Shippen, author of *The Testosterone Syndrome*, also emphasizes eating more soy, as it contains phytoestrogens that can block the action of the body's own estrogen, which is more powerful. He recommends eating plenty of cruciferous vegetables, such as cabbage, cauliflower, and broccoli, as these vegetables help rid the body of excess estrogen.[43] Maintaining an adequate level of dietary fiber is also important for clearing estrogen from the body.

Since environmental estrogens and other toxins are a factor in male hormonal imbalances, you should reduce your exposure to these substances. Minimize intake of animal products, especially milk and eggs, and choose organic meats whenever possible. Since many pesticides and herbicides are estrogenic, it's ideal to buy and eat organic foods whenever possible, including fruits and vegetables.

Testosterone Replacement Therapy

According to Dr. Julian Whitaker, easing andropause requires its own hormone therapy: testosterone replacement. Studies have shown that testosterone replacement can heighten sex drive, increase bone density, and improve mood and sleep patterns, among other effects. If you are considering testosterone replacement, the first step is a blood or saliva test to assess your current levels of the hormone, says Dr. Whitaker. If your levels are low or even average for your age, testosterone therapy can help alleviate andropause symptoms and improve overall health.

The goal of supplementation is to restore blood testosterone levels to those of a healthy 25- to 30-year-old man. For this, Dr. Whitaker recommends weekly injections of testosterone cypionate (100 mg) or biweekly injections of testosterone enanthate (200 mg). These long-acting versions of the hormone are considered the safest and most effective preparations for use in testosterone replacement, says Dr. Whitaker. Because injection guarantees consistent absorption, he considers this to be the best method of testosterone supplementation. Skin patches and oral lozenges can also be effective, he reports. However, Dr. Whitaker advises against oral testosterone in pill form. "With oral testosterone, there is a potential for liver dysfunction and a decrease in protective HDL or 'good' cholesterol levels," he cautions. In addition to the benefits of testosterone replacement cited above, Dr. Whitaker believes there are further positive effects, including increased

Supplements for Male Hormone Support

Sandra Cabot, MD, author of *Smart Medicine for Menopause*, offers a nutritional strategy that men can apply to start improving the functioning of their endocrine system (the source of all hormones). Here are Dr. Cabot's recommended daily supplements for andropause:

- Vitamin E: 500 IU

- Magnesium: 500 mg

- Zinc: 50 mg

- Selenium: 50 mcg

- Manganese: 5 mg

- Ginseng: 2 to 4 grams

These supplements, taken daily, are designed to help the male body cope with the natural decline of testosterone. Vitamin E and magnesium strengthen the heart and circulation, including blood supply to the pelvic region. Zinc can boost male virility and reduce prostate problems such as swelling. Ginseng, for example, acts as a glandular tonic, helping to improve the function of the testicles.[44]

lean muscle mass and protection for the heart, as certain forms of testosterone can improve the ratio between "good" and "bad" cholesterol and lower cholesterol levels overall.[45]

Another option is a gel called Libidex, which can be applied to the skin to stimulate testosterone production and support the endocrine system. Developed by Michael Borkin, DC, NMD Libidex contains DHEA, androstenedione (a testosterone precursor), alpha-liopoic acid, oat extract, saw palmetto, colloidal silver, vitamins A, B_{12}, and E, plus homeopathic support and 10 flower remedies. The typical daily dosage is ⅛ to ½ teaspoon, depending on age, applied to areas of soft skin, preferably upon rising in the morning.

Caution: Men who supplement with testosterone should closely monitor their prostate-specific antigen (PSA) levels, as excess testosterone has been linked to prostate cancer. Also, be warned that searching for this product on the Internet is not recommended for the faint of heart.

Herbal Therapy

The herb ginseng has been used since ancient times and has accumulated much folklore about its actions and uses. One variety, Oriental ginseng (*Panax ginseng*), has received a great deal of attention as a potential aid to virility, and animal studies have indeed shown that *Panax ginseng* increases testosterone levels.[46] Ginseng should not be abused, however, as serious side effects can occur, including headaches, skin problems, and other reactions. For this reason, the proper dosage for the individual should be determined and respected.

Studies indicate that Chinese wolfberry may be able to boost testosterone levels.[47] Oats, which have traditionally been used as an energy and nerve tonic, may be useful for boosting levels of male hormones. As an accompaniment to andropause treatment, Dr. Whitaker generally suggests taking the herb saw palmetto (120 to 360 mg daily).

Homeopathic Remedies

"The first step in andropause treatment is to balance and correct the hormone deficiencies," says endocrinologist Gary Ross, MD. To this end, he finds certain complex homeopathic remedies helpful, either alone or in conjunction with prescribed hormones, including the following:

- Testis Compositum: Stimulates male sexual function, brain function, adrenal function and reduces fatigue

- Coenzyme Compositum: A multiple vitamin in homeopathic form, containing vitamin C and several B vitamins needed for metabolism

- Cerebrum Compositum: Enhances brain and nervous system function and memory and reduces anxiety and depression

- Galium-Heel: For body detoxification and reduction of inflammation

Depending upon the individual, any or all of these homeopathic preparations can be used in all the treatment plans, says Dr. Ross. Response time can vary from quickly to several months, he adds.[48]

success story

Raising Hormone Levels for Better Sleep

CYRIL, A 55-YEAR-OLD PROFESSIONAL WRITER, turned out to be "dreadfully low" in the key male hormones when he went to see Gary Ross, MD. Cyril wasn't sleeping well and complained of a slump in his mental abilities; he wanted his mind to feel sharper.

Using an analysis of Cyril's hormones based on urine collected over 24 hours, Dr. Ross found that Cyril's DHEA (a key adrenal hormone) was very low, at 0.11 (normal is 0.2 to 2.0); his testosterone was also in the basement at 4.95. A blood test also showed his plasma levels of testosterone were also low, at 319. In addition, Cyril had a low level of human growth hormone. This hormone, made in the brain, naturally declines with age, but Cyril's levels were so low as to be worrisome: only 138, whereas 250 and higher is considered the norm for optimal functioning.

Based on all of this information, Dr. Ross developed the following treatment protocol for Cyril: the amino acid tryptophan to help regulate his sleeping; Sexativa, a green oat extract, to release and elevate the level of free testosterone; Libidex (a transdermal gel containing nutrients, herbs, hormones, and flower essences); and homeopathic growth hormone stimulator called Vital, given in liquid form to encourage the body to produce its own growth hormone. After only a short time on this regimen, Cyril started sleeping better and his other symptoms improved as well.

nine

Step 7: Correct Structural Imbalances

In chapter 6, we explored how stress and emotional tension can disturb sleep. Similarly, physical stress and muscular tension may be keeping you awake at night. While exercise and physical activity are important components of any healthy lifestyle, they are an absolute necessity for people who suffer from sleep disorders. Your exercise program should target flexibility, circulation of blood and lymph fluid, and relaxation. You don't need to run marathons or lift weights to benefit from regular exercise. Exercises from the East, such as qigong and yoga, increase flexibility and also help relax an anxious mind.

Daily exercise should be augmented by various forms of bodywork, such as chiropractic, massage, acupressure, or other physical therapies that promote relaxation and improve the circulation of nerve impulses, blood, and lymphatic fluid. In this chapter, we'll take a look at some of the most widely available physical therapies to help you decide which you might prefer or which would be most beneficial for your particular sleep problem.

Structural Imbalances and Sleep Disturbances

Hans Selye, MD, a pioneering researcher on stress, determined that any neurological pressure, at any location in the body, affects the function of the entire spinal cord. As a result, the overall functioning of the human body is affected by any kind of neurological blockage or impingement. Some postulate that this means almost any symptom can be fully or partially caused by spinal dysfunction.

Alternative Medicine Plan to Correct Structural Imbalances

- Exercise
- Chiropractic
- Neuro-Emotional Technique
- Bodywork

The spinal column, or backbone, is made up of the vertebrae, 24 bones that surround and protect the spinal cord. Between the vertebrae, pairs of spinal nerves exit and extend to every part of the body—skin, muscles, bones, organs, glands, and more. The nervous system itself is comprised of three overlapping systems: the central nervous system, which includes the brain and spinal cord; the autonomic nervous system, which controls involuntary functions such as heart rate, digestion, and glandular functions; and the peripheral nervous system, which connects the central nervous system to all of the body's tissues and voluntary muscles.

Health relies upon the balance and equilibrium of these three interrelated components of the nervous system—a balance that can be easily disrupted by spinal injury, misalignment, stress, or illness. When vertebrae get out of alignment (a condition referred to as subluxation), it places pressure on the nerves in that area. As a result, the nerves function less than optimally, which can lead to imbalances and eventually disease.

Chiropractic, like traditional Chinese medicine (TCM), espouses the notion that disease reflects a lack of homeostasis (a state of equilibrium characterized by optimal functioning and balance between interdependent systems). This may be due to either an excess or a deficiency of energy (qi in TCM, and nerve energy in chiropractic). Chiropractors speak of the parasympathetic and sympathetic "tone" of the autonomic nervous system. The sympathetic nervous system controls the fight-or-flight stress response and activates the body; the parasympathetic calms the body and conserves energy. Subluxations can throw this system out of balance. "Subluxations restricting the parasympathetic or exciting the sympathetic nerve flow would result in sympathetic dominance," explains chiropractor Tim Leasenby. "Sympathetic dominance leads to too much energy in the legs in restless legs syndrome and too much energy in the mind/brain in insomnia."

Subluxations of the spinal vertebrae can also affect the body in less obvious ways. A subluxation can have a direct effect on an organ's function when it impedes nerve flow to that organ. When the vertebrae are properly aligned, the spine remains mobile, allowing electrical impulses from the brain to travel freely along the spinal cord to the organs, thus maintaining healthy function. However, when subluxations occur, they interrupt the normal flow in the nerve structures which, in turn, affects the normal functioning of the organ.

Factors other than subluxations can also have far-reaching effects in the body. Muscle tension, whether from normal activity, awkward movement, lack of exercise, or stress, contributes to muscle fatigue and pain by compressing nerve fibers in the muscle that's tense. If not addressed, these body tensions have a tendency to build into chronic patterns of stress, potentially leading to sleep disturbances. Prolonged contraction also interferes with the elimination of chemical wastes in the affected muscles and surrounding tissues and can cause nerve and muscle pain. To understand why this is the case, let's take a moment to understand the lymphatic system, an underappreciated physiological system that plays an enormous role in maintaining health.

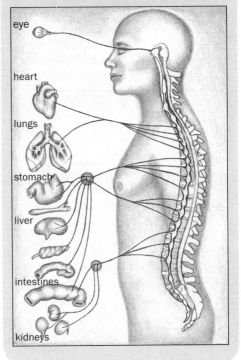

The Spinal Vertebrae and Related Organ Systems

The lymphatic system consists of lymph fluid and the structures (vessels, ducts, and nodes) involved in transporting it from tissues to the bloodstream. Lymphatic fluid fills the spaces between cells in the body. This fluid contains nutrients to be delivered to cells and cellular debris (bacteria, dead cells, heavy metals, and waste products) to be removed. The purpose of the lymphatic system is to carry toxins away from the cells by collecting and filtering lymph fluid. Lymph fluid flows slowly through the body to the abdomen and chest, where it drains into the bloodstream through large ducts. Unlike the circulatory system, which relies on the heart to move its fluid, the lymphatic system doesn't have a pump; it relies on physical activity and movement to circulate lymphatic fluid and thereby eliminate wastes from the body. If the lymph stagnates, serious problems can result as the body becomes overburdened with toxins.

A regular program of exercise can help keep your lymphatic system functioning optimally. It can also help you sleep better and improve your overall health. Researchers have consistently found that people leading more sedentary lives have a higher incidence of insomnia. One of the reasons for the higher incidence of sleep disorders in older people may be a decreased level of physical activity. By addressing subluxations, tension, and lymphatic stagnation, chiropractic, massage, and other forms of bodywork can help relieve physical tension and structural imbalances that may be contributing to disrupted sleep.

Exercise

Though exercise is one of the last topics we address, it's certainly not the least important strategy for enhancing sleep—and overall health and well-being. Most health-care professionals endorse exercise for promoting sleep—if it is done at the right level, at the right time of day. "I don't think there's a single thing in life that's as therapeutic as the right kind of exercise program applied over time," says naturopath John Hibbs, "but misapplied, it can be just another stressor."

As early as 1978, researchers were crediting exercise with producing more restful sleep.[1] In a more recent study, 50 men and women over the age of 67 were split into two groups: Half did 45 minutes of aerobic exercise three times a week and the other half did stretching exercises with the same frequency. After six months, they all came to a sleep lab for testing. Those in aerobics group were getting 33% more deep sleep than before the study began. Also, some of the exercisers picked at random were found to be secreting 30% more human growth hormone (HGH), a hormone secreted by the pituitary gland in very brief pulses during the early hours of sleep. Not one person in the stretching group showed any changes in levels of either deep sleep or HGH.[2] The release of HGH is closely tied to the circadian rhythm of sleep. The reason for increased production of HGH with exercise is that muscle tissue requires more HGH for maintenance than fat does.

Other researchers speculate that exercise later in the day raises body temperature very slightly until bedtime, and the extra heat seems to drop the body into deeper sleep. That's one of the reasons that a hot bath (researchers call it "passive heating") before bedtime can induce deeper sleep. Karla A. Kubitz, professor of kinesiology and sports psychology expert, says that the beneficial effect is dependent on the time of day you exercise as well as the intensity and duration of the exercise. "I find that many more patients have normalization of sleep patterns with regular exercise than disruption of their patterns," says Dr. Kubitz. "When there is a disruption, it is usually related to timing, such as exercising just before bedtime." Dr. Kubitz has found exercise can increase slow wave (deep) sleep and total sleep time.

Exercise may also decrease the time it takes to fall asleep and reduce REM (dream) sleep time.[3]

Experiments in South Africa have found that exercise significantly improves sleep quality. In one study, nine young women entered a 12-week aerobic training program. The program involved cycling three times a week on a bicycle at a heart-rate intensity of 155 to 165 beats per minute, 15 minutes per session initially, increasing to 60 minutes for the last four weeks. Also, the women participated in sprints of 100, 200, 400, and 800 meters, and a 4-kilometer road run once a week, increasing to 8 kilometers in the last two weeks. The exercise, which was done between 4 p.m. and 7 p.m., shortened the time it took for the women to fall asleep. However, the study found that the women had decreased levels of deep sleep as the result of exercising before bedtime. The women exercised at about 70% of their maximum energy output, or what is called a submaximal level.[4]

The timing of exercise seemed to be a factor in the improvement of sleep quality in a study in Finland involving a random sample of 1,600 people, aged 36 to 50. Light to moderate exercise early in the evening was found to promote sleep and improve its quality. A walk after dinner is a perfect way to get a bit of exercise, wind down, and improve digestion all at the same time. However, exercise late in the evening was found to be less beneficial. In the study, 65% of the respondents said they felt better in the morning when they had exercised the previous evening. When asked their feelings on sleep-promoting activities, 33% of the respondents said evening exercise promoted sleep and improved its quality.[5]

How to Start Exercising

The most important thing is to get moving. This may mean developing a workout schedule or simply returning to regular participation in your favorite physical activity or sport. Before beginning any exercise program, consult your physician and have a thorough exam to rule out any health conditions that may need attention. If you have heart disease or diabetes, or are at high risk for these or other serious illnesses, begin an exercise program only with your physician's approval. If you have been physically inactive for some time, consult with your physician to determine whether you need to undergo a detoxification program before you begin exercising. It's especially important for inactive men over the age of 40 and women over 50 to consult their physician.

According to the President's Council on Physical Fitness and Sports, a balanced physical fitness program incorporates the following elements:[6]

Warm up: Begin gradually. Start with 5 to 10 minutes of basic warm-up exercises, which can include gentle stretching or a short, slow walk.

Cardiorespiratory fitness: Endurance athletes, such as long-distance runners or swimmers, have the stamina for their physically demanding sports because they have good cardiorespiratory fitness. Their heart and lungs are able to deliver oxygen and nutrients to the tissues and remove wastes over sustained periods of activity. After you have warmed up your muscles and are breathing more deeply, begin your activity and gradually pick up the pace. This may mean moving from a slow walk to a brisker pace or increasing the speed on a treadmill. If it has been a long time since you've exercised regularly, begin slowly. Your first session may consist of 5 minutes of warming up and another 5 to 10 minutes of walking.

Muscular strength: A muscle's capacity to exert force for a brief period of time can be developed by participating in sports or by specific weight-training exercises. By regularly working individual muscle groups, they increase in strength. Join your local gym and learn how to use the free weights, or incorporate activities that require regular lifting into your daily routine, such as chopping wood and gardening. Be certain you use proper lifting stances to protect your back and joints from injury. Strive for at least two 20-minute sessions of strength-building exercises per week.

Muscular endurance: This involves extending a muscle's ability to undergo repeated contractions or to continue applying force against resistance; doing 100 push-ups requires this kind of endurance. Try to incorporate at least three 30-minute sessions of exercise such as push-ups, sit-ups, and similar calisthenics to develop endurance in all of your major muscle groups. Some public parks often have a "par course" that includes many of these exercises at designated stations. Again, other activities involving vigorous work around the house, such as washing the car, can provide similar benefits.

Flexibility: Flexibility is the ability to move your muscles freely through a full range of movement. Dancers rely on their excellent flexibility, but everyone can benefit from increased flexibility, as it can prevent injury. Try to incorporate about 10 to 15 minutes of gentle, nonbouncing stretching exercises into your workouts. This can be done before you set off on a walk or bike ride and also at the end of the session. If you are familiar with yoga or tai chi, both are excellent for increasing flexibility.

Cool down: Always be sure to cool down afterward; don't stop exercising abruptly without giving your body a chance to slow down. If you've just walked a mile in 20 minutes, take another 5 minutes to slow down and allow your body to gradually shift into low gear.

Exercises for Specific Parts of the Body

These exercises target the head, neck, shoulders, and back. For many people, stress and tension tend to build up in these areas, causing muscle contractions and pain. Do these exercises two to three times per day to stretch contracted muscles. When doing these stretches, concentrate on breathing to provide a deeper, more relaxed stretch.[7]

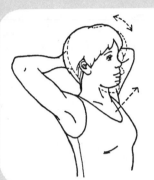

Base of head and neck

1. With your chest up, tuck your chin down and in, rocking your head down. Do not bend your neck, bob your head, or hold your breath while nodding.

2. Turn your head to the left and repeat step 1, then turn your head to the right and repeat again.

Neck, shoulders, and upper back

1. This is the starting and ending position. This exercise can be done sitting or standing.

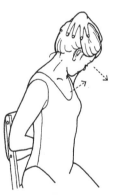

2. While exhaling, turn your head slightly to the left and use your left hand to and pull head and neck down in a diagonal direction.

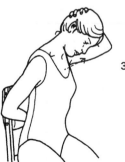

3. Maintain pressure and rotate your head to the right, away from your left arm about 40 degrees. Repeat this rotation motion several times before returning to the starting position. Repeat several times on the left side, then do the exercise on the right side.

Reprinted by permission from Visual Health Information

Exercises for Specific Parts of the Body

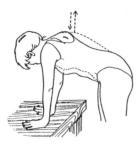

Upper back stretch

With your chin in and arms straight, raise your upper back toward the ceiling and inhale. Relax, exhale, and lower your spine, letting your shoulder blades come close to each other.

Upper chest and shoulders

Stand facing the corner of a room with your hands against the two walls at the level shown. Exhale and lean in toward the corner, keeping your chest up.

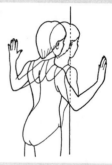

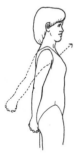

Shoulders and middle back

Interlock your fingers behind your back and raise your arms as high as possible while exhaling. Keep your chest up and your chin in.

Shoulder rotation

Hold a length of stretchy rubber tubing with your hands about shoulder width apart. Move your hands apart while exhaling and pinch your shoulder blades together slightly. Keep your elbows bent at a 90-degree angle and close to your sides.

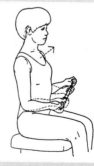

Increase Activity in Day-to-Day Life

For many people, it's more realistic to get exercise by incorporating activities of moderate exertion in their day-to-day lives, such as walking the dog or taking stairs instead of the elevator. While a dedicated exercise program is preferable, including more physical activity throughout your day can help you maintain a basic level of fitness. Park your car a block away from your destination and walk. If you can do certain errands, such as going to the post office or the grocery store, by walking or biking, do so. Walking more frequently and using fewer labor-saving devices can burn additional calories and help keep you active.

For many years, the prescription for health maintenance included three to five 30-minute sessions of exercise per week. Current recommendations from the American College of Sports Medicine and the U.S. Centers for Disease Control and Prevention state that nearly everyone should strive for 30 minutes daily; if it's more convenient, you can divide that amount into three 8- to 10-minute bouts per day.[8] Research has shown that people who exercise in shorter, more frequent sessions reap the same health benefits as those who do all of their exercising at once. Even if you are seriously short of time, set a minimum goal of three daily walking sessions of 10 minutes each.

Calories Burned by Moderate Activities

In the table below, the calories burned are for a 150- to 160-pound person. A lighter person would burn fewer calories, and a heavier person more.

Calories Burned by Day-to-Day Activities	
Activity	**Calories Burned**
Raking leaves for 30 minutes	150
Washing and waxing the car for 45–60 minutes	150
Stair walking for 15 minutes	150
Walking for 15 minutes	75
Social dancing for 30 minutes	150
Shooting baskets for 30 minutes	150
Shoveling snow for 30 minutes	300

From the Department of Health and Human Services, Centers for Disease Control and Prevention, "Physical Activity for Everyone." 2006. Available at www.cdc.gov/nccdphp/dnpa/physical/recommendations/adults.htm.

Qigong: Good for Insomnia, and for Overall Health

Qigong (also referred to as chi-kung) is like acupuncture without doctors, says Roger Jahnke, OMD, author of *The Healer Within*, because you can use it to manipulate and enhance your own energy. Qigong has three aspects: regulating the body through posture and movement, regulating the breath, and regulating the mind through meditation and relaxation. *Qigong*, which means "cultivating vital energy," involves working with one's own qi, or life force. "The presence of healthy qi is obvious," says Dr. Jahnke. "It is what produces radiance and vitality. Its absence is also obvious: fatigue, pain, and disease."

Qigong practice can range from simple calisthenic-type movements with coordinated breathing to complex exercises where brain wave frequency, heart rate, and other organ functions are altered intentionally by the practitioner. When practiced regularly, qigong's combination of movement, deep relaxation, and breathing can improve strength and flexibility, reverse damage caused by prior injuries and disease, and promote relaxation, awareness, and healing. Traditional Chinese medicine holds that qigong stimulates and nourishes the body's internal organs by aiding in the circulation of qi. It can break down energy blocks and facilitate the free flow of energy throughout the body, promoting the flow of blood and lymph, and the even flow of nerve impulses necessary for good health. "The overall benefit of qigong is to mobilize and harmonize the body's naturally occurring healing resource (qi)," according to Dr. Jahnke.

Like acupuncture, qigong activates the energy currents that flow along the meridian pathways in the body. This affects the entire body and can help maintain the function of the organs and tissues. For example, one qigong exercise involves controlled breathing and deep relaxation while lifting the arms and rising upward on the toes. According to Dr. Jahnke, this exercise can help prevent tension headaches, constipation, insomnia, and other disorders by improving circulation of the cardiovascular and lymphatic systems, as well as modulating brain chemistry.

Dr. Jahnke recommends a daily qigong practice of 30 minutes to 1 hour. In addition to helping eradicate insomnia, regular practice can reduce stress, improve circulation, and provide increased resistance to disease. Dr. Jahnke says that qigong produces the following health-promoting effects:

- Initiates the "relaxation response," which decreases the sympathetic function of the autonomic nervous system. This decreases heart rate and blood pressure, dilates the capillaries, and optimizes delivery of oxygen to all of the body's tissues.

- Alters the neurochemistry profile (neurotransmitters bond with receptor sites on cells to excite or inhibit their function). This moderates pain, depression, and addictive cravings and optimizes immune function.

- Improves resistance to disease and infection by accelerating the elimination of toxic metabolic by-products from the tissues, organs, and glands via the lymphatic system.

- Coordinates communication between the right and left hemispheres of the brain. This promotes deeper sleep, reduced anxiety, and mental clarity.

- Induces alpha and theta brain waves. This reduces heart rate and blood pressure, facilitating relaxation.

- Moderates the function of the hypothalamus, pituitary, and pineal glands, as well as the cerebrospinal fluid of the brain and spinal cord. This mediates pain and mood, facilitates immune function, and regulates sleep.

Yoga

One of the most ancient systems of self-healing practiced today, yoga teaches a basic principle of mind-body unity: if the mind is chronically restless and agitated, the health of the body will be compromised. Similarly, if the body is in poor health, mental clarity will be adversely affected. The practice of yoga can help integrate mind, body, and spirit.

Classical ashtanga yoga is divided into eight branches (*ashtanga* means "eight limbs") that give guidance on the proper diet, hygiene, detoxification regimes, and physical practices to help the individual integrate their personal, psychological, and spiritual awareness. The most well-known type of yoga is hatha yoga, which teaches certain asanas (postures) and breathing techniques to create profound changes in the body and mind. An important aspect of yoga is harnessing and increasing the flow of prana, or life energy (similar to the Chinese qi). The blockage of prana, whether due to improper diet, lifestyle stressors, or imbalance in one's physical, emotional, or spiritual health, can lead to illness. Breathing techniques and the duration certain postures are held can help remove blockages in the flow of prana.

Breathing Awareness with Yoga

Well-known yoga teacher Beryl Bender Birch says one of the gifts of yoga is that it trains you to pay attention to your breath. "As long as you can stay focused on your breath, you're in the present moment," says Bender Birch. "You can't be with your breath and also be worried about a fight you had this morning, and you can learn to use yoga breathing techniques to loosen that stranglehold, that stress." For people with stress and anxiety, she recommends a yoga breathing technique called *ujjayi* breathing. *Ujjayi* breathing is deep-chest breathing that lengthens the breath through glottal control, a slight conscious constriction of the throat that creates a unique hissing sound. Here are her step-by-step instructions for *ujjayi* breathing:[9]

1. Begin by whispering an "ahh" or "urr" sound with your mouth open on an exhalation. Completely empty your lungs as you make the sound.

2. Inhale while making the same "ahh" or "urr" sound. Completely fill your lungs.

3. Repeat this process with your mouth closed. You will notice a soft aspirant sound as you inhale, and a throaty sibilant sound as you exhale, much like a closed-mouth whisper. Continue to breathe with your mouth closed, inhaling and exhaling through the nose only. You should feel your diaphragm rising and falling and notice an increasing sensation of relaxation as you continue to breathe this way.

The main reason yoga can help people with sleep disorders, in addition to its ability to relax tight muscles, is that regular practice restores the connection between mind and body, says Beryl Bender Birch, author of *Power Yoga*. As this happens, your brain waves begin to slow down, fostering more relaxation. "Yoga is about learning to pay attention," she says. "*Yoga* means "to unite," and it's about joining the mind and body." When people are integrated in this way, they are relaxed and their stress is reduced, she says. Regular yoga practice can have therapeutic, balancing, and purifying effects on metabolism, and particularly the endocrine system. According to Birch, this can help sleep disorders that are caused by hormone imbalances, poor digestion, or malnutrition.

The safest and most reliable way to use yoga therapeutically is to follow a balanced program of postures to achieve an overall normalizing and health-inducing effect. It is best for the beginner to start with a simple program of basic postures. A structured course can teach the fundamental breathing techniques and postures, which you can then practice on your own. Find a local teacher or use yoga tapes or books as a guide.

success story

Yoga Transforms Sleep by Transforming Life

BRAD, A 51-YEAR-OLD HIGH-PROFILE ATTORNEY, was unable to turn off his mind when he went home at night. The details of his cases and the intensity, drama, and stress of mediating battles in other people's lives churned over and over in his mind, preventing him from relaxing. Despite a heavy exercise routine that included running marathons and weight training, only rarely could Brad could fall asleep easily or sleep through the night. He also suffered from hypertension and poor circulation.

Brad's osteopath was treating him for numerous running injuries, such as inflammation and tightness in his leg muscles and knee problems. The osteopath suggested to Brad that he start doing yoga as a preventive measure to keep his muscles and joints flexible and thereby avoid further injuries, so Brad signed up for a class.

At first, Brad was unable to let go during yoga class, even during the relaxation session at the end of class. Unable to lie down, he instead paced around the room. His teacher felt this tied into his profession, and that discord and intensity of his job were preventing him from relaxing in class—and from sleeping at night. She believed that no matter what the reason for his insomnia, it was the imbalance in his life that was the main problem. She counseled Brad to pay attention to what his sleeping difficulties might be telling him about his life.

After several weeks, Brad began to unwind. Friends who knew him as an attorney said they couldn't believe he was the same person when they saw him in yoga class. Brad started going to yoga class three to five times a week. Over the course of a year, he gradually began making changes in his lifestyle and relationships, adding more balance and finding a new partner who supported him in learning to relax. He noticed that he slept better when he was out of town and away from the telephones, so Brad began scheduling more vacations and treating himself better. He continues to attend yoga classes and is sleeping through the night on a regular basis.

Kegel Exercises

You may be a little surprised to see Kegel exercises recommended for improving sleep. What's the connection? Kegel exercises can help maintain the health of the bladder and urinary tract. The benefit in terms of sleep is that this can translate into less frequent awakening due to a need to urinate. The benefits of Kegel exercises for women have been publicized for many years, but they can also be immensely helpful for men. It's time to close the gender gap and encourage men to do these exercises too.

Although enlargement of the prostate (benign prostatic hypertrophy, or BPH) is not considered to be a sleep disorder, we would be remiss if we didn't address this condition, which is so common in men, especially as they age. Some men wake up in order to urinate as many as 10 times a night. This can be highly disruptive to sleep, even if it isn't a true sleep disorder. While there are natural herbal products that work to diminish frequent nighttime urination, the best approach is to strengthen the pelvic floor muscles, which can reduce the frequency of the need to urinate. Women who suffer from disturbed sleep due to frequent nighttime urination may also benefit from Kegel exercises. But because there are so many educational resources on Kegel exercises for women, we'll focus here on Kegel exercises for men, with a set of exercises I call "Prostate Aerobics."

The pelvic floor muscles are generally ignored by men, with many unfortunate repercussions, including poor urinary control, prostate dysfunction, and diminished sexual performance. In early adulthood, men tend to be highly motivated to achieve orgasm, which is a good thing, as orgasms actually exercise the prostate and surrounding muscles. But for most men, frequency of orgasms diminishes in midlife, which can allow these vital pelvic floor muscles to atrophy and become weak. But this need not be the case, and in fact, exercising the pelvic floor muscles may be the most effective thing a man can do to ensure prostate health and enhance sexual performance. You may be wondering what exactly the pelvic floor is. It's a hammocklike array muscles that supports the internal organs within the pelvis and abdomen. So, now you're probably wondering how to exercise these muscles. Simply put, you exercise these muscles by squeezing and relaxing them. That sounds straightforward enough, but first you have to find the right muscles. To identify the correct muscles, try stopping your urine stream and then allowing it to start again. The muscles you use to do this are the ones you should be exercising. Until you're sure you're exercising the correct muscles, continue to check in by stopping your stream of urine. Here's another way to make sure you're using the correct muscles: If you contract your pelvic floor muscles while standing, you should see your penis move slightly.

When doing the following exercises, don't tighten your buttock or thigh muscles, and relax your stomach muscles as much as possible. To do Prostate Aerobics, begin by squeezing your pelvic floor muscles for a count of four, then relax for a count of four. At first, you may only be able to contract the muscles for 1 to 2 seconds and your control will be minimal, but as your muscles get stronger you'll be able to hold four a count of four. Have no doubts; you will be able to feel the difference when a you achieve a full, healthy contraction and relaxation. Work up to repeating these exercises for 5 minutes twice a day. Remember to relax between each contraction. Just let the muscles go loose; don't push down. Keep your other muscles relaxed, and be sure to breathe while doing the exercises; holding your breath may put excessive pressure on the muscles. You can do these exercises anytime, anywhere. As you become more toned and proficient, you may find all manner of creative times when these can be done: while watching TV, standing in line, or driving. Though the effects are powerful, there's no outward sign of what you're doing, so no one but you will be the wiser. Because this muscle strengthens quickly, you'll soon notice that you're waking up with more solid erections (and that's always a good thing).

It usually takes about 6 to 12 weeks to see results, in terms of nighttime urination. For optimum prostate and genitourinary health, always contract your pelvic floor muscles whenever you sit up from lying down, stand from a sitting position, or lift something heavy.

Once they learn about the benefits of these exercises, some men exercise more than they should, hoping this will help them more rapidly regain bladder control and achieve prostate health (or maybe it's the lure of enhanced sexual performance). Be aware that if you do these exercises too intensively too soon, your bladder control may get worse for awhile. Start slowly and increase the amount of time gradually.

Prostate Aerobics

Exercise 1: Quickly clench and release your pelvic floor muscles over the course of a 10-second period, then take a 10-second break. Do three sets, then take a 30-second break. Then, clench and unclench for 5 seconds with 5-second breaks in between. Do this 10 times in a row. Next, contract for 30 seconds and then release for 30 seconds. Do this 3 times in a row. Repeat the first step (three sets of quick contractions for a 10-second period) and you're done for the day.

Exercise 2: Tighten your pelvic floor muscles and hold for a count of 5, then release. Repeat 10 times. Then, contract and release the muscle 10 times quickly. Repeat 3 times. Next, contract and release in long and short intervals for counts of 10. Repeat 3 times. Finally, contract and hold for as long as you can. Try to work your way up to 120 seconds (relax, that's only 2 minutes).

Exercise 3: Fully contract and release your pelvic floor muscles over and over again. Begin with one set of 30, and then slowly work your way up to over 100. Squeeze as tightly as you possibly can, making sure that you're contracting only your pelvic floor muscles. Hold for 20 seconds, then rest for 30 seconds. Repeat 5 times.

Exercise 4: This one's simple: Just contract and release your pelvic floor muscles for 2 minutes a day, and gradually work your way up to doing it for 20 minutes at least 3 times a day. You should eventually be able to perform at least 200 repetitions per session.

Chiropractic

Osseous manipulation is the repositioning of bones, including the joints of the spinal column, cranium, and other movable joints. Chiropractors, as well as naturopathic doctors and qualified osteopathic physicians, are trained and licensed to practice this type of therapy. Chiropractic is concerned with the relationship of the spinal column and musculoskeletal structures to the nervous system. Because the nervous system controls the functions of all other systems of the body, it holds the key to the body's incredible potential to heal itself. The spinal column acts as a switchboard for the nervous system, and when slight misalignments of the spine (called subluxations) interfere, the transmissions of the nervous system can be altered, as when an electrical wire that has been crimped. This can not only cause localized pain in the spine, it can also interfere with neurological information being transmitted to the major organs and cause dysfunction or disease. By adjusting the spine joints to remove subluxations, normal nerve function can be restored.

Types of Chiropractic Treatment

The primary feature of chiropractic treatment is chiropractic adjustments. If an examination reveals localized areas of dysfunction, treatment is begun to restore proper alignment to the spine. The chiropractic physician may accomplish the adjustment using various methods: touch (palpation), active motion (having the patient bend or stretch in different ways), and passive movement (in which the doctor assists the patient), or some combination of these.

One type of adjustment is a maneuver in which the joint is gently and precisely stretched to just beyond its normal range of motion. An audible, painless click is often heard, which is caused by the release of gases from the joint fluid. The patient will usually notice an increased range of movement in the joint, and any soreness should rapidly disappear.

Some chiropractors prefer to use methods known as nonforce techniques, applying gentle touch along the spine, skull, and pelvis. No forceful adjustments are used, and there are no popping sounds when the vertebral subluxations are corrected. Another option is the use of a handheld instrument called an activator, a small instrument with a rubber tip used to gently and painlessly move the vertebrae.

Applied kinesiology deals not only with the placement of bones, but with the muscles that hold them in position. Chiropractors employing applied kinesiology use special techniques to help balance opposing muscles attached to a misaligned bone. Their approach restores normal muscle function in order to allow osseous adjustments to be more effective.

Network Spinal Analysis (NSA) is a new method of chiropractic developed by groundbreaking chiropractor Donald M. Epstein, who observed from clinical experience that not all subluxations of the spine are the same. NSA combines a variety of chiropractic techniques to enable the practitioner to adjust subluxations with the precise amount and type of force suggested by clinical findings. "This is different from attempting to match the vertebra being adjusted to a specific technique," Dr. Epstein explains. "The difference lies in the sequence of the adjustments and the 'networking' of the various methods."

Just as there are several types of adjustments, there are also several types of chiropractic physicians. Though they are usually split into two groups—those who combine chiropractic with other modalities (mixers) and those who deal only with locating and removing subluxations (straight chiropractors)—in reality, chiropractors exist along a spectrum between these two extremes.

Chiropractic Brings Relief from Insomnia

JERRY, A 35-YEAR-OLD WRITER, had been self-treating his insomnia with all types of natural products—herbs, vitamins, minerals, and homeopathic remedies—for years, but with no success. He had difficulty both falling asleep and staying asleep; in fact, there were long periods of time when he got no sleep at all. His episodes of insomnia had recurred regularly for 15 years. Because natural treatments hadn't helped him, Jerry had resigned himself to living with the insomnia. Little did he know that he had finally found a solution when he visited chiropractor David Waldman, for chronic upper and middle back pain.

During the exam, Jerry told the chiropractor about his unsuccessful experiments with natural products to cure his sleep problems. When Jerry described his doses, the doctor said that he was actually taking toxic levels of the sedative herbs valerian and St. John's wort, L-tryptophan, and other substances. Not surprisingly, given his history of poor sleep and overuse of supplements, Jerry had problems with his digestion, including frequent indigestion after meals, gas and bloating, and a queasy stomach.

The chiropractor evaluated Jerry's spinal function through an exam and other tests, and found that he had inflammation and joint dysfunction in his middle and upper spine. The doctor began a series of spinal manipulations, or adjustments, in that area and also used therapeutic touch in the middle part of the spine, using his hands to unblock energy in Jerry's back.

Jerry discontinued the array of herbal remedies that he was taking for sleep and saw the chiropractor six times over the next three weeks. At the end of the three weeks, Jerry's pain was reduced and all of his sleep and digestive problems were gone. Since that time, he's experienced a few isolated episodes of insomnia, but as soon as those arise, he goes back for treatment and his sleep is restored.

The chiropractor's assessment was that there were two factors involved in Jerry's inability to sleep. One was that he couldn't get into a comfortable position, so he was feeling physical discomfort, which created an inability to relax and fall asleep. And, less obviously, he was impacted by neurological compression due to subluxations, which can affect the functioning of the entire nervous system in innumerable ways. One of the effects can be neurological irritation and irritability, which can interfere with sleep.

Craniosacral Therapy

Craniosacral therapy refers to correcting imbalances in the relationship among breathing, the sacrum (the base of the backbone, attached to the pelvis), and the bones of the skull (cranium), especially the occiput. The sacrum acts as a pump to propel cerebrospinal fluid up the spine to the brain; the cranial bones contract and pump it back down. Health depends on a smoothly functioning sacro-occipital pump. Restrictions that result from injury, inflexibility of the joints of the spine and cranium, or dysfunctions in other parts of the body can all cause abnormalities in the craniosacral system that can contribute to dysfunction and poor health, especially in the brain and spinal cord.

The purpose of craniosacral therapy is to enhance the functioning of this important system. Usually delivered by a chiropractor or other trained practitioner, craniosacral adjustments require only a light touch to restore the sacrum to full motion and balance with respect to the cranial bones. The proper functioning of the craniosacral system implies health for the central nervous system and allows it to rest at a more stress-free level.

People who experience craniosacral treatment describe profound states of relaxation and feeling lighter and more integrated. "When there is synchronous movement in the craniosacral system, the physiology of the central nervous system functions more efficiently and the nerve tissue is, in general, healthier," says chiropractor Robert Norett.

Neuro-Emotional Technique

Neuro-Emotional Technique (NET) is a process developed by chiropractor Scott Walker using principles from chiropractic and acupuncture. In NET theory, physical problems are almost always caused by a neuro-emotional complex (NEC), which consists of a combination of several or all of the following: a spinal vertebra out of alignment; an acupuncture meridian out of balance; a specific emotion being activated; a memory picture of an event in the past; and conditioned responses of various muscle or body systems. NET practitioners, who are mostly chiropractors, identify NECs through case history, physical examination, and applied kinesiology, which evaluates the health of various organs or body parts by using a simple strength resistance on a muscle related to that organ or body part. The practitioner then performs a spinal adjustment along with manipulation of reflex points, thereby releasing the NEC and the emotional pattern that goes with it. Once the NEC is released, the physical problem usually clears up.

Dr. Walker estimates that he has about a 90% success rate using NET to treat people with insomnia. It may be that sleep disorders respond well to NET because they frequently entail an emotional component, such as anxiety, fear, worry, sadness, or depression. In diagnosing some types of insomnia, Dr. Walker uses the Chinese clock, which states that qi (life force energies) run through the 12 major meridians on a daily cycle. By asking people what time they usually wake up at night, he can determine what meridian is affected. Often it is during liver time (1 A.M. to 3 A.M.) or gallbladder time (11 P.M. to 1 A.M.).

According to Dr. Walker, the Chinese clock can be a useful starting place for identifying reflex points that need treatment. For example, if a person always wakes up at midnight, the practitioner knows to check the gallbladder reflex points. If muscle testing finds a weakness in the gallbladder reflex points, this confirms that the gallbladder meridian is disrupted. Next, the practitioner will hold a reflex point for emotional issues, located on the forehead, to see if the imbalance has an emotional component. If the muscle tests weak while the practitioner is holding the emotional reflex point, this indicates that emotions are involved and that NET can be useful.

The person is encouraged to relax and let any memories surface while answering questions from the practitioner, a process Dr. Walker calls "semantic testing." This phase of treatment involves stirring up concepts in the patient's memory in an effort to stimulate memories associated with the NEC. When a clear picture of a painful memory emerges, the patient describes it to the practitioner. Then the patient holds the memory picture in their mind and touches the relevant reflex points while the practitioner gives the patient a spinal adjustment, simultaneously releasing both the body memory and the emotional picture. Sometimes just one memory release can cure insomnia, but there are often layers of memories to be released. Dr. Walker estimates the typical insomnia patient gets significant relief in three to seven visits.[10]

Dr. Walker explains that NET is based on a "triad of health," like an equilateral triangle where one side is structure or spinal alignment, the second is biochemistry, and the third is emotions. A person's health is dependent on each side of the triangle being sound, and on all three existing in harmony. The biochemistry side refers mainly to informational messenger molecules that circulate in the body fluids, such as hormones and neuropeptides, and mediate emotions.

What this means, Dr. Walker says, is that emotions aren't necessarily generated in the mind and that they can be accessed in various parts of the body via neuropeptides. When a specific emotional trauma takes place, the body chemistry takes a "picture" of that trauma and memorizes the physiological responses; in other words, the body preserves the biochemical response to the emotional trauma through the neuropeptides. Over time, that traumatized body response pattern will weaken the meridians and other body structures associated with the event, ultimately causing symptoms or a disease, until the traumatic response pattern is released. "NET is really about the physiological aspects of emotions," Dr. Walker says.

Bodywork

The term *bodywork* refers to therapies such as massage, reflexology, and acupressure, which are employed to improve the structure and functioning of the human body. Bodywork in all its forms helps to reduce pain, soothe injured muscles, stimulate circulation of both the blood and lymphatic fluid, and promote deep relaxation—all helpful for sleep disorders.

Massage

Massage is used for general well-being, stress reduction, resolution of embedded emotional issues or psychological problems, recovery from sports injuries or muscle soreness, or as an adjunct therapy for various medical conditions. In recent decades, an overwhelming amount of scientific evidence has accumulated in support of the claim that massage therapy is beneficial.[11] According to John Yates, Ph.D., author of *A Physician's Guide to Therapeutic Massage*, massage can benefit such conditions as muscle spasm and pain, spinal curvatures, soreness related to injury and stress, headaches, whiplash, temporomandibular joint (TMJ) syndrome, and tension-related respiratory disorders such as bronchial asthma or emphysema. Massage can also help reduce swelling, correct posture, improve body motion, and facilitate the elimination of toxins from the body.[12] Lymphatic massage, for example, can move metabolic waste through the body to promote rapid recovery from illness or disease. Other studies show that massage can be used as an adjunct in the treatment of cardiovascular disorders and neurological and gynecological problems, and can often be used in place of pharmacological drugs.[13]

Tim Silva, a licensed massage therapist, says massage is a natural way to treat sleep disorders because it already has the goal of releasing muscle tension and helping the person relax. When you consider the benefits of massage—improved circulation of blood and lymphatic fluid, release of toxins, release of tension, mind-body integration, and reduction of stress—you can see that all of these would be beneficial for easing sleep disorders.[14]

The Therapeutic Effects of Massage

Gertrude Beard, author of the classic *Massage: Principles and Techniques*, summarizes the findings of numerous research studies on the therapeutic effects of massage. Studies indicate that massage has the following benefits:

- Sedates the nervous system and promotes voluntary muscle relaxation
- Relieves certain types of pain
- Provides effective treatment of chronic inflammatory conditions by increasing lymphatic circulation
- Improves circulation through the capillaries, veins, and arteries, and increases blood flow through the muscles
- Triggers reflex actions in the body to stimulate various organs
- Promotes recovery from fatigue

Beard adds that therapeutic massage should be applied only by a skilled practitioner trained in appropriate methods.

Reflexology

Reflexology is based on the idea that there are reflex areas in the hands and feet that correspond to every part of the body, including the organs and glands. Practiced in Asia for thousands of years, it was introduced in the United States by Dr. William H. Fitzgerald in 1913; his method was further developed by Eunice Ingham, a physiotherapist, who mapped out reflexes on the feet and developed techniques for inducing healing effects in areas of the body that correspond to the reflex points. Practitioners often focus on breaking up lactic acid and calcium crystals accumulated around any of the 7,200 nerve endings in each foot. By applying gentle but precise pressure to these reflex points, reflexologists can release blockages that inhibit energy flow and cause pain and disease. This pressure is believed to affect internal organs and glands by stimulating the parts of the body associated with the reflex points. Typically, practitioners use their thumbs to press on the various zones, or areas of the feet, that correspond to organs or other structural components of the body. For sleep disorders, reflexology can help to detoxify organs such as the kidneys and liver, as well as stimulate sluggish glands, like the thyroid and adrenals.

Reflexology Resolves
Multiple Symptoms

BARBARA, 44, WAS DIAGNOSED with multiple sclerosis. Around the same time, as part of that crippling disease, she developed constant foot pain that was so severe she had trouble walking and had to use a cane. The foot pain prevented her from sleeping, even though Barbara bought a metal lift to put under her bed covers to keep the sheets and blankets off her feet. She also tried chiropractic treatments, special shoes, heel lifts, and podiatrist visits, all to no avail. "They took X-rays of my feet to see if there was something wrong, but they couldn't find anything," she say. Barbara also suffered from constipation and leg cramps as part of her multiple sclerosis. Finally, she decided to consult with a licensed massage therapist and foot reflexologist.

During the first visit, a 30-minute session where the therapist kneaded, massaged, and pressed on the many knots of muscle tension on the bottom of her feet, Barbara felt a great deal of discomfort. But after three treatments, Barbara's foot pain was substantially reduced. She saw the reflexologist two or three times a week for the next six months and massaged her feet at home as well. By the end of that time, Barbara's foot pain was gone and she was able to sleep again. She also began having more regular bowel movements and her leg cramps disappeared. The relief has lasted, with occasional tune-ups, ever since.

Oriental Bodywork

Oriental body therapies, such as acupuncture and acupressure, work to balance the flow of qi (vital energy) throughout energy meridians. These meridians run throughout the body and are associated with different organs. If a blockage exists in a meridian, it will be expressed as health problems in the organs associated with that meridian. Blocked qi can be released by applying pressure to specific points along the meridians. Acupuncture uses needles for this purpose, while acupressure (for example, shiatsu or Jin Shin Do) uses rubbing, kneading, or other types of pressure from the fingers and hands.

Reflexology Massage to Promote Sleep

For a better night's rest, here's a simple self-massage to do before bed. For the best effect, take a relaxing soak in a hot tub with a few drops of calming essential oils, such as lavender, rose otto, patchouli, Roman chamomile, sandalwood, or most citrus, before you do the self-massage. You can also rub diluted essential oils directly on your skin to help you further relax.[15]

1. Sit comfortably with your left leg crossed over the right so you can easily reach your left foot.

2. Use the knuckles of your right hand to massage the sole of your left foot. Press firmly, moving slowly in small circles. Pay particular attention to any areas that are tender.

3. After massaging the sole, massage the top of your foot up to the ankle, using only the tips of your fingers, not the fleshy pads; press gently but firmly. Use your thumb to massage firmly between the long tendons that run from your ankle to each toe.

4. Massage the bottom of the heel with your thumb and forefinger.

5. Grasp your foot with both hands and press hard top and bottom, sliding out to the edge of the foot.

6. Grasp your big toe with your thumb and forefinger, pull gently, then shake the toe; repeat with the other toes.

7. Repeat the entire procedure on your right foot.

Foot Reflexology Chart

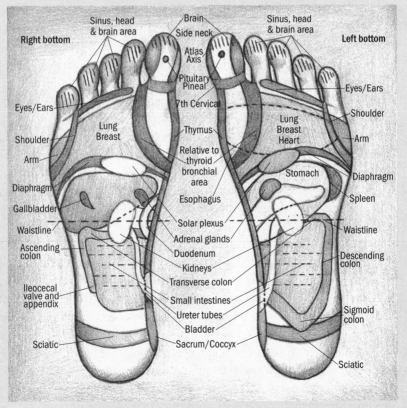

Acupressure Points for Better Sleep

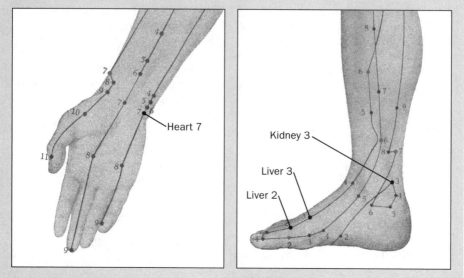

Heart 7

Kidney 3

Liver 3

Liver 2

From An Outline of Chinese Acupuncture, *copyright 1975 by Pergamon Press, Inc.*

Shiatsu, which means "finger pressure" in Japanese, was originally developed from ancient Chinese acupressure techniques. It uses a sequence of firm rhythmic pressure applied to specific points for 3 to 10 seconds and, like acupuncture, is designed to awaken, calm, and harmonize the meridians. Shiatsu affects not only the acupressure points, but the entire mind and body, making it one of the most effective forms of bodywork for sleep disorders. *Jim Shin Do*, another Japanese bodywork technique, is based on *Jim Shin Jyutsu*, a technique developed by Jiro Murai. Master Murai based his system on moving qi through the meridians by using certain combinations of acupressure points in a special sequence. Pressure is held for a minute or more, until the practitioner can feel the flow of blood and qi through the point. Specific opening and releasing sequences are important for moving the qi in the proper direction.

The simplest approach to doing acupressure on yourself to help with insomnia is to work what the Chinese call the microsystems, according to Dr. Roger Jahnke. There are three microsystems in the body: the ears, the feet, and the hands. The whole body is represented by and can be affected at specific points in the microsystems. You start the massage by rubbing the whole microsystem (each ear, for example) vigorously for a few minutes. Then, you begin the massage again, this time going more slowly and looking for areas of particular soreness. When you find sore spots, spend a few minutes focusing on them, using firm and steady pressure. Dr. Jahnke says you can do a good total body treatment using the three microsystems in about 15 minutes. He recommends that people with insomnia try to do at least one 15-minute session each day.

Here are some specific acupuncture points to massage if you can't sleep:

- Liver 2 or 3: Find the fleshy space on the top of your foot between your big toe and second toe. Feel for the sorest spot and massage or press firmly for 1 or 2 minutes.

- Heart 7: Find the bony prominence on the inside of your wrist, opposite the thumb. Massage or press firmly just inside the prominence.

- Kidney 3: Find the fleshy part on the inside of your ankle just behind the bony prominence and massage or press firmly.

Good Night

Hopefully some of the therapies described in this book have helped you sleep better. In fact, it's our hope that they've helped you so much that you didn't even need to read all the way to this conclusion. If you're still struggling with sleep problems, have patience with yourself. The factors that combined to produce the problem were probably at work for quite some time; it might not be realistic to expect to be able to erase them in a few short weeks. Keep in mind the three basic "goods" from the introduction: a good night's sleep, a good morning elimination, and a good breakfast. While you're working on the specific therapies recommended in the book, you can simultaneously implement these basic good practices: go to bed and wake up on time, give yourself time for a morning bowel movement, and eat a nutritionally sound breakfast. Making the time to implement these basic daily changes is the best investment you can make to jump-start your path to health.

Be aware of which therapies and approaches seem to have helped your sleep. If they've benefited you even just a bit, chances are you can achieve more improvement by continuing with that therapy or fine-tuning it. If you've resisted certain approaches we've advocated, give them a fair chance and see what happens. You have very little to lose and a great deal to gain—not just sound, restorative sleep, but overall health and well-being. Most of all, we wish you peaceful sleep and pleasant dreams. Good night.

Quick Definitions

Acupuncture Meridians

Acupuncture meridians are specific pathways in the human body for the flow of life force, or the subtle energy known as qi (pronounced CHEE). In most cases, these energy pathways run up and down both sides of the body and correspond to individual organs or organ systems, designated as lung, small intestine, heart, and so on. There are 12 principal meridians and 8 secondary channels.

Advanced Sleep Phase Syndrome

In advanced sleep phase syndrome (ASPS), the person tends to always fall asleep very early in the evening, usually between 6 p.m. and 9 p.m., and wake up before dawn, sometimes as early as 1 a.m.

Amino Acids

Amino acids are the basic building blocks of the tens of thousands of different proteins in the body, including enzymes, hormones, and the key messenger molecules of the nervous system, called neurotransmitters. Some amino acids cannot be made by the body and must be obtained through the diet; these are known as essential amino acids. Others are produced in the body but not always in sufficient amounts.

Antioxidant

An antioxidant is a natural biochemical substance that protects living cells against damage from harmful free radicals. Antioxidants work against the process of oxidation—the robbing of electrons from substances. Oxidation can lead to cellular aging, degeneration, arthritis, heart disease, cancer, and other illnesses. Antioxidants react with free radicals and neutralize them before they can damage the body. Antioxidant nutrients include vitamins A, C, and E, beta-carotene, selenium, coenzyme Q10, L-glutathione, superoxide dismutase, and bioflavonoids.

Bed-Wetting

Clinically known as sleep enuresis, bed-wetting is an uncontrollable loss of bladder control during the night. It happens in all sleep stages and is believed to be hereditary.

Bruxism

Bruxism is characterized by grinding the teeth during sleep.

Cortisol

Cortisol is a hormone secreted by the adrenal glands. Secretion of cortisol occurs in daily cycles, peaking in the morning and having the lowest values at night.

Delayed Sleep Phase Syndrome

Delayed sleep phase syndrome (DSPS) is a condition in which the person chronically stays up quite late, usually until 3 a.m. to 4 a.m., and then sleeps all morning, getting up at 10 a.m. to 11 a.m.

Endocrine Glands

Endocrine glands, including the testicles, ovaries, pancreas, adrenals, thyroid, parathyroid, and pituitary, are central to the regulation and normalization of all the body's complex, interconnected systems, from metabolism and heat production to spermatogenesis and uterine preparations for pregnancy.

Environmental Estrogens

Environmental estrogens, or xenoestrogens, are foreign compounds or chemical toxins that mimic the effects of estrogen in the body.

Essential Fatty Acids

Essential fatty acids (EFAs) are unsaturated fats required in the diet. Omega-3 and omega-6 fatty acids are the two principal types. Once in the body, omega-3 and omega-6 fatty acids are converted to prostaglandins, hormonelike substances that regulate many metabolic functions, particularly inflammatory processes.

Free Radical

A free radical is an unstable molecule with an unpaired electron that steals an electron from another molecule and produces harmful effects.

Hormones

Hormones, the chemical messengers of the endocrine system, impose order through an intricate communication system among the body's estimated 50 trillion cells. Examples include sex hormones (such as testosterone, estrogen, and progesterone), melatonin, growth hormone, and DHEA.

Human Growth Hormone

Human growth hormone (HGH), which is secreted by the pituitary gland in the brain, is a small, proteinlike hormone similar to insulin. HGH is secreted in very brief pulses during the early hours of sleep and remains in circulation for only a few minutes.

Hypersomnia

Hypersomnia describes sleep disorders in which people sleep too much, either for prolonged periods at night or during the day. Seasonal affective disorder (SAD) is a type of hypersomnia in which people sleep in late, among other symptoms.

Immune System

The immune system guards the body against foreign, disease-producing substances. Its workers are various white blood cells, including 1 trillion lymphocytes and 100 million trillion antibodies produced and secreted by the lymphocytes. Lymphocytes are found in high numbers in the lymph nodes, bone marrow, spleen, and thymus gland.

Insomnia

Insomnia is a broad term casually used to describe the inability either to fall asleep or to remain asleep during the course of the night.

Lymphatic system

The lymphatic system consists of lymph fluid and the structures (vessels, ducts, and nodes) involved in transporting it from tissues to the bloodstream. The lymphatic system is the body's master drain, collecting and filtering the lymph fluid and conveying it to the bloodstream, thereby clearing waste products and cellular debris from the tissues.

Melatonin

Melatonin is the hormone secreted by the pineal gland, located in the center of the brain. Melatonin does the pineal gland's work of controlling the cycle of sleeping and waking and regulating the body's internal time clock, or circadian rhythm. The pineal gland adjusts its melatonin output based primarily on the body's exposure to light, although many other factors, including EMFs, can influence melatonin production.

Narcolepsy

Narcolepsy is a chronic sleep disorder in which patients experience daytime sleepiness so extreme that they fall asleep at inappropriate times for anywhere from a few seconds to 30 minutes.

Neuropeptides

Neuropeptides are chains of amino acids formed in the DNA of neurons and released into the extracellular fluid. To date, approximately 609 neuropeptides have been discovered. These substances, which are part of a larger group of messenger molecules called informational substances, are the carriers and mediators of emotions as well as other neurological functions. Neuropeptides are also manufactured by other tissues in the body and can be transported to the brain. When manufactured and released by endocrine system cells they are called hormones, and when released from the immune system they are called immunotransmitters.

Neurotransmitter

A neurotransmitter is a brain chemical with the specific function of enabling communication between brain cells.

Night Terrors

People experiencing night terrors (also called sleep terrors) suddenly let out a piercing scream or cry and may even jump out of bed, run out of the house, or do bodily harm to themselves or others. Though the sleeper may appear conscious of their acts because their eyes are open and their pupils are dilated, the person may not awaken until after the episode.

Periodic Limb Movement Disorder

Periodic limb movement disorder (PLMD) often coexists with restless legs syndrome. It is characterized by sudden, involuntary, and repetitive leg jerking that occurs at the onset of sleep as well as during the course of sleep.

REM Behavior Disorder

REM behavior disorder occurs during the REM (dream) stage of sleep. Normally, most of our muscles become paralyzed during the REM phase to prevent us from acting out our dreams. In RBD, however, it appears the brain does not properly signal the paralysis function, so sleepers physically engage in their dreams without being actively conscious of their behavior.

Restless Legs Syndrome

Restless legs syndrome (RLS) is an unpleasant sleep disorder in which sufferers often feel creeping, crawling, prickling, burning, itching, or tugging sensations in their legs while resting or sitting for extended periods of time. Sometimes the arms may be affected as well. At night, the sensations can be so bothersome that people with RLS feel the need to move their legs and often cannot get to sleep until the discomfort subsides.

Rhythmic Movement Disorder

Rhythmic movement disorder (RMD) involves head banging, head rolling, body rocking, body rolling, or other repetitive movements. It typically occurs immediately prior to sleep onset and is sustained into light sleep (stages 1 and 2).

Sleep Apnea

Sleep apnea is a potentially life-threatening disorder in which the sleeper involuntarily stops breathing for 10 to 60 seconds, resulting in decreased blood levels of oxygen and increased amounts of carbon dioxide. This change in blood gases alerts the brain to begin breathing. To do so, the brain must awaken the body from deep sleep. The sleeper then resumes breathing, usually with a loud snort or gasp, and then quickly falls back into light sleep.

Somnambulism

Also known as sleepwalking, somnambulism usually occurs in stage 4, the deepest stage of sleep, during the first third of the night. As its name suggests, it typically involves walking, but sitting or other repetitive, routine motions may also occur. Sleepwalkers are not actively conscious of their actions and don't recall the episode upon waking.

Traditional Chinese Medicine

Traditional Chinese medicine (TCM) is a comprehensive system of medical practice that heals the body according to the principles of nature and balance. A Chinese medicine physician considers the flow of vital energy (qi) in a patient through close examination of the patient's pulse, tongue, body odor, voice tone and strength, and general demeanor, among other elements. Underlying imbalances and disharmony in the body are described in terminology analogous to the natural world (heat, cold, dryness, dampness, or wind).

Resources

Bedding and Sleepwear

Natural Bedding Products
Gaiam, 360 Interlocken Boulevard, Broomfield, CO 80021 tel: 303-222-3600
fax: 303-222-3700 website: www.gaiam.com

Garnet Hill, 231 Main Street, Franconia, NH 03580, tel: 800-870-3513
fax: 888-842-9696, website: www.garnethill.com

Vivetique, 11134 Rush Street, South El Monte, CA 91733, tel: 800-365-6563
fax: 626-357-3248, website: www.vivetique.com

Therapeutic Magnets and Mattress Pads
American Health Service, 13822 West Boulton Boulevard, Mettawa, IL 60045,
tel: 800-422-4733, website: www.americanhealthservice.com

Philpott Medical Services, 17171 Southeast 29th Street, Choctaw, OK 73020,
tel: 405-390-3009

Wicking J Sleepwear, Inc., P.O. Box 1179, Evergreen, CO 80437, tel: 303-674-0309
fax: 303-679-2646, website: www.wickingsleepwear.com

Complementary Therapies

Aromatherapy
American Alliance of Aromatherapy, P.O. Box 750428, Petaluma, CA 94975-0428,
tel: 707-778-6762

Ayurveda
Virender Sodhi, MD, ND, 2115 112th Avenue NE, Bellevue, WA 98004,
tel: 425-453-8022 fax: 425-451-2670, email: ayurvedicnews@ayurvedicscience.com,
website: www.ayurvedicscience.com

Biofeedback
Association for Applied Biofeedback and Physiopsychology, 10200 W. 44th Avenue, Suite
304, Wheat Ridge, CO 80033, tel: 800-477-8892 or 303-422-8436 fax: 303-422-8894,
email: AAPB@resourcecenter.com, website: www.aapb.org

Chiropractic Care

American Chiropractic Association, 1701 Clarendon Boulevard, Arlington, VA 22209, tel: 703-276-8800, email: memberinfo@acatoday.org, website: www.acatoday.com

Association for Network Care, 444 N. Main Street, Longmont, CO 80501, tel: 303-678-8101, website: www.associationfornetworkcare.com

International Chiropractic Association, 1110 N. Glebe Road, Suite 650, Arlington, VA 22201, tel: 800-423-4690 or 703-528-5000, website: www.chiropractic.org

Michael Borkin, DC, NMD, 2233 Faraday Avenue, Suite K, Carlsbad, CA 90402, tel: 760-448-2750, email: drb@sabresciences.com

Tim Leasenby, DC, 4260 Westbrook Drive, Suite 106, Aurora, IL 60504, tel: 630-851-9222, website: www.leasenbyclinic.com

Cognitive Therapy

The American Institute for Cognitive Therapy, 136 E. 57th Street, Suite 1101, New York, NY 10022, tel: 212-308-2440, website: www.cognitivetherapynyc.com

University of Pennsylvania Center for Cognitive Therapy, 3600 Market Street, 2nd Floor, Philadelphia, PA 19104, tel: 215-898-4100 fax: 215-898-1865, website: www.uphs.upenn.edu/psycct/

Colon Therapists

International Association for Colon Hydrotherapy (I-ACT), P.O. Box 461285, San Antonio, TX 78246-1285, tel: 210-366-2888 fax: 210-366-2999, website: www.i-act.org

Cranial Electrical Stimulation

PATH Medical, 304 Park Avenue South, 6th Floor, New York, NY 10010, tel: 212-213-6155 fax: 212-213-6188, website: www.pathmed.com

Electromedical Products International, 2201 Garrett Morris Parkway, Mineral Wells, TX 76067, tel: 800-367-7256 or 940-328-0788, website: www.alpha-stim.com

Craniosacral Therapy, The Upledger Institute, 11211 Prosperity Farms Road, Suite D-325, Palm Beach Gardens, FL 33410-3487, tel: 800-233-5880 or 561-622-4334 fax: 561-622-4771, email: upledger@upledger.com, website: www.upledger.com

Enemas

Colema Boards of California, P.O. Box 1879, Cottonwood, CA 96022, tel: 800-544-8147 or 916-347-5868, email: info@colema.com, website: www.colemaboard.com

Flower Remedies

Flower Essence Services, P.O. Box 1769, Nevada City, CA 95959, tel: 800-548-0075 fax: 530-265-6467, website: www.fesflowers.com

The Flower Essence Society, P.O. Box 459, Nevada City, CA 95959, tel: 800-736-9222 or 530-265-9163 fax: 530-265-0584, email: mail@flowersociety.org, website: www.flowersociety.org

Guided Imagery

Academy for Guided Imagery, 30765 Pacific Coast Highway, Suite 369, Malibu, CA 90265, tel: 800-726-2070 fax: 800-727-2070, website: www.academyforguidedimagery.com

Homeopathic Practitioners

Homeopathic Academy of Naturopathic Physicians, P.O. Box 126, Redmond, WA 98075, tel: 253-630-3338 fax: 815-301-6595, email: info@hanp.net, website: www.hanp.net

National Center for Homeopathy, 801 N. Fairfax, Suite 306, Alexandria, VA 22314, tel: 703-548-7790 fax: 703-548-7792, email: info@homeopathic.org, website: www .homeopathic.org

National Certification Commission for Acupuncture and Oriental Medicine (NCCAOM), 11 Canal Center Plaza, Suite 300, Alexandria, VA 22314, tel: 703-548-9004 fax: 703-548-9079, email: info@nccaom.org, website: www.nccaom.org

Hypnotherapy
Bryan Knight, The International Registry of Professional Hypnotherapists, 7306 Sherbrooke Street West, Montreal, Quebec, Canada H4B 1R7, tel: 514-827-4673, website: www.hypnosis.org

Massage
American Massage Therapy Association, 500 Davis Street, Suite 900, Evanston, IL 60201, tel: 877-905-2700 or 847-864-0123 fax: 847-864-1178, email: info@amtamassage .org, website: www.amtamassage.org

Neuro-Emotional Technique
ONE Research Foundation, 144 West D Street, Encinitas, CA 92024, tel: 760-944-7383 fax: 760-944-7816, website: www.onefoundation.org

Nutritional Medicine
American College for Advancement in Medicine, 24411 Ridge Route, Suite 115, Laguna Hills, CA 92653, tel: 949-309-3520 fax: 949-309-3538, email: info@acam.org, website: www.acamnet.org

Reflexology
International Institute of Reflexology, 5650 First Avenue North, P.O. Box 12642, St. Petersburg, FL 33733-2642, tel: 727-343-4811 fax: 727-381-2807, email: iir@tampabay .rr.com, website: www.reflexology-usa.net

TCM Practitioners
American Association of Oriental Medicine, P.O. Box 162340, Sacramento, CA 95816, tel: 866-455-7999 or 916-443-4770 fax: 916-443-4766, website: www.aaom.org

Maoshing Ni, DOM., Ph.D., L.Ac, 1131 Wilshire Boulevard, Suite 300, Santa Monica, CA 90401, tel: 310-917-2200 fax: 310-917-2267, email: contact@taoofwellness.com, website: www.taoofwellness.com

Electromagnetic Fields

Computer Screens
Technology Alternatives Corporation, 1950 NE 208 Terrace, Miami, FL 33179, tel: 800-222-3003 or 305-933-2026 fax: 305-933-8858, website: www.safelevel.com

Information on EMF Exposure
National Institute of Environmental Health Sciences, P.O. Box 12233, Research Triangle Park, NC 27709, tel: 800-363-2383, website: www.niehs.nih.gov

Protective Products
Block EMF, 2120 Las Palmas Drive, Suite E, Carlsbad, CA 92011, tel: 800-578-5939 fax: 760-431-0126, email: customerservice@healthstores.com, website: www.blockemf.com

QLink ClearWave Products
Pure Energies, 1 Century Lane, Miami Beach, FL 33139, tel: 800-700-5537 fax: 801-469-6569, website: www.qlinkworks.com

Exercise

Fitness Tips
The President's Council on Physical Fitness and Sports, 200 Independence Avenue SW, Room 738-H, Washington, DC 20201, tel: 202-690-9000 fax: 202-690-5211, website: www.fitness.gov

Qigong
American Foundation of Traditional Chinese Medicine, 505 Beach Street, San Francisco, CA 94133, tel: 415-766-0502 fax: 415-392-7003

Yoga
International Association of Yoga Therapists, 115 S. McCormick Street, Suite 3, Prescott, AZ 86303, tel: 928-541-0004 fax: 928-541-0182, email: mail@iayt.org, website: www.iayt.org

Beryl Bender Birch, Hard and Soft Yoga Institute, P.O. Box 5009, East Hampton, NY 11937, tel: 631-324-8409, email: yoga@power-yoga.com, website: www.power-yoga.com

Full-Spectrum Lighting and Light Boxes

BioLight Group, 28 Parker Way, Santa Barbara, CA 93101, tel: 805-965-1867, email: info@biolightgroup.com, website: www.biolightgroup.com

Ott-Lite Technology, P.O. Box 172425, Tampa, FL 33672-0425 tel: 800-842-8848 or 813-621-0058 fax: 813-626-8790, website: www.ott-lite.com

Seventh Generation, 60 Lake Street, Burlington, VT 05401-5218, tel: 800-456-1191 or 802-658-3773 fax: 802-658-1771, website: www.seventhgeneration.com

Verilux, 340 Mad River Park, Suite 1, Waitsfield, VT 05673, tel: 888-544-4865 or 802-496-3101 fax: 802-496-3105, email: info@verilux.net, website: www.verilux.net

Enviro-Med, 1600 SE 141st Avenue, Vancouver, WA 98683, tel: 800-222-3296 or 360-256-6989, website: www.bio-light.com

Organizations for Sleep Information

American Sleep Apnea Association, 1424 K Street NW, Suite 302, Washington, DC 20005, tel: 202-293-3650 fax: 202-293-3656, website: www.sleepapnea.org

Associated Professional Sleep Societies, One Westbrook Corporate Center, Suite 920, Westchester, IL 60154, tel: 708-492-0930 fax: 708-273-9354, website: www.apss.org

Better Sleep Council, 501 Wythe Street, Alexandria, VA 22314-1917, tel: 703-683-8371, website: www.bettersleep.org

National Center on Sleep Disorders Research; National Heart, Lung, and Blood Institute; NIH, 6701 Rockledge Drive, Bethesda, MD 20892, tel: 301-435-0199, website: www.nhlbi.nih.gov/sleep

National Sleep Foundation, 1522 K Street NW, Suite 500, Washington, DC 20005, tel: 202-347-3471 fax: 202-347-3472, website: www.sleepfoundation.org

Restless Legs Syndrome Foundation, 14th Street NW, Suite 300, Rochester, MN 55902-2985, tel: 507-287-6465 fax: 507-287-6312, email: rlsfoundation@rls.org, website: www.rls.org

Physicians and Practitioners

American College of Advancement in Medicine (ACAM), 23121 Verdugo Drive, Suite 204, Laguna Hills, CA 92653, tel: 800-532-3688 or 949-583-7666 , email: info@acam.org, website: www.acam.org

Lita Lee, Ph.D., 4826 Mahalo Drive, Eugene, OR 97405, tel: 541-431-1099, website: www.litalee.com

Gary S. Ross, MD, 500 Sutter Street, Suite 300, San Francisco, CA 94102, tel: 415-398-0555 fax: 415-398-6228., website: www.rosshealth.com

Supplements

5-HTP
NutriCology, 2300 North Loop Road, Alameda, CA 94502, tel: 800-545-9960 or 510-263-2000 fax: 510-263-2100, website: www.nutricology.com

Life Enhancement Products, P.O. Box 751390, Petaluma, CA 94975, tel: 800-543-3873 or 707-762-6144 fax: 707-769-8016, email: info@life-enhancement.com, website: www.life-enhancement.com

BioSynergy Health Alternatives, P.O. Box 16833, Boise, ID 83715, tel: 800-554-7145 fax: 208-342-0880, email: email@biosynergy.com, website: www.biosynergy.com

Chinese Patent Remedies
Mayway Corporation, 1338 Mandela Parkway, Oakland, CA 94607, tel: 800-262-9929 or 510-208-3113 fax: 510-208-3069, email: info@mayway.com, website: www.mayway.com

Cleanse 28
Arise and Shine Herbal Products, P.O. Box 400, Medford, OR 97501, tel: 800-688-2444 fax: 541-773-8866, email: admin@ariseandshine.com, website: www.ariseandshine.com

Ginseng
Nature's Herbs, 600 East Quality Drive, American Fork, UT 84003, tel: 800-437-2257 or 801-763-0700, website: www.naturesherbs.com

Futurebiotics, 70 Commerce Drive, Hauppauge, NY 11788, tel: 800-645-1721 or 631-273-6300, website: www.futurebiotics.com

Glandular Supplements
Standard Process Laboratories, 1200 West Royal Lee Drive, P.O. Box 904, Palmyra, WI 53156, tel: 800-848-5061 or 262-495-2122, email: info@standardprocess.com, website: www.standardprocess.com

Herbs
Herb Research Foundation, 4140 15th Street, Boulder, CO 80304, tel: 303-449-2265 fax: 303-449-7849, website: www.herbs.org

Homeopathic Remedies
National College of Naturopathic Medicine, 049 SW Porter Street, Portland, OR 97201, tel: 503-552-1555, website: www.ncnm.edu

Heel/BHI, P.O. Box 11280, Albuquerque, NM 87192, tel: 800-621-7644 or 505-293-3843, email: info@heelusa.com, website: www.heelusa.com

Liquid Calcium and Magnesium
Integrative Therapeutics, 9 Monroe Parkway, Suite 250, Lake Oswego, OR 97035, tel: 800-931-1709 fax: 800-380-8189, website: www.integrativeinc.com

Melakava
Shakti Enterprises, tel: 847-475-1900 fax: 847-729-3237, email: customerservice@ chineseherbs.net, website: www.chineseherbs.net/china/index.html

Melatonin
Life Extension Foundation, P.O. Box 229120, Hollywood, FL 33022, tel: 800-678-8989 or 954-766-8433, website: www.lef.org

Source Naturals, Threshold Enterprises, 3 Janis Way, Scotts Valley, CA 95066, tel: 800-815-2333 or 831-438-1144, website: www.sourcenaturals.com

Parasite Formulas
Uni Key Health Systems, 181 West Commerce Drive, P.O. Box 2287, Hayden Lake, ID 83835, tel: 800-888-4353 or 208-762-6833, email: unikey@unikeyhealth.com, website: www.unikeyhealth.com

Allergy Research Group, 2300 North Loop Road, Alameda, CA 94502, tel: 800-545-9960 or 510-263-2000 fax: 510-263-2100, email: info@allergyresearchgroup.com, website: www.allergyresearchgroup.com

Thorne Research, P.O. Box 25, Dover, ID 83825, tel: 800-228-1966 or 208-263-1337 fax: 208-265-2488, email: info@thorne.com, website: www.thorne.com

Enzymatic Therapy, 825 Challenger Drive, Green Bay, WI 54311, tel: 800-783-2286, website: www.enzy.com

Hulda Regehr Clark, ND, Ph.D., Self Health Resource Center, 1055 Bay Boulevard, Suite A, Chula Vista, California 91911, tel: 866-372-5275 fax: 619-409-9501, email: Service@DrClarkStore.com, website: www.herbalparasitecleanse.com

SuperGarlic 6000
Metagenics, 971 Calle Negocio, San Clemente, CA 92673, tel: 800-877-1703 fax 949-366-0818, website: www.metagenics.com

Triple Yeast Defense
Imhotep, P.O. Box 183, Ruby, NY 12475, tel: 800-677-8577 fax: 845-336-5446, website: www.imhotepinc.com

Ultimate Cleanse
Nature's Secret, 5310 Beethoven Street, Los Angeles, CA 90066, tel: 800-297-3273, email: info@naturessecret.com, website: www.naturessecret.com

UltraFlora Plus and Probioplex
Metagenics, 971 Calle Negocio, San Clemente, CA 92673, tel: 800-877-1703 fax 949-366-0818, website: www.metagenics.com

Vital (homeopathic growth hormone stimulator)
Liddell Laboratories, 1036 Country Club Drive, Moraga, CA 94556, tel: 800-460-7733 or 925-377-3000 fax: 925-631-7948, email: info@liddell.net, website: www.liddell.net

Whole Body and Colon Program
Pure Body Institute, 230 S. Olive, Ventura, CA 93001, tel: 805-653-5448 fax: 805-653-2458, email: info@pbiv.com, website: www.pbiv.com

Yeast Formula
PhytoPharmica, 825 Challenger Drive, Green Bay, WI 54311, tel: 800-376-7889, website: www.phytopharmica.com

Testing and Screening Services

Adrenal Stress Index (ASI)
Diagnos-Techs, 6620 South 192nd Place, J-104, Kent, WA 98032, tel: 800-878-3787 or 425-252-0596 fax: 425-251-0637, email: diagnos@diagnostechs.com, website: www.diagnostechs.com

Anti-Candida Antibody Profile
Genova Diagnostics, 63 Zillicoa Street, Asheville, NC 28801, tel: 800-522-4762 or 828-253-0621 fax: 828-252-9303, website: www.gdx.net/home

ELISA Tests
Immuno Laboratories, 6801 Powerline Road, Fort Lauderdale, FL 33309, tel: 800-231-9197 or 954-691-2500 fax: 954-691-2505, website: www.immunolabs.com

Meridian Valley Clinical Laboratory, 801 SW 16th, Suite 126, Renton, WA 98055, tel: 425-271-8689 fax: 425-271-8674, email: info@meridianvalleylab.com, website: www.meridianvalleylab.com

Individualized Optimal Nutrition Profile
Metametrix Clinical Laboratory, 4855 Peachtree Industrial Boulevard, Suite 201, Norcross, GA 30092, tel: 800-221-4640 or 770-446-5483 fax: 770-441-2237, email: inquiries@metametrix.com, website: www.metametrix.com

Functional Intracellular Analysis
SpectraCell Laboratories, 10401 Town Park Drive, Houston, TX 77072, tel: 800-227-5227 or 713-621-3101, email: spec1@spectracell.com, website: www.spectracell.com

Functional Liver Detoxification Profile and Oxidative Stress Profile
Genova Diagnostics, 63 Zillicoa Street, Asheville, NC 28801, tel: 800-522-4762 or 828-253-0621 fax: 828-252-9303, website: www.gdx.net/home

Hair Analysis
Omegatech, 24700 Center Ridge Road, Cleveland, OH 44145, tel: 800-437-1404 fax: 440-835-2177, email: HeadQuarters@kingjamesomegatech-lab.com, website: www.kingjamesomegatech-lab.com

ION Panel
Metametrix Clinical Laboratory, 4855 Peachtree Industrial Boulevard, Suite 201, Norcross, GA 30092, tel: 800-221-4640 or 770-446-5483 fax: 770-441-2237, email: inquiries@metametrix.com, website: www.metametrix.com

Stool Analysis
Uni Key Health Systems, 181 West Commerce Drive, P.O. Box 2287, Hayden Lake, ID 83835, tel: 800-888-4353 or 208-762-6833, email: unikey@unikeyhealth.com, website: www.unikeyhealth.com

Genova Diagnostics, 63 Zillicoa Street, Asheville, NC 28801, tel: 800-522-4762 or 828-253-0621 fax: 828-252-9303, website: www.gdx.net/home

Meridian Valley Clinical Laboratory, 801 SW 16th, Suite 126, Renton, WA. 98055, tel: 425-271-8689 fax: 425-271-8674, email: info@meridianvalleylab.com, website: www .meridianvalleylab.com

Endnotes

Chapter 1. *The Basics of Sleep*

1. National Institute of Neurological Disorders and Stroke. "Brain Basics: Understanding Sleep." 2006. Available at www.ninds.nih.gov/disorders/brain_basics/understanding_sleep.htm.
2. R. J. Reiter. "Oxidative Processes and Antioxidative Defense Mechanisms in the Aging Brain." *FASEB Journal* 9:7 (1995), 526–533.
3. Ibid.
4. Dun-Xian Tan et al. "Melatonin: A Potent Endogenous Hydroxyl Radical Scavenger." *Endocrine Journal* 1 (1993), 57–60.
5. R. J. Reiter. "The Indoleamine Melatonin as a Free Radical Scavenger, Electron Donor, and Antioxidant: In Vitro and In Vivo Studies." *Advances in Experimental Medicine and Biology* 398 (1996), 307–313.
6. R. J. Reiter et al. "Melatonin in Relation to Cellular Antioxidative Defense Mechanisms." *Hormonal and Metabolic Research* 29 (1997), 363–372.
7. Ibid.
8. R. J. Reiter. "Novel Intracellular Actions of Melatonin: Its Relation to Reactive Oxygen Species." In: *Frontiers of Hormone Research*, Vol. 21 (1996), 160–166.
9. E. Reimund. "The Free Radical Flux Theory of Sleep." *Medical Hypotheses* 43 (1994), 231–233.
10. G. J. Maestroni. "T-Helper-2 Lymphocytes as Peripheral Target of Melatonin Signaling." *Journal of Pineal Research* 18 (1995), 84–89.
11. R. J. Reiter et al. "The Role of Melatonin in the Pathophysiology of Oxygen Radical Damage." In: M. Müller and P. Pévet, eds., *Advances in Pineal Research*, Vol. 8 (London: John Libbey, 1994), 278.
12. K. M. Morrey, J. A. McLachian, and O. Bakouche. "Activation of Human Monocytes by the Pineal Hormone Melatonin." *Journal of Immunology* 153 (1994), 2671–2680.
13. L. A. Toth. "Sleep, Sleep Deprivation, and Infectious Disease: Studies in Animals." *Advances in Neuroimmunology* 5:1 (1995), 79–92. See also: J. M. Krueger et al. "Sleep, Microbes and Cytokines." *Neuroimmunomodulation* 1:2 (March/April 1994), 100–109.

14. A. Rechtschaffen et al. "Physiological Correlates of Prolonged Sleep Deprivation in Rats." *Science* 221:4606 (July 8, 1983), 182–184.

15. D. Mueller-Wieland, B. Behnke, and W. Krone. "Melatonin Inhibits LDL Receptor Activity and Cholesterol Synthesis in Freshly Isolated Human Mononuclear Leukocytes." *Biochemical and Biophysical Research Communications* 203:1 (1994), 416–421. See also: N. Birau, U. Peterssen, C. Meyer, and J. Gottschalk. "Hypotensive Effect of Melatonin in Essential Hypertension." *IRCS Medical Science* 9 (1981), 906.

16. U.S. Department of Health and Human Services. *Your Guide to Healthy Sleep* (Washington: U.S. Department of Health and Human Services, 2005), 14. Available at www.nhlbi.nih.gov/health/public/sleep/healthy_sleep.pdf.

17. S. H. Kennedy, S. Tighe, and G. M. Brown. "Melatonin and Cortisol 'Switches' during Mania, Depression, and Euthymia in a Drug-Free Bipolar Patient." *Journal of Nervous and Mental Disease* 177:5 (1989), 300–303. See also: P. Monteleone et al. "Depressed Nocturnal Plasma Melatonin Levels in Drug-Free Paranoid Schizophrenics." *Schizophrenia Research* 7 (1992), 77–84.

18. Arthur C. Guyton, MD, and John E. Hall, Ph.D. *Textbook of Medical Physiology*, 9th edition (Philadelphia: W. B. Saunders, 1996), 761.

19. Ibid.

20. S. Gabel. "Information Processing in Rapid Eye Movement Sleep: Possible Neurophysiological, Neuropsychological, and Clinical Correlates." *Journal of Nervous and Mental Disorders* 175 (April 1987), 193–200.

21. P. Maquet et al. "Functional Neuroanatomy of Human Rapid-Eye-Movement Sleep and Dreaming." *Nature* 383 (September 12, 1996), 163–166.

22. U. D. McCann et al. "Sleep Deprivation and Impaired Cognition: Possible Role of Brain Catecholamines." *Biological Psychiatry* 31:11 (June 1, 1992), 1082–1097. See also: C. P. Maurizi. "The Function of Dreams (REM Sleep): Roles for the Hippocampus, Melatonin, Monoamines, and Vasotocin." *Medical Hypotheses* 23:4 (August 1987), 433–440.

23. A. Karni et al. "Dependence on REM Sleep of Overnight Improvement of a Perceptual Skill." *Science* 265 (July 29, 1994), 679–682.

24. J. De Koninck et al. "Language Learning Efficiency, Dreams, and REM Sleep." *Psychiatric Journal of the University of Ottawa* 15:2 (June 1990), 91–92.

25. M. Nesca and D. Koulack. "Recognition Memory, Sleep, and Circadian Rhythms." *Canadian Journal of Experimental Psychology* 48:3 (September 1994), 359–379.

26. S. Gabel. "Information Processing in Rapid Eye Movement Sleep: Possible Neurophysiological, Neuropsychological, and Clinical Correlates." *Journal of Nervous and Mental Disorders* 175 (April 1987), 193–200.

27. Roger Fritz, Ph.D. *Sleep Disorders: America's Hidden Nightmare* (Naperville, IL: National Sleep Alert, 1993), 30.

28. C. P. Maurizi. "The Function of Dreams (REM Sleep): Roles for the Hippocampus, Melatonin, Monoamines, and Vasotocin." *Medical Hypotheses* 23:4 (August 1987), 433–440.

29. William Dement, MD, Ph.D., with Christopher Vaughan. *The Promise of Sleep* (New York: Delacorte Press, 1999), 271.

30. National Sleep Foundation. *Summary of Findings: 2005 Sleep in America Poll* (Washington: National Sleep Foundation, 2005), 7.

31. National Institute of Neurological Disorders and Stroke. "Brain Basics: Understanding Sleep." 2006. Available at www.ninds.nih.gov/disorders/brain_basics/understanding_sleep.htm.

32. N. Ishida, M. Kaneko, and R. Allada. "Biological Clocks." *Proceedings of the National Academy of Sciences of the United States of America* 96:16 (August 3, 1996), 8819–8820.

33. Ibid.

34. Russel J. Reiter and Jo Robinson. *Melatonin: Your Body's Natural Wonder Drug* (New York: Bantam Books, 1995), 17.

35. J. Z. Nowak and J. B. Zawilska. "Melatonin and Its Physiological and Therapeutic Properties." *Pharmacy World and Science* 20:1 (1998), 18–27.

36. Ray Sahelian, MD. 5-HTTP: Nature's Serotonin Solution (Garden City Park, NY: Avery Publishing, 1998), 29.

37. Russel J. Reiter and Jo Robinson. *Melatonin: Your Body's Natural Wonder Drug* (New York: Bantam Books, 1995), 161.

38. A. J. Lewty, T. A. Wehr, and F. K. Goodwin. "Light Suppresses Melatonin Secretion in Humans." *Science* (December 1980), 210.

39. M. L. Rao, B. Muller-Oerlinghause, and H. P. Volz. "Blood Serotonin, Serum Melatonin and Light Therapy in Healthy Subjects and in Patients with Nonseasonal Depression." *Acta Psychiatrica Scandinavica* 86 (1992), 127–132.

Chapter 2. *Sleep Disorders and Their Causes*

1. National Sleep Foundation. *Summary of Findings: 2005 Sleep in America Poll* (Washington, DC: National Sleep Foundation, 2005), 7.

2. Ibid.

3. National Institute of Neurological Disorders and Stroke. "Brain Basics: Understanding Sleep." 2006. Available at www.ninds.nih.gov/disorders/brain_basics /understanding_sleep.htm.

4. National Sleep Foundation. *Summary of Findings: 2005 Sleep in America Poll* (Washington, DC: National Sleep Foundation, 2005), 8.

5. National Commission on Sleep Disorders Research. *Wake Up America: A National Sleep Alert*, Vol. 1 (Bethesda, MD: National Institutes of Health, 1993).

6. National Sleep Foundation. "2000 Omnibus Sleep in America Poll." Available from National Sleep Foundation, 1522 K Street NW, Suite 500, Washington, DC 20005; www.sleepfoundation.org.

7. Ibid.

8. Ibid.

9. U.S. Department of Health and Human Services. *Your Guide to Healthy Sleep* (Washington, DC: U.S. Department of Health and Human Services, 2005). Available at www.nhlbi.nih.gov/health/public/sleep/healthy_sleep.pdf. See also National Heart, Lung, and Blood Institute. "Insomnia." 2006. Available at www .nhlbi.nih.gov/health/dci/Diseases/inso/inso_whatis.html.

10. William C. Dement, MD, Ph.D., with Christopher Vaughan. *The Promise of Sleep* (New York: Delacorte Press, 1999), 308; Stanford Sleepiness Scale, www.stanford.edu/~dement/sss.html.

11. National Heart, Lung, and Blood Institute. "Sleep Apnea." 2006. Available at www.nhlbi.nih.gov/health/dci/Diseases/SleepApnea/SleepApnea_WhoIsAtRisk. html.

12. Christensen Damarais. "Allergies May Be Linked to Obstructive Sleep Apnea." *Medical Tribune* (February 1997), 3.

13. U. Koehler and H. Shäfer. "Is Obstructive Sleep Apnea (OSA) a Risk Factor for Myocardial Infarction and Cardiac Arrhythmias in Patients with Coronary Heart Disease?" *Sleep* 19:4 (1995), 283.

14. National Institutes of Health and National Heart, Lung, and Blood Institute. "Sleep Apnea." 2006. Available at www.nhlbi.nih.gov/health/dci/Diseases /SleepApnea/SleepApnea_Treatments.html.

15. Derek S. Lipman, MD. *Snoring from A to ZZZZ* (Portland, OR: Spencer Press, 1996), 71–72.

16. Victor Hoffstein. "Is Snoring Dangerous to Your Health?" *Sleep* 19:6 (1995), 506. See also: Paul L. Enright et al. "Prevalence and Correlates of Snoring and Observed Apneas in 5,201 Older Adults." *Sleep* 19:7 (1997), 529.

17. National Institute of Neurological Disorders and Stroke. "Restless Legs Syndrome Fact Sheet." 2007. Available at www.ninds.nih.gov/disorders/restless_legs /detail_restless_legs.htm.

18. Restless Legs Syndrome Foundation. "Pregnancy and RLS." 2006. Available at: www.rls.org/NetCommunity/Document.Doc?&id=183.

19. Jacques Montplaisir et al. "Persistence of Repetitive EEG Arousals (K-Alpha Complexes) in Patients Treated with L-DOPA." *Sleep* 19:3 (1995), 200.

20. National Institute of Neurological Disorders and Stroke. "Narcolepsy Fact Sheet." 2007. Available at www.ninds.nih.gov/disorders/narcolepsy/detail _narcolepsy.htm#58833201

21. Ibid.

22. Martin Moore-Ede, MD, Ph.D., and Suzanne LeVert. *Complete Idiot's Guide to Getting a Good Night's Sleep* (New York: Alpha Books, 1998), 184.

23. James Perl, Ph.D. *Sleep Right in Five Nights* (New York: William Morrow, 1993).

24. James B. Maas, Ph.D. *Power Sleep* (New York: HarperPerennial, 1999), 194.

25. Jane Brody. "Personal Health." *New York Times* (January 17, 1996), B8.

26. Roger Fritz, Ph.D. *Sleep Disorders: America's Hidden Nightmare* (Naperville, IL: National Sleep Alert, 1993), 106.

27. Martin Moore-Ede, MD, Ph.D., and Suzanne LeVert. *Complete Idiot's Guide to Getting a Good Night's Sleep* (New York: Alpha Books, 1998), 175.

28. Michael S. Aldrich. *Sleep Medicine* (New York: Oxford University Press, 1999).

29. John F. Simonds and Humberto Parragio. "Prevalence of Sleep Disorders and Sleep Behaviors in Children and Adolescents." *Journal of the American Academy of Child Psychiatry* 21 (1982), 383–388.

30. Michael S. Aldrich. *Sleep Medicine* (New York: Oxford University Press, 1999).

31. Martin Moore-Ede, MD, Ph.D., and Suzanne LeVert. *Complete Idiot's Guide to Getting a Good Night's Sleep* (New York: Alpha Books, 1998), 176.

32. American Sleep Disorders Association. Diagnostic Classification Steering Committee. *The International Classification of Sleep Disorders: Diagnostic and Coding Manual* (Rochester, MN: American Sleep Disorders Association, 1990).

33. Terry Chisholm and Rachel L. Morehouse. "Adult Headbanging: Sleep Studies and Treatment." *Sleep* 19:4 (1995), 343.

34. Ibid.

35. Martin Moore-Ede, MD, Ph.D., and Suzanne LeVert. *Complete Idiot's Guide to Getting a Good Night's Sleep* (New York: Alpha Books, 1998), 176.

36. American Sleep Disorders Association. Diagnostic Classification Steering Committee. *The International Classification of Sleep Disorders: Diagnostic and Coding Manual* (Rochester, MN: American Sleep Disorders Association, 1990).

37. K. Hjalmas. "Nocturnal Enuresis: Basic Facts and New Horizons." *European Urology* 33:suppl 3 (1998), 53–57.

38. William C. Dement, MD, Ph.D.,and Christopher Vaughan. *The Promise of Sleep* (New York: Delacorte Press, 1999), 310.

39. Russel J. Reiter and Jo Robinson. *Melatonin: Your Body's Natural Wonder Drug* (New York: Bantam, 1995), 124.

40. Ibid., 125.

41. H. Vafi, MD, and Pamela Vafi. *How to Get a Great Night's Sleep* (Holbrook, MA: Bob Adams, 1994).

42. Dian Dincin Buchman, Ph.D. *The Complete Guide to Sleep* (New Canaan, CT: Keats Publishing, 1997), 43.

Chapter 3. *Step 1: Improve Your Diet*

1. National Institute of Neurological Disorders and Stroke. "Restless Legs Syndrome Fact Sheet." 2007. Available at www.ninds.nih.gov/disorders/restless_legs /detail_restless_legs.htm.

2. T. Chou. "Wake Up and Smell the Coffee: Caffeine, Coffee, and the Medical Consequences." *Western Journal of Medicine* 157:5 (1992), 544–553.

3. Elson M. Haas, MD. *Staying Healthy with Nutrition* (Berkeley, CA: Celestial Arts, 1992), 941.

4. J. Warner. "Coffee Is No. 1 Source of Antioxidants." *WebMD Medical News*, August 28, 2005. Available at www.webmd.com/content/Article/110/109786.htm.

5. Elliot D. Abravanel, MD, and Elizabeth King. *Dr. Abravanel's Anti-Craving Weight Loss Diet* (New York: Bantam, 1990), 53–57.

6. H. J. Rinkel et al. *Food Allergy* (Springfield, IL: Charles C. Thomas, 1950).

7. Stephen Langer, MD, with James F. Scheer. *Solved: The Riddle of Weight Loss* (Rochester, VT: Healing Arts Press, 1989), 39.

8. J. E. Pizzorno and M. T. Murray. *A Textbook of Natural Medicine* (Seattle, WA: John Bastyr University, 1989).

9. B. M. Stone. "Sleep and Low Doses of Alcohol." *Electroencephalography and Clinical Neurophysiology* 48:6 (1980), 706–709.

10. H. P. Landoit et al. "Late-Afternoon Ethanol Intake Affects Nocturnal Sleep and the Sleep EEG in Middle-Aged Men." *Journal of Clinical Psychopharmacology* 16:6 (1996), 428–436.

11. Elson M. Haas, MD. *Staying Healthy with Nutrition* (Berkeley, CA: Celestial Arts, 1992), 952.

12. Dian Dincin Buchman, Ph.D. *The Complete Guide to Sleep* (New Canaan, CT: Keats Publishing, 1997), 45.

13. National Sleep Foundation. "1999 Omnibus Sleep in America Poll." Available from National Sleep Foundation, 1522 K Street NW, Suite 500, Washington, DC 20005; www.sleepfoundation.org.

14. Stanley Coren. *Sleep Thieves* (New York: Free Press, 1996), 135.

15. R. Sandyk. "L-Tryptophan in the Treatment of Restless Legs Syndrome." *American Journal of Psychiatry* 143:3 (1986), 554–555.

16. G. S. Kelly. "Folates: Supplemental Forms and Therapeutic Applications." *Alternative Medicine Review* 3:3 (1998), 208–220.

17. S. Ayres and R. Mihan. "Restless Legs Syndrome: Response to Vitamin E." *Journal of Applied Nutrition* 25 (1973), 8–15.

18. H. S. Pall et al. "Restless Legs Syndrome." *Neurology* 37:8 (1987), 1436. See also: S. T. O'Keefe, K. Gavin, and J. N. Lavan. "Iron Status and Restless Legs Syndrome in the Elderly." *Age and Aging* 23:3 (1994), 200–203.

19. Arthur Winter, MD, FICS, and Ruth Winter, MS. *Smart Food* (New York: St. Martin's Griffin, 1999), 77.

20. Stephen Langer, MD, with James F. Scheer. *Solved: The Riddle of Weight Loss* (Rochester, VT: Healing Arts Press, 1989), 51.

21. Stephen Langer, MD, with James F. Scheer. *Solved: The Riddle of Weight Loss* (Rochester, VT: Healing Arts Press, 1989), 52.

22. Ralph Golan, MD. *Optimal Wellness* (New York: Ballantine Books, 1995).

23. Peter Hauri, Ph.D., and Shirley Linde, Ph.D. *No More Sleepless Nights* (New York: John Wiley and Sons, 1990), 52.

24. Ann Louise Gittleman, MS. "Perimenopause—When Signs of 'The Change' Come Too Early." *Alternative Medicine* 26 (October/November 1998), 84–92.

25. Richard N. Podell, MD, FACP, and William Proctor. *The G-Index Diet* (New York: Warner, 1993).

26. Ann Louise Gittleman, MS. *Supernutrition for Women* (New York: Bantam, 1991), 68.

27. A. Kahn et al. "Insomnia and Cow's Milk Allergy in Infants." *Pediatrics* 76:6 (1985), 880–884.

28. James Braly, MD. *Dr. Braly's Food Allergy and Nutrition Revolution* (New Canaan, CT: Keats Publishing, 1992), 60.

29. Roger J. Williams, Ph.D. *Biochemical Individuality* (New Canaan, CT: Keats Publishing, 1998).

30. Judith J. Wurtman, with Margaret Danbrot, Ph.D. *Managing Your Mind and Mood Through Food* (New York: Harper and Row, 1986), 18–23.

31. Roger Fritz, Ph.D. *Sleep Disorders: America's Hidden Nightmare* (Naperville, IL: National Sleep Alert, 1993), 122–123.

32. M. R. Werbach, MD. *Nutritional Influences on Illness* (Tarzana, CA: Third Line Press, 1993).

33. J. Martineau et al. "Vitamin B_6, Magnesium, and Combined B_6-Magnesium: Therapeutic Effects in Childhood Autism." *Biology Psychiatry* 20 (1985), 467–468.

34. M. Cohen and A. Bendich. "Safety of Pyridoxine: A Review of Human and Animal Studies." *Toxicology Letters* 34 (1986), 129–139.

35. L. M. Tierney Jr., MD, et al. *Current Medical Diagnosis and Treatment* (Norwalk, CT: Appleton and Lange, 1993).

36. S. Ayres and R. Mihan. "Leg Cramps and 'Restless Leg' Syndrome Responsive to Vitamin E (Tocopheral)." *California Medicine* 111:2 (1969), 87–91.

37. J. Penland. "Effects of Trace Element Nutrition on Sleep Patterns in Adult Women." *FASEB Journal* 2 (1988), A434.

38. J. Thom et al. "The Influence of Refined Carbohydrate on Urinary Calcium Excretion." *British Journal of Urology* 50 (1978), 459–464.

39. R. P. Heaney and C. M. Weaver. "Calcium Absorption from Kale." *American Journal of Clinical Nutrition* 51 (1990), 656–657.

40. B. P. Bourgoin et al. "Lead Content in 70 Brands of Dietary Calcium Supplements." *American Journal of Public Health* 83 (1993), 1155–1160.

41. J. A. Harvey et al. "Superior Calcium Absorption from Calcium Citrate Than Calcium Carbonate Using External Forearm Counting." *Journal of the American College of Nutrition* 9 (1990), 583–587.

42. C. Zhou et al. "Clinical Observation of Treatment of Hypertension with Calcium." *American Journal of Hypertension* 7 (1994), 363–367.

43. B. M. Altura. "Basic Biochemistry and Physiology of Magnesium: A Brief Review." *Magnesium and Trace Elements* 10 (1991), 167–171.

44. T. Bohmer et al. "Bioavailability of Oral Magnesium Supplementation in Female Students Evaluated from Elimination of Magnesium in 24-Hour Urine." *Magnesium and Trace Elements* 9 (1990), 272–278. See also L. Gullestad et al. "Oral

versus Intravenous Magnesium Supplementation in Patients with Magnesium Deficiency." *Magnesium and Trace Elements* 10 (1991), 11–16.

45. J. S. Lindberg et al. "Magnesium Bioavailability from Magnesium Citrate and Magnesium Oxide." *Journal of the American College of Nutrition* 9 (1990), 48–55.

46. Betty Kamen, Ph.D. *The Chromium Connection* (Novato, CA: Nutrition Encounter, 1992), 118.

47. W. W. Campbell and R. A. Anderson. "Effects of Aerobic Exercise and Training on the Trace Minerals Chromium, Copper, and Zinc." *Sports Medicine* 4 (1987), 9–18.

48. Jeffrey S. Bland, Ph.D. "Take Your Vitamins." *Delicious!* 8:7 (October 1992), 61.

49. E. B. Finley and F. L. Cerklewski. "Influence of Ascorbic Acid Supplementation on Copper Status in Young Adult Men." *American Journal of Clinical Nutrition* 47 (1988), 96–101.

50. Michael A. Schmidt, DC, CNS, and Jeffrey Bland, Ph.D. "Thyroid Gland as Sentinel: Interface between Internal and External Environment." *Alternative Therapies* 3:1 (January 1997), 78–81.

51. S. T. O'Keefe, K. Gaavin, and J. N. Lavan. "Iron Status and Restless Legs Syndrome in the Elderly." *Age and Aging* 23 (1994), 200–203.

52. V. Gordeuk et al. "Iron Overload: Causes and Consequences." *Annual Review of Nutrition* 7 (1987), 485–508. See also: P. Biemond et al. "Intra-Articular Ferritin-Bound Iron in Rheumatoid Arthritis." *Arthritis and Rheumatism* 29 (1986), 1187–1193. See also: J. T. Salonen et al. "High Stored Iron Levels are Associated with Excess Risk of Myocardial Infarction in Eastern Finnish Men." *Circulation* 86 (1992), 803–811.

53. Eric R. Braverman, MD. *P.A.T.H. Wellness Manual* (Princeton, NJ: Princeton Associates for Total Health, 1995), 124.

54. James Perl, Ph.D. *Sleep Right in Five Nights* (New York: William Morrow, 1993), 236.

55. T. C. Birdsall. "5-Hydroxytryptophan: A Clinically Effective Serotonin Precursor." *Alternative Medicine Review* 3:4 (1998), 271–280.

56. R. Ursin. "The Effects of 5-Hydroxytryptophan and L-Tryptophan on Wakefulness and Sleep Patterns in the Cat." *Brain Research* 106:1 (1976), 105–115.

Chapter 4. *Step 2: Detoxify Your Body*

1. R. Steinzor and M. Clune. *Paper Tigers and Killer Air* (Washington, DC: Center for American Progress, 2006).

2. Colin Ingram. *The Drinking Water Book* (Berkeley, CA: Celestial Arts, 2006).

3. Environmental Working Group. "A National Assessment of Tap Water Quality." 2005. Available at www.ewg.org/tapwater/findings.php.

4. Burton Goldberg Group. *Alternative Medicine: The Definitive Guide* (Tiburon, CA: Future Medicine Publishing, 1993), 3.

5. Ibid., 4.

6. Joseph Pizzorno, ND. *Total Wellness* (Rocklin, CA: Prima Publishing, 1996), 105.

7. William Lee Cowden, MD. "Is Your Shower Toxic? Some Pollution Solutions." *Alternative Medicine* 29 (April/May 1999), 69.

8. D. N. Taylor et al. "Effects of Trichloroethylene in the Exploratory and Locomotor Activity in Rats Exposed during Development." *Science Total Environment* 47 (1985), 415–420. See also: H. N. Arito, T. Suruta, K. Nakagaki, and S. Tanaka. "Partial Insomnia, Hyperactivity and Hyperdipsia Induced by Repeated Admin-

istration of Toluene in Rats: Their Relation to Brain Monoamine Metabolism." *Toxicology* 37:1–2 (1985), 99–110.

9. W. Melillo. "How Safe Is Mercury in Dentistry?" *Washington Post Weekly Journal of Medicine, Science and Society* (September 1991), 4. See also: World Health Organization. *Environmental Health Criteria for Inorganic Mercury* (Geneva, Switzerland: World Health Organization, 1991), 118.

10. William J. Rea, MD. *Chemical Sensitivity*, Vol. 3 (Boca Raton, FL: C.R.C. Lewis, 1996), 1555–1579.

11. S. Ziff. "Consolidated Symptom Analysis of 1,569 Patients." *Bio-Probe Newsletter* 9:2 (March 1993), 7–8.

12. Jack Tips, ND, Ph.D. *Your Liver . . . Your Lifeline* (Ogden, UT: Apple-A-Day Press, 1995), 13–15.

13. William G. Crook, MD. *The Yeast Connection and the Woman* (Jackson, TN: Professional Books, 1995), 25. See also: Simon Martin. *Candida: The Natural Way* (Boston, MA: Element Books, 1998), 7.

14. Burton Goldberg Group. *Alternative Medicine: The Definitive Guide* (Tiburon, CA: Future Medicine Publishing, 1993), 587.

15. Hal Huggins, DDS. "Dental Toxins: Your Teeth May Be Making You Sick." *Alternative Medicine* 23 (April/May 1998), 48–54.

16. R. L. Siblerud, J. Motl, and E. Kienholz. "Psychometric Evidence That Mercury from Silver Dental Fillings May Be an Etiological Factor in Depression, Excessive Anger, and Anxiety." *Psychological Reports* 74:1 (1994), 67–80.

17. L. A. Toth and J. M. Krueger. "Effects of Microbial Challenge on Sleep in Rabbits." *FASEB Journal* 3:9 (1989), 2062–2066.

18. Jeffrey Bland, Ph.D. "Drugs and Liver Overload." *Delicious!* (May 1995), 48.

19. Stephen Langer, MD, with James F. Scheer. *Solved: The Riddle of Weight Loss* (Rochester, VT: Healing Arts Press, 1989), 24.

20. Burton Goldberg Group. *Alternative Medicine: The Definitive Guide* (Tiburon, CA: Future Medicine Publishing, 1993), 588.

21. Simon Martin. *Candida: The Natural Way* (Boston, MA: Element Books, 1998), 10–11. This information is adapted from a candida questionnaire developed by William Crook, MD, and included in his book, *The Yeast Connection Handbook* (Jackson, TN: Professional Books, 1996), 15–19.

22. Stephen Langer, MD, with James F. Scheer. *Solved: The Riddle of Weight Loss* (Rochester, VT: Healing Arts Press, 1989), 24.

23. Jack Tips, ND, Ph.D. *Conquer Candida and Restore Your Immune System* (Austin, TX: Apple-A-Day Press, 1995), 68–69.

24. Ann Louise Gittleman, MS. *Guess What Came To Dinner: Parasites and Your Health* (Garden City Park, NY: Avery Publishing Group, 1993), 80–86. See also: Hermann Bueno, MD. *Uninvited Guests* (New Canaan, CT: Keats: 1996), 33.

25. Ann Louise Gittleman, MS. *Guess What Came to Dinner: Parasites and Your Health* (Garden City Park, NY: Avery Publishing Group, 1993), 94–95. See also: Gary Null, Ph.D. *The Woman's Encyclopedia of Natural Healing* (New York: Seven Stories, 1996), 285. See also: Pavel I. Yutsis, MD. "Intestinal Parasites at Large." *Explore!* 7:1 (1996), 27–31.

26. Ann Louise Gittleman, MS. *Guess What Came to Dinner: Parasites and Your Health* (Garden City Park, NY: Avery Publishing Group, 1993), 96.

27. Christopher Hobbs, L.Ac. *Foundations of Health* (Capitola, CA: Botanica Press, 1992).

28. L. K. T. Lam et al. "Isolation and Identification of Kahweol Palmitate and Cafestol Palmitate as Active Constituents of Green Coffee Beans That Enhance

Glutathione-S-Transferase Activity in the Mouse." *Cancer Research* 42 (1982), 1193–1198.

29. Howard Straus. "Coffee Corner." *Gerson Healing Newsletter* 11:5 (1996), 9–11.

30. Eugene Zampieron, ND, and Ellen Kamhi, Ph.D., RN. *The Natural Medicine Chest* (New York: M. Evans, 1999), 52–54.

31. Ann Louise Gittleman, MS. *Guess What Came to Dinner: Parasites and Your Health* (Garden City Park, NY: Avery Publishing Group, 1993).

32. Giovanni Maciocia, C.Ac. *The Practice of Chinese Medicine* (London: Churchill Livingstone, 1994), 285.

Chapter 5. *Step 3: Reset Your Body Clock*

1. Richard M. Coleman. *Wide Awake at 3:00 A.M.* (New York: W. H. Freeman, 1986), 6.

2. Roberto Refinetti, Ph.D. *Circadian Physiology* (Boca Raton, FL: CRC Press, 2000), 140.

3. T. H. Monk, M. L. Moline, and R. C. Graeber. "Inducing Jet Lag in the Laboratory: Patterns of Adjustment to an Acute Shift in Routine." *Aviation Space and Environmental Medicine* 59 (1998), 703–710. See also: A. R. Wever. "Phase Shifts of Human Circadian Rhythms Due to Shifts of Artificial Zeitgebers." *Chronobiologia* 7 (1980), 303–327.

4. Angela Lorio. "Shift Workers Must Defy Their Circadian Rhythm." *Medical Tribune* (November 27, 1997), 7.

5. Richard M. Coleman. *Wide Awake at 3:00 A.M.* (New York: W. H. Freeman, 1986), 59.

6. R. R. Rosa and Michael J. Colligan. *Plain Language About Shiftwork* (Washington, DC: U.S. Department of Health and Human Services, 1997). Available at www.cdc.gov/niosh/pdfs/97-145.pdf. See also: U.S. Department of Health and Human Services. *Your Guide to Healthy Sleep* (Washington, DC: U.S. Department of Health and Human Services, 2005). Available at www.nhlbi.nih.gov/health/public/sleep/healthy_sleep.pdf.

7. R. R. Rosa and Michael J. Colligan. *Plain Language About Shiftwork* (Washington, DC: U.S. Department of Health and Human Services, 1997). Available at www.cdc.gov/niosh/pdfs/97-145.pdf.

8. P. D. Peneve et al. "Chronic Circadian Desynchronization Decreases the Survival of Animals with Cardiomyopathic Heart Disease." *American Journal of Physiology* 275 (1998), H2334–H2337.

9. R. J. Reiter. "Static and Extremely Low Frequency Electromagnetic Field Exposure: Reported Effects on the Circadian Production of Melatonin." *Journal of Cellular Biochemistry* 51:4 (April 1993), 394–403.

10. R. C. Espiritu, D. F. Kripke, and O. J. Kaplan. "Low Illumination Experienced by San Diego Adults: Association with Atypical Depressive Symptoms." *Biological Psychiatry* 35 (1994), 403–407.

11. M. Koller et al. "Personal Light Dosimetry in Permanent Night and Day Workers." *Chronobiology International* 10 (1993), 143–155.

12. Russel J. Reiter and Jo Robinson. *Melatonin: Your Body's Natural Wonder Drug* (New York: Bantam Books, 1995), 162.

13. Ibid.

14. M. L. Roa, B. Muller-Oerlinghausen, and H. P. Volz. "Blood Serotonin, Serum Melatonin and Light Therapy in Healthy Subjects and in Patients with Nonseasonal Depression." *Acta Psychiatrica Scandinavica* 86 (1992), 127–132.

15. M. Koller et al. "Different Patterns of Light Exposure in Relation to Melatonin and Cortisol Rhythms and Sleep of Night Workers." *Journal of Pineal Research* 16:3 (April 1994), 127–135.

16. James Perl, Ph.D. *Sleep Right in Five Nights* (New York: William Morrow, 1993), 231.

17. W. F. Byerley et al. "Biological Effect of Bright Light." *Progress in Neuro-Psychopharmacology and Biological Psychiatry* 13:5 (1989), 683–686.

18. D. J. Kennaway et al. "Phase Delay of the Rhythm of 6-Sulphatoxy Melatonin Excretion by Artificial Light." *Journal of Pineal Research* 4:3 (1987), 315–320. See also: A. J. Lewy, T. A. Wehr, and F. K. Goodwin. "Light Suppresses Melatonin Secretion in Humans." *Science* (December 1980), 210.

19. Russel J. Reiter and Jo Robinson. *Melatonin: Your Body's Natural Wonder Drug* (New York: Bantam Books, 1995), 165.

20. D. G. M. Murphy et al. "Seasonal Affective Disorder: Response to Light as Measured by Electroencephalogram, Melatonin Suppression, and Cerebral Blood Flow." *British Journal of Psychiatry* 163 (1993), 327–331.

21. M. L. Laakso et al. "One-Hour Exposure to Moderate Illuminance (500 Lux) Shifts the Human Melatonin Rhythm." *Journal of Pineal Research* 15:1 (August 1993), 21–26.

22. G. Copinschi, O. Van Reeth, and E. Van Cauter. "Biologic Rhythms: Effect of Aging on the Desynchronization of Endogenous Rhythmicity and Environmental Conditions." *Presse Medicale* 28:17 (May 1–8, 1999), 942–946.

23. I. Haimov et al. "Sleep Disorders and Melatonin Rhythms in Elderly People." *British Medical Journal* 309 (1994), 167.

24. Dorothy Castor, PAC, et al. "Effect of Sunlight on Sleep Patterns of the Elderly." *Journal of the American Academy of Physician Assistants* 4:4 (June 1991), 321–326.

25. P. Semm, T. Schneider, L. Vollrath. "Effects of an Earth-Strength Magnetic Field on Electrical Activity of Pineal Cells." *Nature* 288 (1980), 607–608.

26. T. Schneider et al. "Melatonon Is Crucial for the Migratory Orientation of Pied Flycatchers (*Ficedula hypoleuca Pallas*)." *Journal of Experimental Biology* 194:1 (September 1994), 255–262.

27. S. Reuss, P. Semm, and L. Vollrath. "Different Types of Magnetically Sensitive Cells in the Rat Pineal Gland." *Neuroscience Letters* 40:1 (September 19, 1983), 23–26.

28. R. Dubbels et al. "Melatonin Determination with a Newly Developed ELISA System: Inter-Individual Differences in the Response of the Human Pineal Gland to Magnetic Fields." In: G. J. Maestroni, A. Conti, and R. J. Reiter, eds., *Advances in Pineal Research*, Vol. 7 (London: John Libbey, 1994), 27–33.

29. M. Kato. "Biological Influences of Electromagnetic Fields." *Hokkaido Igaku Zasshi* 70:4 (July 1995), 551–560.

30. M. Karasek et al. "Chronic Exposure to 2.9 mT, 40 Hz Magnetic Field Reduces Melatonin Concentrations in Humans." *Journal of Pineal Research* 25:4 (December 1998), 240–244.

31. D. H. Pfluger and C. E. Minder. "Effects of Exposure to 16.7 Hz Magnetic Fields on Urinary 6-Hydroxymelatonin Sulfate Excretion of Swiss Railway Workers." *Journal of Pineal Research* 21:2 (September 1996), 91–100.

32. Russel J. Reiter and Jo Robinson. *Melatonin: Your Body's Natural Wonder Drug* (New York: Bantam Books, 1995), 173.

33. R. Luboshitzky. "Endocrine Activity during Sleep." *Journal of Pediatric Endocrinology and Metabolism* 13:1 (January 2000), 13–20.

34. I. Modai et al. "Blood Levels of Melatonin, Serotonin, Cortisol, and Prolactin in Relation to the Circadian Rhythm of Platelet Serotonin Uptake." *Psychiatry Research* 43:2 (August 1992), 161–166.

35. O. Van Reeth et al. "Nocturnal Exercise Phase Delays Circadian Rhythms of Melatonin and Thyrotropin Secretion in Normal Men." *American Journal of Physiology* 266:6 Part 1 (June 1994), E964-E974.

36. P. J. Murphy, B. L. Myers, and P. Badia. "Nonsteroidal Anti-Inflammatory Drugs Alter Body Temperature and Suppress Melatonin in Humans." *Physiology and Behavior* 59:1 (January 1996), 133-139.

37. P. J. Murphy et al. "Nonsteriodal Anti-Inflammatory Drugs Affect Normal Sleep Patterns in Humans." *Physiology and Behavior* 55:6 (June 1994), 1063-1066.

38. K. Surrall et al. "Effect of Ibuprofen and Indomethacin on Human Plasma Melatonin." *Journal of Pharmacy and Pharmacology* 39:10 (October 1987), 840-843.

39. P. J. Murphy et al. "Nonsteriodal Anti-Inflammatory Drugs Affect Normal Sleep Patterns in Humans." *Physiology and Behavior* 55:6 (June 1994), 1063-1066.

40. A. C. Meyer, J. J. Nieuwenhuis, and B. J. Meyer. "Dihydropyridine Calcium Antagonists Depress the Amplitude of the Plasma Melatonin Cycle in Baboons." *Life Sciences* 39 (1986), 1563-1569.

41. M. Kabuto, I. Namura, and Y. Saitoh. "Nocturnal Enhancement of Plasma Melatonin Could Be Suppressed by Benzodiazepines in Humans." *Endocrinologia Japonica* 133:3 (1986), 405-414.

42. P. Monteleone et al. "Preliminary Observations on the Suppression of Nocturnal Plasma Melatonin Levels by Short-Term Administration of Diazepam in Humans." Journal of Pineal Research 6:3 (1989), 253-258.

43. I. McIntyre, G. D. Burrows, and T. R. Norman. "Suppression of Plasma Melatonin by a Single Dose of the Benzodiazepine Alprozolam in Humans." *Biological Psychiatry* 24 (1988), 105-108. See also: P. P. Hubain et al. "Alprazolam and Amitriptyline in the Treatment of Major Depressive Disorder: A Double-Blind Clinical and Sleep EEG Study." *Journal of Affective Disorders* 18:1 (January 1995), 67-73.

44. M. Kabuto, I. Namura, and Y. Saitoh. "Nocturnal Enhancement of Plasma Melatonin Could Be Suppressed by Benzodiazepines in Humans." *Endocrinologia Japonica* 133:3 (1986), 405-414.

45. Kenneth P. Wright, Jr., et al. "Caffeine and Light Effects on Nighttime Melatonin and Temperature Levels in Sleep-Deprived Humans." *Brain Research* 747 (1997), 78-84. See also: A. M. Babey, R. M. Palmour, and S. N. Young. "Caffeine and Propranolol Block the Increase in Rat Pineal Melatonin Production Produced by Stimulation of Adenosine Receptors." *Neuroscience Letters* 176:1 (July 18, 1994), 93-96.

46. S. Rojdmark et al. "Inhibition of Melatonin Secretion by Ethanol in Man." *Metabolism* 42:8 (August 1993), 1047-1051. See also: C. L. Chik and A. K. Ho. "Ethanol Reduces Norepinephrine-Stimulated Melatonin Synthesis in Rat Pinealocytes." *Journal of Neurochemistry* 4:4 (October 1992), 1280-1286.

47. K. Honma, M. Kohsada, and S. Honma. "Effects of Vitamin B_{12} on Plasma Melatonin Rhythm in Humans: Increased Light Sensitivity and Phase-Advances the Circadian Clock." *Experientia* 48 (1992), 716-720. See also: Hiroshi Itoh et al. "Effects of Vitamin B_{12} and Bright Light on Circadian Rhythms." *Japanese Journal of Psychiatry and Neurology* 48:2 (1994), 502-505.

48. J. Daniel Kanofsky, MD, MPH. "Magnesium Deficiency in Chronic Schizophrenia." *International Journal of Neuroscience* 61 (1991), 87-90.

49. Russel J. Reiter and Jo Robinson. *Melatonin: Your Body's Natural Wonder Drug* (New York: Bantam Books, 1995), 197.

50. James Perl, Ph.D. *Sleep Right in Five Nights* (New York: William Morrow, 1993), 232.

51. National Sleep Foundation. "2000 Omnibus Sleep in America Poll." Available from National Sleep Foundation, 1522 K Street NW, Suite 500, Washington, DC 20005; www.sleepfoundation.org.

52. M. A. Carskadon, ed. *Encyclopedia of Sleep and Dreaming* (New York: Macmillan, 1993), 703.

53. Hiroshi Itoh et al. "Effects of Vitamin B_{12} and Bright Light on Circadian Rhythms." *Japanese Journal of Psychiatry and Neurology* 48:2 (1994), 502–505. See also: Satoko Hashimoto et al. "Vitamin B_{12} Enhances the Phase-Response of Circadian Melatonin Rhythms to a Single Bright Light Exposure in Humans." *Neuroscience Letters* 220 (1996), 129–132.

54. R. Sandyk. "Resolution of Sleep Paralysis by Weak Electromagnetic Fields in a Patient with Multiple Sclerosis." *International Journal of Neuroscience* 90:3–4 (August 1997), 145–147.

55. Ron Lawrence, MD, Ph.D., and Paul J. Rosch, MD, FACP. *Magnet Therapy: The Pain Cure Alternative* (Rocklin, CA: Prima Publishing, 1998), 117.

56. Kathryn Reid et al. "Day-Time Melatonin Administration: Effects on Core Temperature and Sleep Onset Latency." *Journal of Sleep Research* 5 (1996), 150–154.

57. Lars Palm et al. "Long-Term Melatonin Treatment in Blind Children and Young Adults with Circadian Sleep-Wake Disturbances." *Developmental Medicine and Child Neurology* 39 (1997), 319–325.

58. J. S. Carman, R. M. Post, and F. K. Goodwin. "Negative Effects of Melatonin on Depression." *American Journal of Psychiatry* 1333:10 (1976), 1181–1186. See also: M. D. Steinhilber, M. Brungs, and C. Carlberg. "The Nuclear Receptor for Melatonin Represses 5-Lipoxygenase Gene Expression in Human B-Lymphocytes." *Journal of Biological Chemistry* 270:13 (1995), 7037–7040. See also: I. Hansson, R. Holmdahl, and R. Mattson. "The Pineal Hormone Melatonin Exaggerates Development of Collagen-Induced Arthritis in Mice." *Journal of Neuroimmunology* 39 (1992), 23–30.

59. B. Voordouw et al. "Melatonin and Melatonin-Progestin Combinations Alter Pituitary-Ovarian Function in Women and Can Inhibit Ovulation." *Journal of Clinical Endocrinology and Metabolism* 74:1 (1992), 108–117.

60. G. J. Maestroni and A. Conti. "Anti-Stress Role of the Melatonin-Immuno-Opioid Network: Evidence for a Physiological Mechanism Involving T-Cell-Derived, Immunoreactive Beta-Endorphin and MET-enkephalin Binding to Thymic Opioid Receptors." *International Journal of Neuroscience* 61 (1991), 289–298.

61. Y. H. Watanabe et al. *Nutrition Reports International* 25 (1982), 733–741.

62. N. Zisapel. "The Use of Melatonin for the Treatment of Insomnia." *Biological Signals* 8:1–2 (January-April 1999), 84–89.

63. K. Petrie et al. "Effect of Melatonin on Jet Lag after Long Haul Flights." *British Medicine Journal* 298 (1989), 705–707.

64. Ray Sahelian, MD. "Melatonin Isn't Just for Sleep Anymore." *Let's Live* (October 1995).

65. A. Lewy et al. "Melatonin, Light and Chronobiological Disorders." In: D. Evered and S. Clark, eds., *Photoperiodism, Melatonin and the Pineal* (London: Pitman, 1985), 231–252.

66. Roger Field. "Melatonin May Relieve Sleep-Cycle Disorders." *Medical Tribune* (April 8, 1993), 2.

67. D. Kunz and F. Bes. "Melatonin as a Therapy in REM Sleep Behavior Disorder Patients: An Open-Labeled Pilot Study on the Possible Influence on REM-Sleep Regulation." *Movement Disorders* 14:3 (May 1999), 507–511.

68. D. Kunz and F. Bes. "Melatonin Effects in a Patient with Severe REM Sleep Behavior Disorder: Case Report and Theoretical Considerations." *Neuropsychobiology* 36:4 (1997), 211–214.

69. L. M. Rosen et al. "Prevalence of Seasonal Affective Disorder at Four Latitudes." *Psychiatry Research* 31 (1989), 131–144.

70. A. Wirz-Justic et al. "Natural Light Treatment of Seasonal Affective Disorder." *Journal of Affective Disorders* 37:2–3 (April 12, 1996), 109–120.

71. Y. Meesters et al. "Light Therapy for Seasonal Affective Disorder: The Effects of Timing." *British Journal of Psychiatry* 166 (1995), 607–612.

72. Alfred J. Lewy, MD, Ph.D. "Treating Chronobiologic Sleep and Mood Disorders with Bright Light." *Psychiatric Annals* 17:10 (October 1987), 664–669.

Chapter 6. *Step 4: Resolve Emotional Issues*

1. A. Perkins. "Saving Money by Reducing Stress." *Harvard Business Review* 72:6 (1994), 12.

2. Harris Interactive. "Attitudes in the American Workplace VII." Poll conducted May 31 to June 17, 2001. Available at www.stress.org/2001Harris.pdf.

3. National Institute for Occupational Safety and Health. *Stress . . . at Work* (Cincinnati, OH: National Institute for Occupational Safetly and Health, 1999). Available at http://www.cdc.gov/niosh/stresswk.html.

4. J. L. Marx. "The Immune System 'Belongs to the Body.'" *Science* 277 (1985), 1190–1192.

5. L. Schindler, E. Hohenberger-Sieber, and P. Pauli. "Correlates of Disordered Sleep: A Replication Study." *Zeitschrift für Klinische Psychologie, Psychopathologie und Psychotherapie* 36:2 (1988), 118–129.

6. W. F. Waters et al. "Attention, Stress, and Negative Emotion in Persistent Sleep-Onset and Sleep-Maintenance Insomnia." *Sleep* 16:2 (1993), 128–136.

7. A. N. Vgontzas et al. "Chronic Insomnia and Activity of the Stress System: A Preliminary Study." *Journal of Psychosomatic Research* 45:1 (1998), 21–31.

8. Hans Seyle, MD. *Stress without Distress* (New York: New American Library, 1975). See also: J. D. Beasley and J. Swift. *Kellogg Report: The Impact of Nutrition, Environment, and Lifestyle on the Health of Americans* (Annandale-on-Hudson, NY: Institute of Health Policy and Practice, The Bard College Center, 1989).

9. Associated Press. "For Chronic Pain, Try to Relax." (October 19, 1995).

10. Brian Tracy. *The Psychology of Achievement* (Niles, IL: Nightingale-Conant Corporation, 1987), 4.

11. R. A. Chalmers et al., eds. *Scientific Research on Maharishi's Transcendental Meditation and TM-Sidih Program: Collected Papers*, Vol. 2–4 (Vlodrop, Netherlands: Maharishi Vedic University Press, 1989).

12. R. K. Wallace et al. "Physiological Effects of Transcendental Meditation." *Science* 167 (1970), 1751–1754. See also: M. C. Dillbeck et al. "Physiological Differences between TM and Rest. *American Physiologist* 42 (1987), 879–881.

13. R. W. Cranson et al. "Transcendental Meditation and Improved Performance on Intelligence-Related Measures: A Longitudinal Study." *Personality and Individual Differences* 12 (1991), 1005–1116.

14. D. H. Shapiro and R. N. Walsh. *Meditation: Classic and Contemporary Perspectives* (New York: Aldine, 1984).

15. N. Miller. "Learning of Visceral and Glandular Responses." *Science* 163:866 (January 1969), 434–445.

16. Jean Callahan. "Relax." *Self* (June 1995), 130.

17. Lara Pizzorno, MA, LMP. "The Healing Power of the Mind." *Delicious!* (May 1995), 20.

18. Peter Hauri, Ph.D., and Shirley Linde, Ph.D. *No More Sleepless Nights* (New York: John Wiley and Sons, 1990, 1991), 98.

19. N. Miller. "Learning of Visceral and Glandular Responses." *Science* 163:866 (January 1969), 434–445, 627.

20. Shad Helmsetter, Ph.D. *What to Say When You Talk to Yourself* (Scottsdale, AZ: Grindle Press/Audio, 1986).

21. Lawrence Paros, Ph.D., and Daniel L. Kirsch, Ph.D., DAAPM. "Cranial Electrotherapy Stimulation (CES): A Very Safe and Effective Non-Pharmacological Treatment for Anxiety." *MedScope Monthly* 3:1, 1–16, 24–27.

22. Eric Braverman, MH. *P.A.T.H. Wellness Manual* (Princeton, NJ: P.A.T.H., 1995), 171.

23. Daniel L. Kirsch, Ph.D., DAAPM, and Fred Lerner, Ph.D., DAAPM. "Electromedicine, the Other Side of Physiology." In: Richard S. Weiner, ed., *Pain Management: A Practical Guide for Clinicians* (Boca Raton, FL: CRC Press, 1998), Chapter 23, 2–3.

24. P. Huard and M. Wong. *Chinese Medicine* (New York: World University Library /McGraw Hill, 1968).

25. Terry Willard. "Insomnia: Wake Up to Ten Simple Solutions." *Herbs for Health* (January/February 1997), 37–39.

26. German Ministry of Health. *Valerian.* Commission E Monographs for Phytomedicines (Bonn, Germany: German Ministry of Health, 1985).

27. European Scientific Cooperative on Phytotherapy. *Valerian Root* (Meppel, Netherlands: European Scientific Cooperative on Phytotherapy, 1990).

28. Simon Y. Mills, MA. *The Dictionary of Modern Herbalism* (Rochester, VT: Healing Arts Press, 1988), 211.

29. Terry Willard. "Insomnia: Wake Up to Ten Simple Solutions" *Herbs for Health* (January/February 1997), 38.

30. Linda White, MD. "No More Tossing and Turning," *Vegetarian Times* (November 1996), 38.

31. Terry Willard. "Insomnia: Wake Up to Ten Simple Solutions." *Herbs for Health* (January/February 1997), 39.

32. Christopher Hobbs. "Valerian: A Literature Review." *HerbalGram* 21 (1989), 19–34.

33. German Ministry of Health. *Passion Flower Leaves.* Commission E Monographs for Phytomedicines (Bonn, Germany: German Ministry of Health, 1985).

34. S. Foster. *Passion Flower.* Botanical Series 314 (Austin, TX: American Botanical Council, 1993).

35. E. Lehmann et al. "Efficacy of a Special Kava Extract (*Piper methysticum*) in Patients with Anxiety, Tension, and Excitedness of Non-Mental Origin." *Phytomedicine* 3 (1996), 113–119.

36. H. P. Volz and M. Kieser. "Kava-Kava Extract WS 14490 versus Placebo in Anxiety Disorders: A Randomized Placebo-Controlled 25-Week Outpatient Trial." *Pharmacopsychiatria* 30 (1997), 1–5.

37. Terry Willard. "Insomnia: Wake Up to Ten Simple Solutions." *Herbs for Health* (January/February 1997), 37.

38. Ibid., 39.

39. Lesley Tierra, L.Ac., Dip.Ac. *Healing with Chinese Herbs* (Freedom, CA: The Crossing Press, 1997).

40. Simon Y. Mills, MA. *The Dictionary of Modern Herbalism* (Rochester, VT: Healing Arts Press, 1988), 58–59.

41. European Scientific Cooperative on Phytotherapy. *Valerian Root* (Meppel, Netherlands: European Scientific Cooperative on Phytotherapy, 1990). See also: S. Foster. *Chamomile*. Botanical Series 307 (Austin, TX: American Botanical Council, 1991).

42. O. Suzuki et al. "Inhibition of Monoamine Oxidase by Hypericin." *Planta Medica* 50 (1984), 272–274. See also: H. Muldner and M. Zoller. "Antidepressive Effect of a *Hypericum* Extract Standardized to an Active Hypericine Complex: Biochemical and Clinical Studies." *Arzneimittel-Forschung* 34:8 (1984), 918–920.

43. Peter De Smet et al. "St. John's Wort as an Antidepressant." *British Medical Journal* 7052:313 (August 3, 1996), 241–242. See also: Klaus Linde et al. "St. John's Wort for Depression: An Overview and Meta-Analysis of Randomized Clinical Trials." *British Medical Journal* 7052:313 (August 3, 1996), 253–258.

44. William Boericke, ND. *Pocket Manual of Homeopathic Materia Medica*, 9th edition (New York: Boericke and Runyon, 1927), 179.

45. Andrew Lockie, MD, and Nicola Geddes, MD. *The Women's Guide to Homeopathy* (New York: St. Martin's 1994), 238.

46. Peter Holmes, MH, L.Ac. "Lavender Oil: A Study in Contradictions." *International Journal of Aromatherapy* 4:2 (Summer 1992), 20.

47. Patricia Kaminski and Richard Katz. *Flower Essence Repertory* (Nevada City, CA: Flower Essence Study, 1994), 203.

Chapter 7. *Step 5: Protect Yourself from Environmental Factors*

1. N. Wertheimer and E. Leeper. "Electrical Wiring Configurations and Childhood Cancer." *American Journal of Epidemiology* 109 (1979), 273–284.

2. J. Wolpay. *Biological Effects of Power Line Fields* (New York: New York State Power Lines Project, Scientific Advisory Panel, 1987).

3. Lita Lee, Ph.D. *Radiation Protection Manual* (Redwood City, CA: Grassroots Network, 1990), 34.

4. National Institute of Environmental Health Sciences and National Institutes of Health. *EMF Electric and Magnetic Fields Associated with the Use of Electric Power* (Washington, DC: National Institute of Environmental Health Sciences, 2002), 24. Available at www.niehs.nih.gov/emfrapid/booklet/emf2002.pdf.

5. Ibid.

6. Robert O. Becker, MD, and Gary Selden. *The Body Electric: Electromagnetism and the Foundation of Life* (New York: William Morrow and Sons, 1985).

7. Robert O. Becker, MD. *Cross Currents: The Perils of Electropollution, the Promise of Electromedicine* (New York: Jeremy P. Tarcher, 1990), 160–166.

8. Robert O. Becker, MD, and Gary Selden. *The Body Electric: Electromagnetism and the Foundation of Life* (New York: William Morrow and Sons, 1985).

9. R. Edwards. "Leak Links Power Lines to Cancer," *New Scientist* 4 (October 7, 1995), 4.

10. C. Ezzell. "Power-Line Static. Debates Rage over the Possible Hazards of Electromagnetic Fields." *Science News* 140 (September 1991), 202–203.

11. B. W. Wilson, C. Wright, and L. E. Anderson. "Evidence for an Effect of ELF Electromagnetic Fields on Human Pineal Gland Function." *Journal of Pineal Research* 9 (1990), 259–269.

12. D. Wartenberg. "EMFs: Cutting Through the Controversy." *Public Health Reports* 111:3 (May/June 1996), 204–217.

13. Robert O. Becker, MD. *Cross Currents: The Perils of Electropollution, the Promise of Electromedicine* (New York: Jeremy P. Tarcher, 1990), 270.

14. Burton Goldberg Group. *Alternative Medicine: The Definitive Guide* (Tiburon, CA: Future Medicine Publishing, 1993), 332.

15. Russel J. Reiter and Jo Robinson. *Melatonin: Your Body's Natural Wonder Drug* (New York: Bantam Books, 1995), 178.

16. B. Holmberg. "Magnetic Fields and Cancer: Animal and Cellular Evidence—An Overview." *Environmental Health Perspectives* 2:Suppl (1995), 63–67. See also: C. Decker. "ELF-Zapped Genes Speed DNA Transcription." *Science News* (April 14, 1990), 229.

17. M. Mevissen, A. Leerchl, and W. Loscher. "Study on Pineal Function and DMBA-Induced Breast Cancer Formation in Rats during Exposure to a 100-mG, 50-Hz Magnetic Field." *Journal of Toxicology and Environmental Health* 48 (1996), 169–185.

18. Jane Thurnell-Read. *Geopathic Stress: How Earth Energies Affect Our Lives* (Rockport, MA: Element Books, 1996).

19. Robert O. Becker, MD. *Cross Currents: The Perils of Electropollution, the Promise of Electromedicine* (New York: Jeremy P. Tarcher, 1990), 71.

20. Gustav Freiherr von Pohl. *Earth Currents: Causative Factor of Cancer and Other Diseases* (Stuttgart, Germany: Frech-Verlag, 1983).

21. Jane Thurnell-Read. *Geopathic Stress: How Earth Energies Affect Our Lives* (Rockport, MA: Element Books, 1996), 38.

22. Robert O. Becker, MD. *Cross Currents: The Perils of Electropollution, the Promise of Electromedicine* (New York: Jeremy P. Tarcher, 1990), 220.

23. Lita Lee, Ph.D. *Radiation Protection Manual* (Redwood City, CA: Grassroots Network, 1990), 39.

24. Robert O. Becker, MD. *Cross Currents: The Perils of Electropollution, the Promise of Electromedicine* (New York: Jeremy P. Tarcher, 1990), 276.

25. Master Lam Kam Chuen. *Feng Shui Handbook* (New York: Henry Holt, 1996), 42.

26. Sarah Rossbach. *Interior Design with Feng Shui* (New York: Penguin Books, 1987), 21.

27. Richard Webster. *101 Feng-Shui Tips for the Home* (St. Paul, MN: Llewellyn, 1998); Master Lam Kam Cheun. *Feng Shui Handbook* (New York: Henry Holt, 1996).

28. Glenda Cassutt. "Energize Your Home for Good Health." *Natural Health* (May/June 1995), 95.

29. Richard Webster. *101 Feng-Shui Tips for the Home* (St. Paul, MN: Llewellyn, 1998). See also: Kirsten M. Lagatree. *Feng Shui: Arranging Your Home to Change Your Life* (New York: Villard, 1996). See also: Li Pak Tin and Helen Yeap. *Feng Shui: Secrets That Change Your Life* (York Beach, ME: Samuel Weiser, 1997).

30. Karen Kingston. *Creating Sacred Space with Feng Shui* (New York: Broadway Books, 1997).

31. Ibid.

32. George Birdsall. *The Feng Shui Companion: A User-Friendly Guide to the Ancient Art of Placement* (Rochester, VT: Inner Traditions, 1997).

33. Norman Ford. *The Sleep Rx: 75 Proven Ways to Get a Good Night's Sleep* (Englewood Cliffs, NJ: Prentice Hall, 1994), 209.

34. Don Eady. "Sleep Easy." *Alive* (January 1996), 32.

35. T. A. Thomas and P. M. Brundage. *Quantitative Assessment of Potential Health Effects from the Use of Fire Retardant (FR) Chemicals in Mattresses* (Bethesda, MD: US Consumer Products Safety Commission, 2006). Available at www.cpsc.gov /library/foia/foia06/brief/matttabd.pdf.

36. R. O. Jenkins et al. "Antimony leaching from cot mattresses and sudden infant death syndrome (SIDS)." *Human and Experimental Toxicology* 17:3 (1998), 138–139.

37. Tina Spangler. "Is Your Bedroom Making You Sick?" *Natural Health* (May/June 1996), 82–85.

Chapter 8. *Step 6: Balance Your Hormones*

1. A. Steiger. "Thyroid Gland and Sleep." *Acta Medica Austriaca* 26:4 (1999), 132–133.
2. J. F. Owens and K. A. Matthews. "Sleep Disturbance in Healthy Middle-Aged Women." *Maturitas* 30:1 (1998), 41–50.
3. D. L. Keefe, R. Watson, and F. Naftolin. "Hormone Replacement Therapy May Alleviate Sleep Apnea in Menopausal Women: A Pilot Study." *Menopause: The Journal of the North American Menopause Society* 6:3 (1999), 196–200.
4. John R. Lee, MD, with Virginia Hopkins. *What Your Doctor May Not Tell You about Menopause* (New York: Warner Books, 1996), 34.
5. Ibid., 131, 184.
6. Giampiero Porzio et al. "HRT as First-Step Treatment of Insomnia in Postmenopausal Women." *European Menopause Journal* 4:4 (1997), 145–148.
7. P. Polo-Kentola et al. "When Does Estrogen Replacement Therapy Improve Sleep Quality?" *American Journal of Obstetrics and Gynecology* 178:5 (1998), 1002–1009.
8. K. P. Wright Jr., and P. Badia. "Effects of Menstrual Cycle Phase and Oral Contraceptives on Alertness, Cognitive Performance, and Circadian Rhythms during Sleep Deprivation." *Behavioral Brain Research* 103:2 (1999), 185–194.
9. Maurice M. Ohayon. "Severe Hot Flashes are Associated with Chronic Insomnia." *Archives of Internal Medicine* 166:12 (2006), 1262–1268.
10. Theresa L. Crenshaw, MD. *The Alchemy of Love and Lust* (New York: G. P. Putnam's Sons, 1996), 205.
11. Eugene Shippen, MD, and William Fryer. *The Testosterone Syndrome* (New York: M. Evans, 1998), 91.
12. H. P. Roffwarg et al. "Plasma Testosterone and Sleep: Relationship to Sleep Stage Variables." *Psychosomatic Medicine* 44:1 (1982), 73–84.
13. R. C. Schiavi, D. White, and J. Mandeli. "Pituitary-Gonadal Function during Sleep in Healthy Aging Men." *Psychoneuroendocrinology* 17:6 (1992), 599–609.
14. Theo Colborn, Dianne Dumanoski, and John Peterson Myers. *Our Stolen Future* (New York: Dutton/Penguin Group, 1996).
15. Betty Kamen, Ph.D. "Thyroid and Stress Connections." *Hormone Replacement Therapy: Yes or No?* (Novato, CA: Nutrition Encounter, 1993), 196.
16. A. W. Meikle et al. "Effects of a Fat-Containing Meal on Sex Hormones in Men." *Metabolism* 39:9 (1990), 943–946.
17. C. D. Hunt et al. "Effects of Dietary Zinc Depletion on Seminal Volume and Zinc Loss: Serum Testosterone Concentrations and Sperm Morphology in Young Men." *American Journal of Clinical Nutrition* 56:1 (1992), 148–157.
18. Joseph Pizzorno, ND. *Total Wellness* (Rocklin, CA: Prima Publishing, 1996), 244.
19. Eugene Shippen, MD, and William Fryer. *The Testosterone Syndrome* (New York: M. Evans, 1998), 49.
20. S. J. Brown. "Environmental Doctors Take Up Pollution Prevention Cause." *Family Practice News* (January 1, 1995), 6.
21. J. Yeh and A. J. Friedman. "Nicotine and Cotinine Inhibit Rat Testis Androgen Biosynthesis In Vitro." *Journal of Steroid Biochemistry* 33:4A (1989), 627–630.
22. Joseph Pizzorno, ND. *Total Wellness* (Rocklin, CA: Prima Publishing, 1996), 242.
23. Ibid., 236–237.
24. K. Spiegel, E. Tasali, P. Penev, and E. Van Cauter. "Brief Communication: Sleep Curtailment in Healthy Young Men Is Associated with Decreased Leptin Levels,

Elevated Ghrelin Levels, and Increased Hunger and Appetite." *Annals of Internal Medicine* 141:11 (2004), 846–850:

25. N. Hellmich. "Sleep Loss May Equal Weight Gain." *USA Today,* December 6, 2004.

26. Albert Einstein Medical Center, Philadelphia, Pennsylvania. *Premier Years* (February 1996), 1–3.

27. Charles Morin, Ph.D. *Relief from Insomnia: Getting the Sleep of Your Dreams* (New York: Doubleday, 1996), 188–189.

28. Ibid., 190.

29. James Perl, Ph.D. *Sleep Right in Five Nights* (New York: William Morrow, 1993), 100–103.

30. Russel J. Reiter and Jo Robinson. *Melatonin: Your Body's Natural Wonder Drug* (New York: Bantam, 1995), 8.

31. L. Haimov and P. Lavie. "Sleep Disorders and Melatonin Rhythms in Elderly People." *British Medical Journal* 309 (1994), 167.

32. John R. Lee, MD, with Virginia Hopkins. *What Your Doctor May Not Tell You about Menopause* (New York: Warner Books, 1996), 300.

33. Michael Murray, ND, and Joseph Pizzorno, ND. *Encyclopedia of Natural Medicine* 2nd edition (Rocklin, CA: Prima Publishing, 1998), 636.

34. E. H. Brown and L. P. Walker, Pharm.D., M.Ac., DHM. *Menopause and Estrogen* (Berkeley, CA: Frog Ltd., 1996), 111–119.

35. Ann Louise Gittleman, MS. "Perimenopause: When Signs of 'The Change' Come Too Early." *Alternative Medicine* (October/November 1998), 84–92.

36. John R. Lee, MD, with Virginia Hopkins. *What Your Doctor May Not Tell You about Menopause* (New York: Warner Books, 1996), 279–317.

37. John R. Lee, MD, with Virginia Hopkins. *What Your Doctor May Not Tell You about Menopause* (New York: Warner Books, 1996), 317.

38. John R. Lee, MD. *Natural Progesterone: The Multiple Roles of a Remarkable Hormone* (Sebastopol, CA: BLL Publishing, 1993), 41.

39. John R. Lee, MD, with Virginia Hopkins. *What Your Doctor May Not Tell You about Menopause* (New York: Warner Books, 1996), 263–278.

40. Jill Stansbury. "Fortifying Fertility with Vitamins and Herbs." *Nutrition Science News* 2:12 (December 1997), 606–612.

41. Linda Ojeda, Ph.D. *Menopause Without Medicine* (Alameda, CA: Hunter House, 1995), 101.

42. Harriet Beinfield, L.Ac. "Menopause East and West." *Body, Mind, Spirit* (June/July 1995), 24–26.

43. Eugene Shippen, MD, and William Fryer. *The Testosterone Syndrome* (New York: M. Evans, 1998), 190–193.

44. "Staying Sexually Fit during Male Menopause." *Alternative Medicine Digest* 10 (1995), 10–13. See also: Sandra Cabot, MD. *Smart Medicine for Menopause* (Garden City Park, NY: Avery, 1995).

45. Julian Whitaker, MD. "A Hormone Replacement Program for Men." *Health and Healing* 8:2 (February 1998), 1–4.

46. M. S. Fahim et al. "Effect of *Panax ginseng* on Testosterone Level and Prostate in Male Rats." *Archives of Andrology* 8:4 (1982), 261–263.

47. James A. Duke, Ph.D. *The Green Pharmacy* (Emmaus, PA: Rodale, 1997), 192.

48. Gary S. Ross, MD. "Men's Health Issues in Clinical Practice: Andropause." *Biomedical Therapy* 15:3 (June 1997), 94–95.

Chapter 9. *Step 7: Correct Structural Imbalances*

1. S. J. Griffin and J. Trinder. "Physical Fitness, Exercise and Human Sleep." *Psychophysiology* 15:5 (1978), 447–450.
2. Benedict Carey. "The Sleep Solution." *Health* (July/August 1996), 74.
3. Karla Kubitz, MD. "The Effects of Acute and Chronic Exercise on Sleep: A Meta-Analytic Review." *Sports Medicine* 21:4 (1996), 277–291.
4. Helen S. Driver et al. "Submaximal Exercise Effects on Sleep Patterns in Young Women before and after an Aerobic Training Programme." *Physiologica Scandinavica* 133:Suppl 574 (1988), 8–13.
5. Ilkka Vuori et al. "Epidemiology of Exercise Effects on Sleep." *Acta Physiologica Scandinavica* 133:Suppl. 574 (1988), 3–7.
6. The President's Council on Physical Fitness and Sports. "Guidelines for Personal Exercise Programs." 2004. Available at www.fitness.gov/fitness.pdf or www.fitness.gov/fitness.htm.
7. This is an adaptation of a program designed by Visual Health Information, P.O. Box 44646, Tacoma, WA 98444; tel: 253-536-4922; fax: 253-536-4944; website: www.vhikits.com.
8. R. Pate et al. "Physical Activity and Public Health: A Recommendation from the Centers for Disease Control and Prevention and the American College of Sports Medicine." *Journal of the American Medical Association* 65 (1995), 312–318.
9. Beryl Bender Birch. *Power Yoga* (New York: Simon and Schuster, 1995), 44–45.
10. For another description of NET treatments, see: K. Peterson. "Two Cases of Spinal Manipulation Performed while the Patient Contemplated an Associated Stress Event: The Effect of the Manipulation/Contemplation on Serum Levels in Hypercholesterolemic Subjects." *Chiropractic Technique* 7:2 (May 1995).
11. The Bodywork KnowledgeBase is an abstracted collection of the world literature on massage compiled by Richard van Why, available from the American Massage Therapy Association: 500 Davis Street, Suite 900, Evanston, IL 60201; 877-905-2700; www.amtamassage.org.
12. John Yates, Ph.D. *A Physician's Guide to Therapeutic Massage* (Vancouver, British Columbia, Canada: Massage Therapists' Association of British Columbia, 1990).
13. The Bodywork KnowledgeBase is an abstracted collection of the world literature on massage compiled by Richard van Why, available from the American Massage Therapy Association: 500 Davis Street, Suite 900, Evanston, IL 60201; 877-905-2700; www.amtamassage.org.
14. William Collinge, MPH, Ph.D. *The American Holistic Health Association Complete Guide to Alternative Medicine* (New York: Warner Books, 1996), 270.
15. Philip Goldberg and Daniel Kaufman. *Everybody's Guide to Natural Sleep* (Los Angeles: Jeremy Tarcher, 1990), 192–193.

Index

A

Accidents, 1, 5, 16
Acetaminophen, 112
Aconite, 150
Acupressure, 222, 224–25
Acupuncture
  hormonal imbalance and,
    195–96
  meridians, 100, 219, 222,
    227
  qi and, 143, 222
  for stress reduction, 143
  success story, 195–96
Adrenal glands, 132–33, 134–
  35, 180–81
Adrenaline, 46, 185
Adrenal Stress Index (ASI),
  134–35, 239
Advanced sleep phase syn-
  drome (ASPS), 29,
  121–22, 188, 227
Affirmations, 139
Aging
  hormone levels and, 19, 182
  melatonin production and,
    109, 188
  sleep disorders and, 36, 188
Alcohol, 37, 46–47, 56, 113, 186
Alfalfa, 194
Alpha-tocopherol, 65
Amino acids, 69–71, 227

Andropause, 181–82, 197–99
Anti-Candida Antibody
  Profile, 84, 239
Antidepressants, 33, 34
Antioxidants, 8, 43, 228
Anxiety. *See also* Stress
  anticipatory, 128–29
  breathing technique for, 211
  CES and, 142
  flower remedies for, 154
  herbal therapy for, 143–47
  meditation and, 124, 136
  prescription medications
    for, 112
  sleep rituals and, 124, 141
Aromatherapy, 152–53, 233
Arsenicum Album, 150
Artemisia absinthium, 99
Artemisia annua, 99
Aspirin, 112
ASPS. *See* Advanced sleep
  phase syndrome
Automatic thoughts, 141
Autonomic nervous system, 204
Ayurvedic medicine, 96, 97, 233

B

Bach Flower Remedies, 153–54
Back, exercises for, 207–8
Barberry, 95
Baths, 115

B cells, 9
Bedding materials, 176–77,
  233. *See also* Mattresses
Bedroom environment
  creating comfortable, 174
  feng shui and, 168–71
  geopathic stress and,
    172–73
Bed-wetting, 32, 228
Belladonna, 151
Benzodiazepine receptor
  agonists (BZRAs), 25
Benzodiazepines, 33, 34,
  112–13
Berberine, 95
Beta-blockers, 112
Betel nut, 101
Bifidobacterium bifidum, 95,
  96
Biofeedback, 137–38, 233
Black cohosh, 194
Blankets, electric, 159
Body clock. *See* Circadian
  rhythms
Bodywork, 220–25
BPH (benign prostatic hyper-
  trophy), 213
Brain
  body clock and, 17
  free radicals and, 8
  waves, 11, 12

Breathing
 diaphragmatic, 129, 131
 ujjayi, 211
Bruxism, 32, 228
Buckwheat, 194
BZRAs. *See* Benzodiazepine
 receptor agonists

C

Caffeine, 37, 42–44, 54, 113
Calcium, 47, 66, 237
Calcium-channel blockers, 112
Candida, 79, 81, 82–87, 94–96
Caprylic acid, 95
Carbohydrates, 58, 60. *See also*
 Sugar
Castor oil packs, 93
Cataplexy, 28
CES. *See* Cranial electrical
 stimulation
Chamomile, 96, 146–47, 153
Chamomilla (homeopathic
 remedy), 151
Chasteberry, 194
Chinese patent remedies, 147,
 237
Chiropractic, 202, 215–18, 234
Chlorophyll, 94
Chocolate, 42, 43
Cholesterol, 10
Chromium, 67
Chronotherapy, 116
Cinnamon, 96
Circadian rhythms
 aging and, 188
 body temperature and, 104
 definition of, 16
 disruption of, 20, 37–38,
  102, 104–13
 free-running and
  entrained, 103–4
 hormone levels and, 104
 light and, 16–17, 19–20,
  114–16
 melatonin and, 17–20
 resetting, 113–26
Citrus seed extract, 99
Cleanse 28, 89, 237
Cobalamin, 64
Cocculus, 151
Coffea Cruda, 151

Coffee
 caffeine in, 37, 42–44, 54,
  113
 enemas, 92, 93
Cognitive therapy, 140–42, 234
Colon
 cleansing, 88–90
 dietary support for, 90–91
 role of, 37
 therapists, 234
Computer screens, 166–67, 235
Copper, 47, 67–68, 77, 173, 186
Cortisol
 circadian rhythms and,
  104, 111
 definition of, 184, 228
 stress and, 71, 104, 111, 132
Counseling, 140–42
CPAP (continuous positive
 airway pressure) device,
 25, 26
Cranial electrical stimulation
 (CES), 142–43, 234
Craniosacral therapy, 218
Cytokines, 9

D

Dandelion root, 94
Darkfield microscopy, 84
Dehydroepiandrosterone. *See*
 DHEA
Delayed sleep phase syndrome
 (DSPS), 28–29, 116,
 121–22, 228
Dental fillings, 77, 78, 81
Detoxification. *See also* Toxins
 approach to, 87–88
 Ayurvedic, 96, 97
 candida, 94–96
 colon, 88–91
 defense system, 74–76
 importance of, 72, 73
 liver, 91–94
 parasites, 96–101
 testing capabilities for, 82
DHEA (dehydroepiandros-
 terone), 184, 186
Diaphragmatic breathing,
 129, 131
Diet. *See also* Food; Food
 allergies; Meals;
 Supplements
 elimination, 50–51

fiber in, 90–91
 hormonal imbalances and,
  191–93, 196–97
 nutritional deficiencies in,
  48–49, 82
 recommendations for, 43,
  53–62
 sleep and, 37, 42–48, 113
 success story, 52–53
Digestive system, 74, 75
Diosgenin, 193
Dong quai, 194
Dreams
 hypnagogic, 11
 memory and, 14
 purpose of, 14
Drugs, 46, 56, 112–13. *See also*
 Sleeping pills
DSPS. *See* Delayed sleep
 phase syndrome
Dysbiosis, 74
Dyssomnias, 22

E

Early birds, 29
EFAs. *See* Essential fatty acids
Electromagnetic fields (EMFs)
 definition of, 155, 157
 effects of, 38, 109–11, 157–
  58, 160–62
 in nature, 158–59
 oscillation rate of, 160–61
 reducing exposure to,
  165–67
 resources for, 235
 sources of, 38, 159–60
 strength of, 161
 success story, 156
Elements, five, 167, 169
Elimination diet, 50–51
ELISA test, 51, 239
EMFs. *See* Electromagnetic
 fields
Endocrine glands, 10, 228
Endotoxins, 79
Enemas, 89–90, 92, 93, 97, 234
Essential fatty acids (EFAs),
 192, 229
Essential oils, 146, 152–53
Estrogen, 179–81, 183–85,
 186, 192. *See also*
 Phytoestrogens;
 Xenoestrogens

Exercise. *See also* Qigong; Yoga
  benefits of, 114, 203, 204–5
  calories burned by, 209
  in day-to-day life, 209
  elements of, 205–6
  Kegel, 213–15
  resources for, 236
  for specific parts of body,
    207–8
  starting, 205
  timing of, 114, 204, 205

F

Feng shui, 40, 158, 164–65,
    167–71
FIA. *See* Functional Intracel-
    lular Analysis
Fiber, 90–91
Fight-or-flight response, 131,
    133
5-HTP (5-hydroxytrypto-
    phan), 19, 70, 237
Flexibility, 206
Flower remedies, 153–54, 234
Folic acid, 65
Food. *See also* Diet; Food
    allergies; Meals
  antiparasitic, 98–99
  to avoid before bedtime,
    61, 62
  chain, eating lower on, 62
  guidelines for, 59
  whole, 57–58
Food allergies
  definition of, 45
  diagnosing, 49–51
  effects of, 37, 45–46, 81
  treating, 56, 57
Foot reflexology, 221–22, 223
Formaldehyde, 177
Free radicals, 7–8, 229
Fructose, 56
Functional Intracellular
    Analysis (FIA), 49, 239
Functional liver detoxification
    profile, 82, 239

G

Garlic, 95, 238
Gas, intestinal, 62
Gastroesophageal reflux dis-
    order (GERD), 62
Genistein, 192

Gentian, 96
Geopathic stress, 38, 155,
    162–64, 172–73
Ghrelin, 187
Ginger, 96
Ginseng, 101, 195, 198, 237
Glycemic index, 54–55
Goldenseal, 95

H

Hair analysis, 48–49, 239
Heartburn, 62
Heavy metals, 37, 76, 81, 186
Helper T cells, 9–10
Herbs. *See also* individual herbs
  for candida, 95
  Chinese patent remedies,
    147, 237
  forms of, 146
  for hormonal balance, 194,
    198
  for liver support, 94
  for parasitic infections,
    99–101
  resources for, 237
  for stress reduction,
    143–48
  success story, 195–96
HGH. *See* Human growth
    hormone
Histamine, 45–46
Homeopathy
  for andropause, 199
  founding of, 149
  principles of, 149–50
  resources for, 234–35, 237
  success story, 148–49
Hops, 144, 194
Hormonal imbalances
  causes of, 182–86
  in men, 181–82, 185–86,
    196–99
  sleep disorders and, 38,
    178–82
  success stories, 189–91,
    195–96, 199–200
  testing for, 186–87, 189
  therapies for, 189, 191–99
  in women, 179–81, 183–85,
    191–95
Hormones. *See also* Hormonal
    imbalances
  aging and, 19, 182

definition of, 178, 229
glossary of, 184
Horsetail, 194
Human growth hormone
    (HGH), 13, 104, 204,
    229
Hypersomnia, 29–30, 229
Hypnic myoclonia, 11
Hypnotherapy, 138–39, 235
Hypoglycemia, 44, 46, 58,
    61, 81
Hypothalamus, 16–17
Hypothyroidism, 178–79, 180

I

Ibuprofen, 112
Ignatia Amara, 151
Imagery, guided, 129, 139–40,
    234
Immune system
  definition of, 230
  function of, 9
  sleep and, 9–10
Individualized Optimal
    Nutrition (ION)
    Profile, 49, 239
Indomethacin, 112
Insomnia
  acupressure for, 224–25
  alcohol and, 46–47
  aromatherapy for, 153
  caffeine and, 43
  in Chinese medicine, 100
  classifications of, 22–23
  conventional treatment of,
    23–24, 33–35
  definition of, 22, 230
  diet and, 47, 48, 61
  drugs and, 46
  flower remedies for, 154
  herbal therapy for, 143–48
  homeopathic remedies for,
    148–49, 150–51
  hormonal imbalances and,
    178–81
  melatonin for, 120, 122–23
  NET and, 219
  nicotine and, 47
  rebound, 34
  success stories, 52–53, 86–
    87, 217–18
  supplements for, 61, 62, 68,
    70

Insomnia (continued)
yin-yang imbalance and, 194
Insulin
glycemic index and, 54–55
rebound, 37
sugar and, 44, 54
Intestines, 74, 75, 96, 97
Iron, 47, 68

J

Jet lag, 105–6, 120–21
Jin Shin Do, 222, 224

K

Kava, 145
Kegel exercises, 213–15
Kleine-Levin syndrome, 29

L

Lactobacillus acidophilus,
95, 96
Lavender, 153
Laxatives, 88
LDL cholesterol, 10
Leaky gut syndrome, 6, 79
Lemon balm, 145
Leptin, 187
Libidex, 198
Licorice, 96, 194
Light
boxes, 115, 125–26, 236
circadian rhythms and, 17,
19–20, 107–9, 114–16
full-spectrum, 115, 236
Ligustri berries, 101
Liver
cleansing, 91–93
nutritional support for,
93–94
role of, 37, 74–75
toxins and, 79
Longan fruit, 195
Lotus seed, 195
Lycii berries, 195
Lycopodium, 151
Lymphatic system, 203, 230

M

Magnesium, 47, 66–67, 113,
198, 237
Magnets
geopathic stress and, 173
therapeutic, 116–18, 233

Manganese, 198
Marjoram, 153
Massage, 220–21, 235
Mattresses, 174–77
Mattress pads, 117, 233
MCS. See Multiple chemical
sensitivity
Meals
size of, 61
timing of, 61
Meditation, 135–37
Melakava, 238
Melatonin
aging and, 109, 188
definition of, 230
EMFs and, 109–11, 161–62
production of, 8, 9, 17–20,
60, 107–9, 161–62
receptor agonists, 34
resources for, 238
role of, 7, 8–9, 10, 17–19
supplementation, 118–23
testing levels of, 108
Meliae seeds, 101
Menopause, 179, 194
Mercury amalgam fillings, 77,
78, 81
Meridians, 100, 219, 222, 227
Microsleep, 16
Milk thistle, 94
Mind-body therapies, 135–42
Mindfulness meditation, 136
Minerals, 65–69
Monitor screens, 166–67
MSG (monosodium
glutamate), 48
Multiple chemical sensitivity
(MCS), 176
Multiple sleep latency test
(MSLT), 33
Muscle tension, 203

N

Narcolepsy, 27–28, 230
Natrum Muriaticum, 151
Natural killer (NK) cells,
9, 10
Neck, exercises for, 207
Neroli, 153
Network Spinal Analysis
(NSA), 216
Neuro-Emotional Technique
(NET), 219–20, 235

Neuropeptides, 230–31
Neurotransmitters, 44, 45–46,
231
Niacin, 63–64
Nicotine, 37, 47, 186
Nightmares, 34, 147, 150, 151
Night owls, 29
Night sweats, 147
Night terrors, 14, 31, 231
Noradrenaline, 185
NREM (non–rapid eye move-
ment) sleep, 11
NSA. See Network Spinal
Analysis
NSAIDs (nonsteroidal anti-
inflammatory drugs),
112
Nutritional deficiencies, 48–
49, 82, 235
Nux Vomica, 151

O

Oats, 198
Obesity, 187
Opium (homeopathic
remedy), 151
Oregano, 95
Oregon grape root, 94, 95
Oxidative stress profile, 82, 239

P

Panchakarma, 96, 97
Pantothenic acid, 64
Parasites, 80, 85–86, 96–101,
238
Parasomnias, 22, 30–32
Passionflower, 144–45
Pau d'arco, 95–96
Pelvic floor muscles, 214–15
Peppermint, 95
Perimenopause, 179–80, 185
Periodic limb movement
disorder (PLMD), 27,
43, 231
Phagocytes, 9, 10
Phosphatidylserine, 71
Phytoestrogens, 183, 192
Pineal gland, 8, 10, 17, 19,
109–10, 161
PLMD. See Periodic limb
movement disorder
Polysomnography, 32–33
Power lines, 159, 160

Pregnenolone, 184
Prick-puncture test, 49
Probioplex, 238
Probiotics, 96
Progesterone, 179–81, 183–85, 193–94
Prostate
    aerobics for, 213–15
    enlargement of, 213
Pulsatilla, 151
Pulse test, 51
Pumpkin seeds, 100–101
Pyridoxine, 64

Q
Qi
    blockages of, 143, 155, 222
    definition of, 155, 158, 167
    feng shui and, 158–59, 167–71
Qigong, 209–11, 236
Quisqualis seeds, 100–101

R
RAST (radioallergosorbent test), 49–50
Rebound insomnia, 34
Reflexology, 221–22, 223, 235
Reishi mushroom, 145–46
Relaxation therapies, 135–54
REM behavior disorder, 31, 122, 231
REM (rapid eye movement) sleep, 11, 14, 15
Restless legs syndrome (RLS), 26–27
    caffeine and, 43
    conventional treatment for, 26
    definition of, 26, 231
    diagnosing, 27
    diet and, 47
    prevalence of, 26
    supplements for, 65, 68
    symptoms of, 26, 27
Rhus Toxicodendron, 151
Rhythmic movement disorder (RMD), 31–32, 232
Riboflavin, 63
RLS. See Restless legs syndrome
RMD. See Rhythmic movement disorder

Rose, 194
Rosemary, 95

S
SAD. See Seasonal affective disorder
Sage, 194
St. John's wort, 147–48
Sarsaparilla, 194
Saw palmetto, 198
Schisandra berries, 101
SCN. See Suprachiasmatic nucleus
Scratch test, 49
Screening. See Testing and screening
Seasonal affective disorder (SAD)
    causes of, 20, 37, 123
    definition of, 123, 229
    light therapy for, 124–26
    prevalence of, 123
    success story, 125–26
    symptoms of, 123
Selenium, 186, 198
Self-hypnosis, 139
Serotonin, 19, 20, 44, 70
Shepherd's purse, 194
Shiatsu, 222, 224
Shift work, 106–7, 121
Shoulders, exercises for, 207–8
Siberian ginseng, 194
Sick building syndrome, 76
Silymarin, 94
Skullcap, 146
Sleep
    average duration of, 15, 21
    benefits of, 4, 7–10
    body weight and, 187
    checklist for, 142
    debt/deprivation, 15–16, 21, 33, 187
    history, assessing, 40
    micro-, 16
    purpose of, 7, 16
    required amount of, 15–16
    rituals for, 124
    stages of, 10–11, 13–15
Sleep apnea
    conventional treatment for, 25–26
    definition of, 24–25, 232
    diagnosing, 33

drugs and alcohol and, 25, 35, 56
    effects of, 25
    food allergies and, 37
    magnet therapy and, 116
    prevalence of, 24
    snoring and, 25, 174
Sleep disorders. See also individual disorders
    aging and, 36
    alternative medicine and, 35–36
    causes of, 22, 35–39
    diagnosing, 32–33
    diet and, 37, 42–48
    effects of, 4
    organizations for, 236
    prevalence of, 21
    primary vs. secondary, 22
    types of, 22–32
Sleep enuresis. See Bed-wetting
Sleeping pills, 21, 33–35, 112–13
Sleep phase disorders, 28–29, 121–22. See also Advanced sleep phase syndrome; Delayed sleep phase syndrome
Sleep terrors. See Night terrors
Sleepwalking (somnambulism), 14, 30–31, 232
Smoking. See Nicotine
Snoring, 25, 174
Soft drinks, 42, 43
Somnambulism. See Sleepwalking
Soy foods, 191–92
Spikenard, 153
Spinal vertebrae, 202, 203
Stanford Sleepiness Scale, 24
Stool analysis, 84–86, 239
Stress
    causes of, 132
    definition of, 131
    effects of, 38, 111, 127, 130–33, 180–81, 185
    geopathic, 38, 155, 162–64, 172–73
    prevalence of, 130
    quiz for, 133–34
    reducing, 135–54

Stress *(continued)*
  symptoms associated with,
    134
Structural imbalances
  correcting, 202, 204–25
  effects of, 38–39, 201–4
Subluxations, 202
Success stories
  acupuncture and herbs,
    195–96
  candida, 86–87
  chiropractic, 217–18
  diet, 52–53
  EMFs, 156
  feng shui, 164–65
  homeopathy, 148–49
  hormonal imbalance, 189–
    91, 195–96, 199–200
  lifestyle changes, 5–7
  light therapy for SAD,
    125–26
  melatonin supplements,
    122–23
  reflexology, 222
  return-to-sleep strategy,
    127–30
  yoga, 212–13
Sugar, 37, 44–45, 54–56
SuperGarlic 6000, 238
Supplements
  anti-candida, 95–96
  glandular, 237
  guide to taking, 69
  for hormonal support, 193,
    198
  list of, 62–71
  melatonin, 118–23
  probiotic, 96
  resources for, 237–38
Suprachiasmatic nucleus
    (SCN), 16–17, 103, 109
Sweetbriar, 194

T
T cells, 9–10
TCM. *See* Traditional Chinese
    medicine
Tea
  caffeine in, 42, 43
  herbal, 146
Teeth grinding. *See* Bruxism
Testing and screening
  for candidiasis, 82–85

  for detoxification
    capabilities, 82
  for food allergies, 49–51
  for hormonal imbalances,
    186–87, 189
  of melatonin levels, 108
  for nutritional deficiencies,
    48–49
  for parasites, 85–86
  resources for, 239
  for sleep disorders, 32–33
Testosterone, 182, 184, 185,
    186, 197–98
Thiamin, 63
Thoughts, negative, 141
Thyme, 95
Thymus gland, 9
Toxicity, loading theory of, 73
Toxins. *See also* Detoxification
  effects of, 80–82
  prevalence of, 72
  sources of, 38, 76–77, 79–80
Traditional Chinese medicine
    (TCM)
  definition of, 232
  disease and, 100, 202
  for hormonal balance,
    194–95
  insomnia and, 100
  parasites and, 99–101
  practitioners of, 235
Transcendental Meditation
    (TM), 136
Travel, 105–6, 120–21
Triple Yeast Defense, 238
Tryptophan, 19, 44, 47, 60–61,
    70, 114
Tyramine, 61
Tyrosine, 60, 61

U
Ujjayi breathing, 211
Ultimate Cleanse, 89, 238
UltraFlora Plus, 238
Unicorn root, 194
Urination, frequent, 62, 213

V
Valerian, 143–44
Vasopressin, 14
Visualization, 139–40
Vital (homeopathic growth
    hormone stimulator),
    238

Vitamins, 63–65
  B_1, 63, 113
  B_2, 63
  B_3, 63–64
  B_5, 64
  B_6, 47, 64, 113
  B_{12}, 64, 113, 115–16
  E, 47, 65, 198

W
White peony root, 195
Whole Body and Colon
    Program, 89, 238
Whole foods, 57–58
Winter blues. *See* Seasonal
    affective disorder
Wolfberry, 198
Worry time, 124, 142

X
Xenoestrogens, 76, 183, 186,
    229

Y
Yam, wild, 194
Yarrow, 194
Yeast, 79, 81, 82–85, 94–96,
    238
Yin and yang, 100, 167, 194
Ylang-ylang, 153
Yoga, 211–13, 236

Z
Zeitgebers, 17, 103, 104
Zinc, 47, 68–69, 186, 198

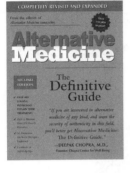
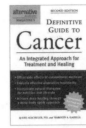

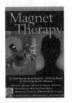

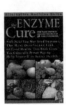
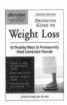

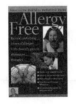
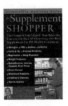
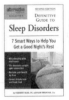

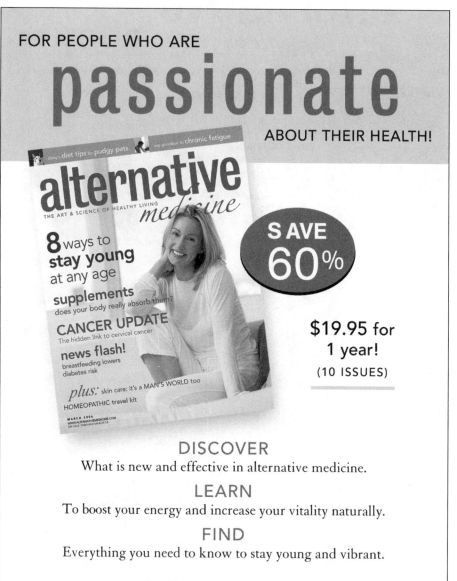